Second Edition

ORTHOPEDIC SURGERY OF THE DOG AND CAT

ELLIS P. LEONARD, B.S., D.V.M.

Fellow of the American College of Veterinary Surgeons;
Professor Emeritus of Small Animal Surgery,
New York State Veterinary College, Cornell University

W. B. SAUNDERS COMPANY

Philadelphia • London • Toronto • 1971

W. B. Saunders Company: West Washington Square
Philadelphia, Pa. 19105

12 Dyott Street
London, WC1A   1DB

1835 Yonge Street
Toronto 7, Ontario

Listed here is the latest translated edition of this book
together with the language of the translation
and the publisher.

Japanese (*1st Edition*) – Ishiyaku, Tokyo, Japan

Orthopedic Surgery of the Dog and Cat   SBN 0-7216-5721-4

Print No.:   9   8   7   6   5   4   3   2   1

Dedicated to

Douglas Pierson Leonard

Preface to Second Edition

Ten years have elapsed since this book first appeared. During the interim, new ideas and the improvement of old ones have brought new sophistication to the field of small animal orthopedics. A new edition, therefore, seemed desirable.

The object of revision is to present the subject matter in its current state and at the same time retain enough of its historical background to make it valid. This places a burden on the author of deciding what to keep and what to delete; what to add and what not to add. There have been both additions and deletions in this edition. Some of the original material has been retained wherever it seemed that it might serve a useful purpose.

This book is not intended as an encyclopedia of all orthopedic materials and methods. It is not even a complete text but rather, is intended to serve as a collateral experience for both student and practitioner.

The general format has been retained and chapters on Amputation, Elbow Dysplasia, Legg-Perthes Disease and Osteochondritis Dissecans have been added. New methods of treatment have been added throughout the book. For those wishing to explore a subject in depth, the reference lists have been expanded but are by no means considered complete.

Many people helped in producing this edition and I would like to gratefully acknowledge their contributions.

Miss Mia Reinap and her coworkers were most helpful in researching the literature at the Flower Library, New York State Veterinary College.

I wish to thank Dr. Bruce Hohn, Professor of Surgery and Radiology, College of Veterinary Medicine, Ohio State University, for permission to use the illustrations on approaches to the hip joint.

Dr. George Ross, Jr., Professor of Small Animal Surgery, New York State Veterinary College, provided material for illustrations as well as technical advice.

Both Dr. Robert Kirk and Dean George Poppensiek were most kind in providing facilities for the work.

Dr. Jack Geary, Professor of Radiology, New York State Veterinary College, advised concerning the radiographic illustrations and provided material on atlanto-axial subluxations.

Dr. Howard Evans, Professor of Anatomy, New York State Veterinary College, provided help and advice on anatomical problems.

Miss Marion Newson, Medical Artist, New York State Veterinary College, made the new line drawings found in Chapter 13.

Miss Mel Scherzer, free lance artist, prepared the schematic line drawings.

The photographs were made by Mr. Martin Bingham and Mr. Frederick Keib of Photo Science Studios, Cornell University.

In addition to their regular duties Mrs. Pauline Lawery and Mrs. Judy McPherson typed the manuscript.

My wife Alice, always a source of encouragement, gave considerable help with the proofreading.

The usual expert advice and cooperation was provided by the staff at W. B. Saunders Company in the final production of this book.

I am, indeed, grateful for the assistance given me by all of these people.

ELLIS P. LEONARD

Preface to
First Edition

The American Board of Orthopedic Surgery has indicated that orthopedic surgery is "that branch of surgery especially concerned with the preservation and restoration of the function of the skeletal system, its articulations, and associated structures." It may be defined as that branch of surgery which deals with the corrective treatment of disease or deformity of the locomotor system.

The word "orthopedic" is a modification through usage of the correctly spelled word "orthopaedic." It originated from two Greek words, *orthos*, meaning straight, and *pais*, meaning child. It could, therefore, be literally translated to mean "the straightening of children."

Professor Nicholas André first used the word "orthopedic" in 1741 when he published *The Art of Preventing and Correcting Deformities in the Bodies of Children*. His approach to the problem was through diet, exercise, and the use of various external appliances. Since that time, orthopedics has taken on a much broader meaning as applied to humans and a less broad and slightly different meaning as applied to animals.

Among the writings of Hippocrates are found the early observations on fractures and their repair. The search for ways and means of correcting fractures and relieving deformities, however, was begun by man centuries before. During the eighteenth century, the dog began to play a part in fracture investigations, and today its role is extremely important in the preliminary investigation of fracture repair.

In veterinary surgery, the application of orthopedic procedures has primarily been one of correction and repair of the skeletal system as it applies to locomotion, and more particularly following fracture or dislocation. It is natural to think of orthopedic surgery in these terms in a profession in which euthanasia is so commonly practiced. Whenever deformity appears, whether it be hereditary or acquired, congenital or degenerative, the usual decision until recent years has been to destroy the patient for economic or humane reasons.

The basic surgery in veterinary orthopedics has been repair of fractures and luxations. Even this has not been extensively practiced in large animals.

Nevertheless, with the advance of knowledge in all phases of medicine and surgery, veterinary orthopedic surgery is gradually encompassing more corrective procedures. Perhaps equally responsible for this change is the fact that there has been tremendous demand for treatment of small animals whose sentimental value far outweighs their economic value.

After twenty-five years of clinical study and observation in the field of orthopedics, the author has recorded as concisely as possible his experiences in orthopedic surgery. For whatever reason seemed important, the experience of others has also been incorporated in this book. For many years it has seemed advisable to bring together into one volume the contributions of many colleagues in this field, beginning with the modern pioneers of orthopedics such as Dibbell, Schroeder, Stader, and Self and including our contemporaries. Much material dealing with orthopedic problems is scattered throughout the veterinary literature and from this the author has drawn heavily; however, the book has been written in the light of his own experience. This book is devoted almost entirely to surgery and principally to that surgery which deals with fractures and luxations. Beginning with bone and cartilage as the two primary tissues involved in such injuries, the basic concepts of bone healing and the aseptic repair of fractures are set forth. The mechanics of reduction and fixation are discussed in some detail, but always with the thought in mind that we are dealing with a living, vital substance, the repair of which requires a sound understanding of all the basic medical sciences.

The mechanics of orthopedics is not difficult to master, and one soon becomes acquainted with the technical details. It cannot be emphasized too strongly, because of this fact, that successful repair depends on good surgical judgment, gentle handling of tissues, and the simplest form of repair consistent with sound recovery.

In composing a book of this kind it is always difficult to know where to discontinue. The principal discussion centers around surgery of the osteochondropathies of the body where locomotion is involved. Hip dysplasia and hypertrophic pulmonary osteoarthropathy are included primarily on the basis of their relationship to locomotion and not because of the surgical aspects of these diseases, even though some slight surgical facet might be found. Other conditions of a surgical or nonsurgical nature, such as sprains, muscular disease, bone tumors, amputations, and bone deformities in general, could have been included for the same reason. They were arbitrarily omitted in the interest of consolidation.

In the interest of clarity, it might be pointed out that the two terms "trauma" and "signs," which are used repeatedly in the text, are used according to their original meanings. For example, the word "trauma" refers to a condition of tissues resulting from violence to those tissues. In contradistinction to the frequent use of the word "trauma" to indicate an etiological factor, i.e., "The injury was caused by trauma," the cause in most cases of trauma is force. In using the word "sign," we are referring to an objective indication of disease, whereas the word "symptom" is subjective and could be used in certain instances when the patient actually complains about his ailment.

The term "epiphyseal separation" has been used sparingly throughout this text, although it is common practice to use it when referring to separations through the epiphyseal line. Nevertheless, most separations at the epiphyseal line show some fracture of adjacent bone. It is for this reason that the term "epiphyseal fracture" has been chosen to denote this condition.

This work has been written as an introduction to small animal orthopedics. It is presented with the student in mind but the practitioner will find it helpful, particularly in the areas of specific treatment. Since the book is of an introductory nature, the references at the end of each chapter are intended to serve as further source material and not as documentary evidence.

In addition to the picayune technicalities of writing a manuscript, there are scores of important tasks which require the assistance of others. I would like to acknowledge with gratitude the considerable help given me in this task by my friends and colleagues.

Valuable assistance in the preparatory research was rendered by Miss Mia Reinap and her staff at the Flower Library of the New York State Veterinary College.

Members of the Anatomy Department were most generous with their help. The late Dr. M. E. Miller furnished several anatomical specimens as well as the information concerning the circulation of the hip joint. Dr. R. E. Habel furnished the microscopic specimens of cartilage and bone, and Dr. H. E. Evans supplied the specimen from which the drawing of ossification centers was made.

Miss Marion Newson, Medical Artist for the New York State Veterinary College, prepared the line drawings with great care and skill. Unfortunately, only a few of her drawings were signed. The roentgenographic prints and other illustrations were prepared by Mr. Martin Bingham of the Photo Science Studios at Cornell University. Mrs. Olga Reidemanis and Mr. Donald Swart assisted me in preparing the material to be photographed and Dr. Robert Kenney, Research Associate of the Department of Pathology and Bacteriology, procured and photographed some of the pathologic specimens.

Mrs. Norma Jordan, Mrs. Pauline Marquis, and Mrs. Marjorie Laughlin spent many hours of diligent work typing the manuscript.

My colleague, Dr. Robert W. Kirk, assumed added responsibilities in the department during my preoccupation, and for this I am grateful. Dr. André Lavignette, Medical Interne in the department, was helpful in assembling case material.

At home I received both encouragement in the writing and help in the proofreading from my wife, Alice, and my son, Lee.

Finally, the help and cooperation given to me by the staff of the W. B. Saunders Company has been outstanding.

To the foregoing people, then, goes a large share of the credit for the production of this work.

ELLIS P. LEONARD

Contents

Part One   General Considerations

Chapter 1

BONE 3

    Cartilage 3
    Bone Composition 6
    Bone Formation 6
    Bone Circulation 8

Chapter 2

BONE HEALING 10

    Normal Healing 10
    Delayed Union and Non-union 12

Chapter 3

ASEPTIC SURGERY IN ORTHOPEDICS 17

    Preparation of Materials 17
    Preparation of the Patient 21
    Preparation of the Surgeon 26

Chapter 4

METHODS AND MATERIALS 30

    Closed Reduction 30
    Open Reduction 32

External Fixation 32
Internal Fixation 55

Part Two   Fractures

Classification of Fractures 90
Diagnosis 94
Treatment 95

Chapter 5

FRACTURES IN THE PELVIC LIMB 97

Fractures of the Femur 97
    Fractures of the Femoral Head and Neck 97
    Fractures of the Proximal Segment 111
    Fractures of the Middle Segment 113
    Fractures of the Distal Segment 120
Fracture of the Patella 127
Fractures of the Tibia and Fibula 128
    Fractures of the Proximal Segment 128
    Fractures of the Middle Segment 131
    Fractures of the Distal Segment 135
Fractures of the Tarsus, Metatarsus and Phalanges 138

Chapter 6

FRACTURES IN THE PECTORAL LIMB 145

Fractures of the Scapula 145
Fractures of the Humerus 147
    Fractures of the Proximal Segment 147
    Fractures of the Middle Segment 148
    Supracondylar and Intercondylar Fractures 152
Fractures of the Radius and Ulna 163
Fractures of the Carpus and Metacarpus 171

Chapter 7

FRACTURES OF THE SKULL, SPINE AND PELVIS 173

Fractures of the Skull 173
Fractures of the Spine 184
Fractures of the Ribs and Sternum 189
Fractures of the Pelvis 191

Part Three   Luxations

Diagnosis 201
Treatment 201

Chapter 8

LUXATIONS IN THE PELVIC LIMB 203

Coxo-femoral Luxation (Luxation of the Hip) 203
Patellar Luxations 218
Femoro-tibial Luxations 226
Luxations of the Hock Joint (Tibio-tarsal Luxations,
    Tarsal Luxations, Tarso-metatarsal Luxations) 242

Chapter 9

LUXATIONS IN THE PECTORAL LIMB 250

Scapulo-humeral Luxations (Luxations of the Shoulder) 250
Humero-radio-ulnar Luxations (Luxations of the Elbow) 253
Luxations of the Carpus, Metacarpus, and Phalanges 256

Chapter 10

LUXATIONS OF THE MANDIBLE AND SPINE 258

Luxation of the Mandible (Temporo-mandibular Luxation) 258
Luxations of the Spine 260

Part Four   Other Orthopedic Diseases

Chapter 11

SOFT TISSUE REPAIR IN COMPOUND FRACTURES 269

Nerve Repair 270
Vascular Repair 271
Tendon Repair 274

Chapter 12

AMPUTATIONS 278

Amputation of the Pelvic Limb 278
Amputation of the Pectoral Limb 282
Amputation of the Digit 286

Chapter 13

INTERVERTEBRAL DISC DISEASE (ENCHONDROSIS INTERVERTEBRALIS)... 288

Chapter 14

HIP DYSPLASIA... 313

Chapter 15

LEGG-PERTHES DISEASE (LEGG-CALVÉ-PERTHES DISEASE, COXA PLANA OSTEOCHONDROSIS, OSTEOCHONDRITIS) 322

Chapter 16

ELBOW DYSPLASIA 327

Chapter 17

OSTEOCHONDRITIS DISSECANS.. 331

Chapter 18

HYPERTROPHIC PULMONARY OSTEOARTHROPATHY (MARIE'S DISEASE, ACROPACHIA, HYPERTROPHIC OSTEOPERIOSTITIS) 338

INDEX.. 343

PART ONE

General Considerations

Chapter 1

Bone

Just as the craftsman who works with wood or metal must know the nature of the material with which he is working before he can expect to achieve success in his field, so the orthopedist must acquaint himself with the character of his "raw material." Too often bone has been looked upon as an inert material and likened to a piece of wood to be sawed, planed, or nailed without thought as to its structure or physical properties. Bone is a living tissue which provides skeletal support to the body and which adapts itself to a variety of situations within the body and its appendages. Instead of being inert, bone is a growing, constantly changing substance of vital importance in sustaining the posture and locomotion of the animal. It is connective tissue of a very specialized type, being closely related to cartilage; the essential difference is that bone is hard. Gradually, the true nature of skeletal tissue cells is becoming more definitive because of newer methods of investigation. It is now possible to study bone in its natural state.

Bone is formed by cells called osteoblasts and resorbed or destroyed by osteoclasts. Both of these cells are active within the skeletal system throughout life. In general, the activity is greatest during the period of growth and more subdued during maturity. Cellular activity in mature bone is stimulated, either locally or in the bony framework as a whole, by disease, mechanical force, or injury.

Since we shall be concerned with cartilage from time to time throughout this book and since cartilage plays an important role in the development of bone, it would therefore be fitting to present a brief discussion of cartilage before proceeding to bone.

CARTILAGE

We recognize three types of cartilage in the body. They are elastic cartilage, fibrocartilage, and hyaline cartilage.

Elastic cartilage (Fig. 1) is so called because of the large number of elastic fibers which make up the framework surrounding the cartilage cells.

3

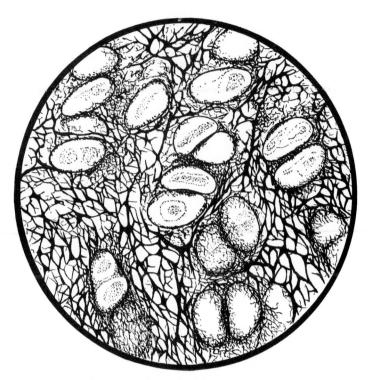

Figure 1. Elastic cartilage. This shows the large cartilage cells with elastic fibers around them. (Drawn from specimen loaned by Dr. R. E. Habel.)

These elastic fibers, while accounting for its great flexibility, also constitute the principal characteristic which distinguishes elastic cartilage from hyaline cartilage. This type of cartilage is found in the external ear and epiglottis and is of little interest to the orthopedist.

Fibrocartilage (Fig. 2) has many collagen fibers arranged in lines parallel to the lines of stress and therefore has great tensile strength. This type of cartilage is found in the capsule (annular cartilage or annulus fibrosus) of the intervertebral disc, the menisci of the stifle, the ligamentum teres of the femur, the symphysis of the pubis, and in the insertion of tendons. Its presence in joints such as the stifle tends to improve the articulation by deepening it (menisci).

Hyaline cartilage (Fig. 3) consists of nests of cartilage cells surrounded by a homogeneous mass composed of collagen fibers and cementing substance which binds the whole together. The cells are nourished by diffusion of tissue fluids through the matrix surrounding them. This cartilage is widely distributed throughout the body and is the precursor of bone in the fetal and growing animal. The trachea, the cartilages of the nose, the costal cartilages, and the articular cartilages are formed of hyaline cartilage.

Perichondrium covers cartilage in the same manner as periosteum covers bone. There is no perichondrium covering the joint surfaces of long

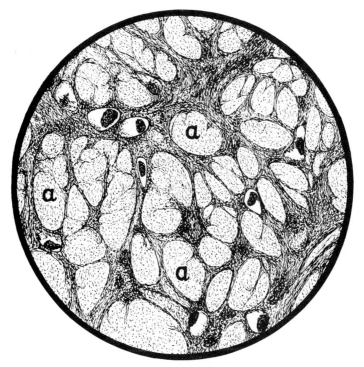

Figure 2. Fibrocartilage; a, collagenous fiber bundles in cross section. (Drawn from specimen loaned by Dr. R. E. Habel.)

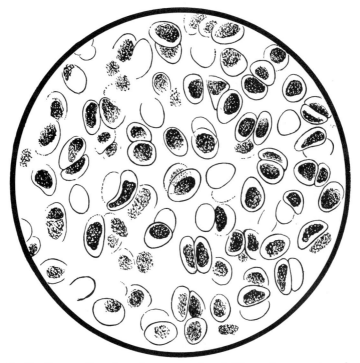

Figure 3. Hyaline cartilage from the carpus of a cat. (Drawn from specimen loaned by Dr. R. E. Habel.)

5

bones, however. The appositional growth of cartilage is from the inner layer of the perichondrium which corresponds to the growth of cortical bone from the deep layer of the periosteum. The outer layer is fibrous and acts as a sheath. Interstitial growth of cartilage occurs only in the young animal, and this is accomplished by the division of chondrocytes.

BONE COMPOSITION

There are three principal components of bone. The first of these is the organic matrix, which is composed of 95 per cent collagen, 4 per cent mucopolysaccharides, and 1 per cent substances that have not been identified. Bone collagen is capable of calcifying, whereas the collagen in soft tissue cannot. Otherwise, the two are quite similar. The mucopolysaccharide is an amorphous jelly exuded by the collagen fibers and serves as a ground substance for them.

Bone mineral, the second component, is hydroxyapatite and consists of about 38 per cent calcium. The term "mineralization" is preferred to "calcification" by Frost because of the low calcium content. Phosphate is the primary element in the deposition of mineral salts. During ossification, bone mineral displaces about 88 per cent of the bone water, which is loosely bound.

The third component is bone water. This is tightly bound to the matrix and remains after ossification.

BONE FORMATION

In the embryo of the dog and cat, bone originates by intramembranous ossification of connective tissue cells or by endochondral bone formation from a hyaline cartilage mold. Bones of the calvarium for the most part arise from intramembranous ossification. Long bones of the body, on the other hand, arise by endochondral formation from cartilage. Recent work by Evans and others tends to indicate that in the very early stages of ossification the centers may arise from intramembranous ossification and later become endochondral.

In the formation, then, of a long bone there is laid down a hyaline cartilage model which develops three centers of ossification, one in the middle of the diaphysis (Fig. 4) and one in each epiphysis. The cartilage cells around these centers calcify and are converted to bone over an ever-widening area until the diaphysis is completely ossified. Circumferential growth then continues from the cambium layer of the periosteum but at a much slower rate. Growth is by apposition and resorption, and although this continues throughout life, it is at a far slower pace during maturity. Longitudinal growth is controlled by the epiphyseal plates, which remain active

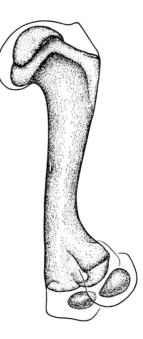

Figure 4. Centers of ossification in a long bone. Ossification begins in the diaphysis before birth. This is taken from a week-old beagle puppy and shows beginning of ossification in the epiphyses. (Drawn from specimen loaned by Dr. H. E. Evans.)

throughout the growing period by producing cartilage cells that are in turn converted to bone cells. Eventually the metaphysis (epiphyseal plate) becomes ossified and longitudinal growth of the bone ceases.

Bone formation may occur directly from connective tissue cells as in the development of the flat bones of the skull. This also occurs in adult life in certain fracture repairs where the space between the fracture segments is not great.

Structurally, bone may be divided into three types, all of which are present to some degree in every bone:

Cortical or Compact Bone

This is the hard bone which is the supporting outside framework and surface. It is composed of layers with longitudinal channels known as Haversian canals, which serve as conduits for nerves and blood vessels. Surrounding the Haversian canals are thin layers or rings of bone known as lamellae. These are concentric and variable in number and have lacunae containing osteocytes interspersed between them. Fine microscopic channels known as canaliculi form the communicating system between the lacunae.

Cancellous Bone

On the inner surface of cortical bone, a latticework of bone called cancellous acts much the same as the cross members in a girder. It is a supporting structure found in all bone and gets its nourishment directly from the bone marrow. It is not as hard as cortical bone and because of its shape does not have an Haversian system.

Medullary Bone

The connective tissue found in the marrow cavity and the interspaces of cancellous bone is sometimes referred to as medullary bone. It supports the marrow and blood vessels within the bone. Marrow, at first red, fills the entire cavity during the period of growth. It gradually becomes fatty and its hematopoietic activity becomes confined to the proximal epiphyses of the femur and humerus insofar as long bones are concerned. Red marrow remains, however, in the sternum, ribs, vertebrae, skull, and pelvis. This is one of the reasons that bone marrow taps are usually made in the sternum or crest of the ilium.

BONE CIRCULATION

Bone is completely covered on the outside by periosteum except for the head of the femur and at the points of articulation; these areas are covered by hyaline cartilage. The inside of the medullary cavity is lined with a membrane called endosteum, which covers all the cancellous bone. This membrane has but a single layer, whereas the periosteum is composed of an inner or cambium layer and an outer fibrous layer. Much of the blood supply

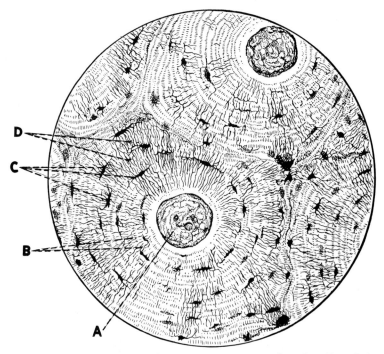

Figure 5. Cross section of a long bone. A, Haversian canal; B, lamellae; C, lacunae; D, canaliculi. (Drawn from specimen loaned by Dr. R. E. Habel.)

to bone is furnished by the endosteum and the periosteum. In long bones the blood circulation is further enhanced by the presence of a nutrient artery which enters the bone along its shaft. This vessel gives off branches to the Haversian system and terminates in the medullary canal in the form of sinusoidal capillaries.

Osteocytes receive their nourishment by way of the Haversian canals, the transverse channels (Volkmann canals), and finally by (Fig. 5) diffusion through the canaliculi. Through the bathing of bone cells in blood and lymph there is a constant exchange of nutritional elements and waste matter comparable to the exchange taking place in any other cells in the body. The process of tearing down and building up goes on throughout life but is particularly noticeable in bone that has been injured or subjected to undue stress.

Although very little information is available about the nerve supply of bone or marrow, we do know that endosteum and periosteum are well supplied with sensory nerve endings.

It is quite evident that bone is a complex substance and under certain circumstances behaves in a most amazing yet logical manner. The orthopedist who handles this substance with understanding will greatly improve his chances of success.

REFERENCES

Aegerter, E., and Kirkpatrick, J. A., Jr.: Orthopedic Diseases. 2nd ed. Philadelphia, W. B. Saunders Co., 1963.

Becker, R. O., Bassett, C. A., and Bachman, C. H.: Bioelectric factors controlling bone structure. *In* Bone Biodynamics (H. M. Frost, ed.). Boston, Little, Brown, 1964, pp 209–232.

Bourne, G. H.: Biochemistry and Physiology of Bone. New York, Academic Press, 1956.

Boyd, J. S.: Radiographic appearance of the centres of ossification of the limb bones of the feline foetus. Br. Vet. Jour. *124*:365–370, 1968.

Chapman, W. L., Jr.: Appearance of ossification centers and epiphyseal closures as determined by radiographic techniques. J.A.V.M.A., *147*:138–141, 1966.

Evans, H.: Personal communication.

Foldes, I.: Importance of Phosphate Esters in Endochondrial Ossification. Budapest, Akademiai Kiado, 1967.

Frost, H. M.: Bone Remodelling Dynamics. Springfield, Ill., Charles C Thomas, 1963.

Horn, V., John, U., and Willie, H.: Sternal marrow biopsy. I. Cell picture in healthy dogs. Arch. Exper. Vet. Med., 7:177, 1953.

Jordan, H. E.: A Textbook of Histology. 5th Ed. New York, D. Appleton & Co., 1930.

McLean, F. C., and Urist, M. R.: Bone. 3rd Ed. Chicago, University of Chicago Press, 1968.

Smith, R. N.: Appearance of ossification centres in the kitten, recorded as individual bones. J. Small Animal Pract., 9:497–511, 1968.

Stein, I., Stein, R. O., and Beller, M. L.: Living Bone in Health and Disease. Philadelphia, J. B. Lippincott Co., 1955.

Sumner-Smith, G.: Observations on epiphyseal fusion of the canine appendicular skeleton. J. Small Animal Pract., *1*:303–311, 1966.

Chapter 2

Bone Healing

NORMAL HEALING

Fracture repair is by cellular growth, which is characteristic of all living tissues. It is therefore highly important that one have a complete understanding of both the physiologic and the pathologic reactions of living tissues before undertaking to assist nature in the repair of these tissues. Whenever bone is injured there is a proliferative reaction on the part of this tissue unlike that of any other tissue in the body. New bone is formed instead of scar tissue through growth originating in the periosteum and the endosteum. In the membranous bones (skull) the growth is by direct extension from the old bone. In the long bones a cartilage mold may first be laid down to fill large gaps in a manner similar to the embryonic formation of bone. Cartilage, therefore, is a precursor of bone, as explained in the previous chapter. In areas where the periosteum is intact or where cancellous bone is in contact across the fracture line, bone healing may take place by direct extension. One should remember that whenever bone is stripped of periosteum the circulation is likely to be cut off and some of the bone cells will die. This will then leave a gap in the fracture even though the ends of bone are in apposition.

Cell proliferation begins after 24 to 48 hours in the soft tissues surrounding the fracture as well as in the periosteum and endosteum. These cells are undifferentiated connective tissue cells at the outset, but quickly develop into osteoblasts, chondroblasts, and fibroblasts.

It is believed that the cells originating from the bony tissues produce osteoblasts and chondroblasts, whereas those from the softer tissues produce fibroblasts. It is further postulated that as the need for more osteoblasts arises, in order to convert fibrous tissue and cartilage to bone, the fibroblasts and chondroblasts transform to osteoblasts.

The first week following a fracture is the most active time of cell proliferation. This is closely related to the extent of the damage to both hard and soft tissues, the degree of motion of the fracture site, the presence or absence of infection, and any other factor which would contribute to an inflammatory state.

10

The periosteal callus is formed early and is composed of hyaline cartilage; the space-occupying cartilage which fills the fracture gap is fibrocartilage. The outer layer of the callus is fibrous connective tissue, which serves as a barrier to keep the callus within bounds. The hyaline cartilage is rapidly replaced by bone, but the fibrocartilage is replaced much more slowly.

During the late stages of repair, remodeling takes place to form the several parts into a single unit of bone. This remodeling is controlled according to Wolff's law, which states that structure and mechanical stress are directly related. The bone, therefore, responds to the mechanical stress put upon it by osteoclastic and osteoblastic activity, which changes the shape and strength of the bone to meet the need. This response is also seen in growing bone and normal adult bone when placed under stress. One theory for this type of response is that there is a change in the electrical potential when stress is applied to bone, so that osteoblastic activity increases under increased work load and osteoclastic activity increases under a decreased load.

At the instant of fracture there is separation of the hard parts, varying in extent and degree depending upon the force factors involved (external and muscular), the fragility of the bone, and, to a lesser degree, upon the location. Hemorrhage follows immediately and fills the space between the bone ends, the medullary canal adjacent to the fracture, spaces under any loosened periosteum, and tissue space in the areas. During the next few days, the serum and blood which has thus collected begins to organize in the way that any traumatic exudate would be expected to organize. This mass of exudate, consisting of blood and serum, completely engulfs the fracture site. The proper repair of the fracture depends entirely on how well histologic organization of this mass takes place.

The blood clot begins to organize within the first 24 hours and granulation tissue makes its appearance. Both the periosteum and the endosteum begin to proliferate and form fibrous connective tissue which gradually extends to bridge the gap between the bone ends. Fibrocartilage and hyaline cartilage also form in the process of organizing the clot. When large fracture spaces occur in long bones, cartilage forms to fill the flaw and acts as a framework for the formation of new bone. When there is little or no displacement of bone, the fracture site will be bridged by fibrous connective tissue which converts directly to bone. In young animals, fractures of the flat bones of the skull heal by extension without callus formation, but spaces left by bone loss in the adult cranium will not be replaced.

Watson-Jones, in his book *Fractures and Joint Injuries*, states that fracture healing is one continuous process, but that it can be divided into three histologic stages, as follows: First stage, the formulation of delicate granulation tissue in which the fragments of bone are still freely movable. Second stage, the growth of cartilage and bone cells with an increased stability at the fracture site, which still requires immobilization. At the end of this stage there is "clinical union." Third stage, formation of mature bone. At this stage we have both clinical and radiographic evidence of sound union.

The first biochemical reaction in all injured tissue is the release of histamine and acetylcholine. When a fracture occurs, the liberation of these substances increases the hyperemia of the area, and this, coupled with the hemorrhage, damaged tissue, and damaged bone, creates a considerable amount of cellular debris in the area. Because of the presence of this cellular debris, there is a lowering of the pH of the tissue fluids in the fracture clot and in the tissue surrounding the fracture site. For a few days following a fracture, there is a decalcification process because of the acidity of the local tissue fluids. This means that the mobilization of calcium for the eventual ossification of the callus is brought about in the first few days of the injury, that it is held in solution so long as the tissue fluids remain acid, and that the calcium for the repair of a fracture is derived from the blood and bone at the site of the fracture. The hematoma surrounding a fracture is rich in calcium and phosphorus, despite the fact that the blood level remains unchanged. This is true whether the animal is old or young, male or female, well-nourished or poorly nourished. There is some question as to whether the bone enzyme, alkaline phosphatase, enters into this reaction to bring about a release of phosphate from the plasma, thus causing a supersaturation of the fracture fluid with calcium phosphate. Alkaline phosphatase is elaborated during the formation of the matrix and is thought to be associated with collagen formation and not with mineralization. The evidence is not complete, however. By whatever method it arrives, it is quite evident that ample calcium is mobilized at the site of the fracture, provided that sufficient injury and hematoma are present. It has been fairly well established that the addition of minerals to the diet following a fracture has little to do with improving the callus.

As soon as the circulation surrounding the fracture becomes reestablished, the pH returns to the alkaline side and the calcium is redeposited within the fibrocartilaginous callus. From a practical clinical viewpoint, this phenomenon is a most important factor to bear in mind when attending a fracture case. It can readily be seen from the foregoing that immobilization is extremely important, because without it there will be constant irritation and hemorrhage at the fracture site, thereby keeping the pH lowered and the calcium in solution. This leads to delayed union and a soft, noncalcified callus. By the same token, the importance of a good blood clot at the fracture site can be readily understood if one realizes the part played by this hematoma in the formation of new bone. In addition, the clot furnishes the framework for the fibrocartilaginous callus during the ossification process. The meticulous clearing away of all blood clots at the site of an open reduction can lead only to delayed union or non-union.

DELAYED UNION AND NON-UNION

Delayed union refers to an exceptionally long healing time; non-union implies that no healing which tends to bridge the fracture site has taken place. The rate of calcification of the callus, therefore, would determine whether one is dealing with delayed union or non-union. In nearly all instances there is some fibrous connective tissue present, but ossification has not taken place or has been considerably delayed. For the most part, delayed union and non-union can be considered together etiologically.

The pH of the tissue fluids about the fracture site is of utmost importance and anything which influences this pH should be considered when dealing with the problems of bone union. Such factors as movement at the fracture site, dead tissue from whatever source, and circulation to the part have a direct bearing on the pH. So long as the tissue fluids remain on the acid side, calcium will remain in solution and calcification will not take place.

Granulation at the fracture site should also be considered. Insufficient granulation may occur as a result of a sparse hematoma or through the destruction of periosteum and/or endosteum. Most of the problems with bone union occur in fractures in the distal third of the radius and tibia, where circulation to the bone is poorest and where surrounding tissue may not be sufficiently damaged to create a good fracture hematoma. When the problem of union has been artificially produced, the trouble usually can be traced to an overzealous operator who has done an excellent job of hemostasis and removal of blood clots during the course of his open repair.

Prevention

Good immobilization is most essential in preventing delayed union. With the part stabilized so that further tissue injury is prevented, the pH will swing to the alkaline side in due course because there will be no further stimulation to acidification by addition of more necrotic cells from hemorrhage or damaged bone.

In addition to stabilizing the fracture, apposition is important from the standpoint of conserving the callus and preventing non-union where callus constituents are scanty.

Attention should be given to the circulation so that it may return to normal as rapidly as possible, thereby enhancing the biochemical reaction of tissue fluids in the area.

Infection is definitely a cause for delay and non-union because of the inflammation which accompanies it. Any inflammatory process will keep the fracture site in a state of flux because of its tendency to lower pH. Such a situation might reasonably exist in the case of a compound fracture, but it is inexcusable following surgical exposure of the bone.

Non-union can be prevented by making certain that sufficient hematoma is at the fracture site and that there is no tissue interposed to prevent bridging of the callus. Perhaps the most common mistake in open reduction of fractures is the removal of the blood clot from the fracture site. To be sure, it is necessary at times to uncover the bone ends in order to appose them properly. It is never necessary, however, to remove all blood from the fracture site. As a matter of fact, the more that can be retained the better, since this is the framework and part of the materials from which the new bone will be built.

The interposition of tissue between fracture segments is a far less common cause of non-union in dogs and cats than we have been led to believe, but it can on occasion be a factor. If it is thought that apposition is being prevented through the interference of muscle or fascia, an open reduction should be performed.

Finally, delayed union and non-union can be prevented by avoiding the use of diathermy or x-ray therapy during the first three weeks of healing. It is quite evident that such procedures promote an inflammatory reaction which results in delay of calcification.

Treatment

Treatment of delayed union and non-union should be aimed at achieving two goals: (1) A new callus must be laid down which will have sufficient calcium to ossify. This can be accomplished in cases of delayed union by mutilating the old soft callus with a sharp instrument, such as an intramedullary pin. This will cause a fresh hematoma to form and calcify. In mild cases, a simple method of producing inflammation and hemorrhage is to allow the dog to go without a splint for a few days. The excessive movement at the fracture site may cause sufficient bleeding and stimulation. In cases of non-union, open reduction should be performed and a thin transverse slice of bone cut from each segment. Usually in these cases the boring of holes in the bone ends is not sufficient. Non-union frequently results in eburnation of the bone ends, and it is therefore necessary to start with fresh exposure of the bone, periosteum and endosteum. The cut ends should bleed freely so that a good hematoma will be formed. Seeding of the site with fresh bone chips, particularly of cancellous bone, has been recommended. The author has used this method to good advantage on several occasions.

(2) The fracture must be rigidly fixed so that movement cannot continue to be a source of irritation interfering with the deposition of calcium. Since many delayed unions and non-unions are seen in the tibia or the radius, it is suggested that some form of half pin splintage be used as fixation. Coaptation alone is insufficient, and conventional intramedullary pinning in these two bones does not overcome all rotational movement. A few successful cases have been reported in which a shuttle pin and coaptation were used. Whatever method is used for this type of case, the operator should assure himself that the immobilization is secure.

When bone healing is delayed because of infection at the fracture site, it goes without saying that the infection must be eliminated before any attempt is made to correct the union. The infection should be dealt with vigorously by making ample exposure of the area so that it can be cleared of debris and drained. Cultures should be made and the patient treated both locally and systemically with a specific antibiotic. Only when it is certain that no infection remains should restorative measures be applied to the fracture.

Bone Graft

The first clinical transplant of bone was made in 1880 by Macewen when he successfully grafted bone from the tibia onto the humerus. Actually, bone transplants are not true grafts, because they do not continue to live in the manner of a true graft. It was pointed out earlier that the injured edges of a fracture die and that these bone cells are replaced by new bone. So it is with the graft. The cut edges as well as all isolated bone cells die and are replaced by new bone. Only the cells of the periosteum and endosteum remain viable to furnish the impetus for new bone formation. Since the cambium layer of the periosteum becomes rather inactive in older dogs, callus formation around bone grafts requires a much longer time in old dogs than it does in young ones.

Grafts can be classified according to their source as: (1) autogenous, bone taken from the same individual; (2) homogenous, bone taken from the same species; or (3) heterogenous, bone taken from another species. Depending on the kind of bone used, transplants may be referred to as *compact* or *cancellous*. Except in the young growing animal, cancellous bone seems to furnish more osteogenetic cells than compact bone.

Regardless of the kind of graft used, there will be constant bone absorption and bone deposition until eventually the entire transplant is replaced by new living bone. It is therefore the function of the bone transplant to act as a framework on which callus can be built, as well as to be utilized in the process by replacement. Homogenous bone fulfills this function in both the fresh and preserved state, but autogenous bone is preferable because it will supply osteogenic impetus from its covering membranes.

The whole subject of bone healing in relation to bone grafts might be summarized by saying that the ideal graft would be performed on a young dog with autogenous cancellous bone. Departing from this ideal healing situation, we would encounter a gradually increasing healing time with various combinations, that of the old dog with a heterogenous compact bone transplant requiring the longest healing time and being the least likely to succeed.

REFERENCES

Allgöwer, M.: Healing of clinical fractures of the tibia with rigid internal fixation. *In* The Healing of Osseous Tissue (R. A. Robinson, ed.). Washington, D.C., National Academy of Sciences—National Research Council, 1967.

Anderson, L. D.: Healing of standard discontinuities of long bones as observed roentgenographically, grossly, and histologically in the adult dog. *In* Healing of Osseous Tissue (R. A. Robinson, ed.). Washington, D.C., National Academy of Sciences—National Research Council, 1967.

Anderson, K. J., and Dingwall, J. A.: The osteogenic repair of long bone defects in the immature and mature cat. *In* The Healing of Osseus Tissue (R. A. Robinson, ed.). Washington, D.C., National Academy of Sciences—National Research Council, 1967.

Bancroft, F. W., and Marble, H. C.: Surgical Treatment of the Motor-Skeletal System. 2nd Ed. Philadelphia, J. B. Lippincott Co., 1951.

Bourne, G. H.: The Biochemistry and Physiology of Bone. New York, Academic Press, 1956.

Davis, L. (ed.): Christopher's Textbook of Surgery. 9th Ed. Philadelphia, W. B. Saunders Co., 1968.

Greville, N. R., and James, J. M.: Surg. Gynec. Obstet., *105*:717, 1957.

Gunn, R. M. C.: Australia Vet. J., *12*:139, 1936.

McLean, F. C., and Urist, M. R.: Bone. 3rd Ed. Chicago, University of Chicago Press, 1968.

Stader, O.: North American Vet., *20*:60, 1939.

Tonna, E. A.: The source of osteoblasts in healing fractures in animals of different ages. *In* The healing of Osseus Tissue (R. A. Robinson, ed.). Washington, D.C., National Academy of Sciences—National Research Council, 1967.

Watson-Jones, R.: Fractures and Joint Injuries, 4th ed. Baltimore, Williams & Wilkins Co., 1952.

Chapter 3

Aseptic Surgery in Orthopedics

Whenever surgery is contemplated for repair of bones, ligaments, joints, or cartilages, the need for asepsis is paramount. Unfortunately, the veterinary profession has not completely outlived the era of antiseptic surgery. It is suggested that those who persist in this antiquated approach refer cases requiring orthopedic surgery to colleagues who are equipped and trained in asepsis. Many poor results in orthopedics can be traced to either a half-way attempt at asepsis or a complete disregard for it. A definite system must be established and a rigorous routine followed if one is to be truly aseptic in surgery. Application of a mask to the face and gloves to the hands does not constitute an aseptic approach. There are no half-way measures in the endeavor to do clean surgery.

Preparation should all be done outside the surgery so that only a clean patient and a clean surgeon enter the operating room. This room should be kept spotlessly clean, paying close attention to cabinet tops, ceiling, floors, and operating lights. If assistants are used, they should be clean and should be made conscious of the bacterial adversaries attending all surgery. Air circulation in an operating room is a definite hazard and should be minimized.

Preparation for aseptic surgery may be divided into three main categories: (1) preparation of materials such as drapes, gowns, gloves, and instruments; (2) preparation of the patient; and (3) preparation of the surgeon.

PREPARATION OF MATERIALS

The first material to consider is that used for drapes. Too often the drape gets little consideration, and yet it is the principal safeguard against contamination during surgery. Various types of materials are used for covering the patient, ranging from plastic to huck towels. A heavy unbleached muslin makes a very satisfactory drape; furthermore, it is easy to obtain, easy to handle, and relatively inexpensive. This material can be torn into sheets of appropriate size and the raw edges hemmed. The cloth can then be dyed

17

green, blue, or gray so that reflected light around the surgical field will be reduced. This adds greatly to the surgeon's ability to see clearly. The drapes should be of adequate size (60 by 36 inches) so that the patient and the table are completely covered. Small drapes are hazardous because they leave too many contaminated areas exposed.

The drapes are placed in bundles of four each after they have been folded four times across the width and an accordion fold applied lengthwise (Fig. 6). The wrapper for the bundle is held in place by pressure-sensitive tape, which is a reasonably good sterile indicator provided the bundles are small. Large bundles require an indicator within the pack.

Thorough cleaning of instruments prior to sterilization is very important. Soaking in a cleaning solution is helpful in removing blood and other surgical debris. The use of a brush on box lock instruments is not recommended because of the tendency for bristles to lodge in the lock and cause it to bind.

Electronic equipment, although rather expensive, is available for instrument cleaning. This equipment is very efficient and much more effective than hand cleaning. High-frequency sound is used with a wetting agent or detergent of low surface tension. Three factors are believed to produce the cleaning effect. They are pressure, temperature, and acceleration. The negative pressure produced by oscillation destroys all cellular material. The passage of sound waves through the solution produces a very high temperature. The acceleration is brought about by the impact of fine cavitation bubbles. There is substantial evidence to show that the electronic method

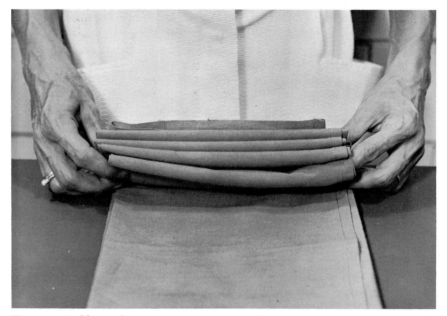

Figure 6. Folding a drape in preparation for sterilization. This is an "accordion" fold.

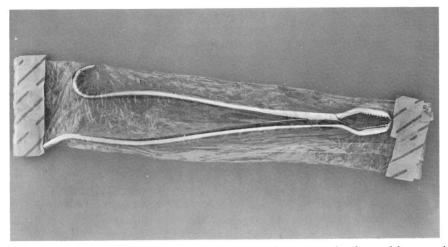

Figure 7. Bone forceps in transparent sterilizing tubing. Note the diagonal lines on the pressure-sensitive tape, indicating that the package has been autoclaved.

not only cleans but also has a bactericidal effect because of the cellular destruction.

All the instruments commonly used in orthopedic procedures can be placed in a metal tray and folded into a large muslin wrapper (double thickness) of such dimensions that it will adequately cover the instrument stand when the bundle is opened. Special instruments can be placed in sterilizing tubing and handled as separate units. These do not require labeling, since the wrapper is transparent (Fig. 7).

Instruments with a cutting edge are likely to be dulled by the use of heat for sterilization. Chemical sterilization can be used for such instruments as knives and scissors. Pentecresol (Upjohn) is a very effective germicide for this purpose and has the further advantage of being noncorrosive and nonirritating. Instruments to be sterilized in germicidal fluids should be thoroughly cleaned and then immersed. Any debris clinging to the metal will reduce the efficiency of the germicide. It is also important that the instruments be allowed to soak in the germicide long enough to kill whatever organisms may be present. Although it is easier to sterilize metal instruments by this method than it is to sterilize the skin or other rough areas, one must not feel so secure that he forgets that these solutions will not kill spores. It is therefore important, if one suspects the presence of spore-formers, that he use a more vigorous type of sterilization for his instruments.

More recently, ethylene oxide gas has been used for the sterilization of sharp or cutting instruments such as knife blades and scissors, disposable articles like syringes and tubing, as well as equipment that cannot be subjected to high temperatures, i.e., plastic trachea tubes and catheters. Some prefer this type of sterilization and use it for all packs instead of heat.

The gas may be purchased in ampules for small sterilizing cannisters or in drums for large sterilizers. Before attempting to use gas sterilization, one should become familiar with the methods of use and the hazards involved. It requires special equipment and should only be used in a well-ventilated room. Contact with the skin can be very irritating and all materials should be given plenty of time to air before using.

The operating gown is folded as one would fold a suit coat, adding two extra lengthwise folds. An accordion fold is then applied starting at the hem of the gown and working toward the collar (Fig. 8). When the folded gown is placed in its wrapper, a disposable professional towel is placed on top before closing the bundle. This is used for drying the hands after scrubbing.

Gloves may be prepared for either the dry glove technique or the wet glove technique by thoroughly washing, drying, and lightly powdering them inside and out with Bio-Sorb (Johnson & Johnson). The cuff of each glove is turned back about two inches and a folded cotton sponge placed in the wrist to keep it open so that steam will circulate inside. The gloves are then placed in a glove wrapper (Fig. 9), along with a small envelope containing Bio-Sorb for dusting the hands before donning the gloves. It is important to place this envelope so that it can be withdrawn without touching the outside surface of the gloves. The glove wrapper is then folded once lengthwise. It is best to autoclave rubber goods separately, and because excessive heat

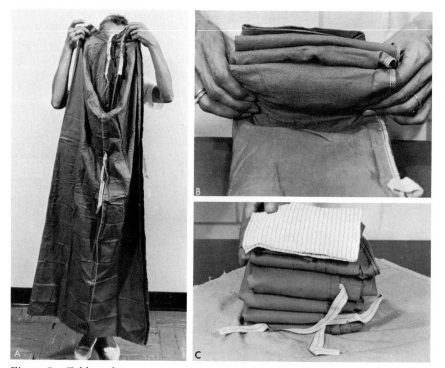

Figure 8. Folding the operating gown. A, The first fold, turning the sleeves inward. B, The "accordion" fold, starting at the bottom. C, A towel is placed on the folded gown. This is a disposable paper towel.

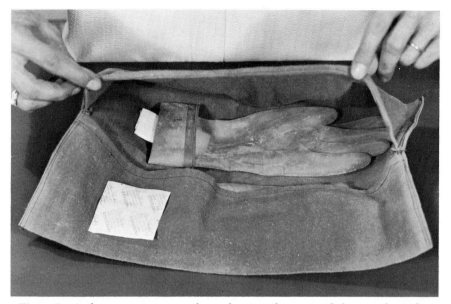

Figure 9.   A glove wrapper or envelope, showing placement of gloves and powder.

tends to weaken them, gloves are usually autoclaved at 15 pounds pressure for 15 minutes.

If Bio-Sorb cream is preferred, this can be purchased in sterile packets. A packet is deposited on the open sterile glove wrapper at the time of surgery by peeling off the outer nonsterile jacket and allowing the packet to fall free. When the cream is applied to the hands, it dries leaving a thin film of powder. It has the advantage of not producing powder dust in the air.

Autoclaving of the surgical bundles should be carried out at 20 pounds pressure for 30 minutes. At the end of this time, if the door to the chamber is left slightly ajar and the steam retained in the jacket, the bundles will dry nicely without danger of contamination. When it becomes necessary to use a pressure cooker in place of an autoclave, only a minimum amount of water should be used and the bundles should be elevated on a frame. With this method the bundles may be dried by loosening the lid and continuing with moderate heat after the sterilizing time has been completed.

PREPARATION OF THE PATIENT

The most thorough preparation of the surgical site can be done only after the patient is anesthetized. Preliminary bathing and clipping may be done in advance, but the actual skin preparation must wait until all movement is under control and the danger of recontamination is past. Preparation of the patient should be carried out in some room outside the surgery, if at

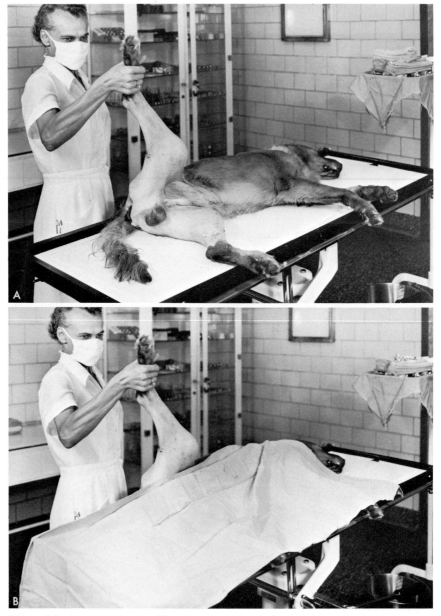

Figure 10. Draping the hind leg in preparation for bone surgery. A, An attendant holds the injured limb vertically. B, The first drape is laid to cover the inside of the opposite thigh and the body.

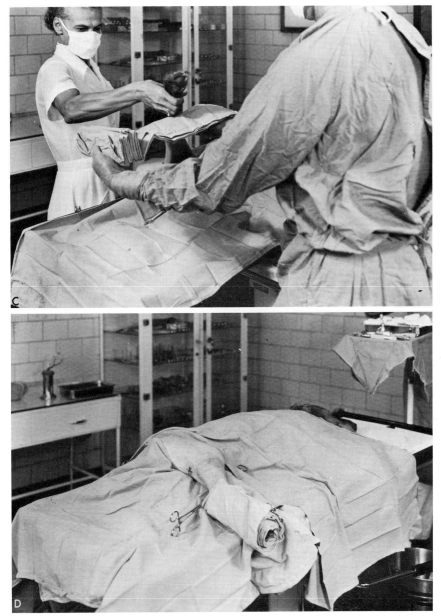

Figure 10 continued.   C, The foot is wrapped with a second drape. D, Two drapes are placed crosswise.

all possible, so that the danger of contamination from hair and skin debris can be reduced. This is especially true of the preliminary stages of preparation such as clipping and scrubbing.

The first step following a generous clipping of the area with No. 40 Oster clippers is a meticulous cleansing of the skin with soap and water or with a germicidal detergent such as hexachlorophene (pHisoHex). Scrubbing should be done with the hand or a sponge, since a brush causes excessive skin erythema and resultant delay in skin healing. When the skin has been scrubbed and rinsed with water, it should be dried with a clean towel.

The next step is to remove as much of the skin oil from the follicles as possible so that the final treatment with antiseptics will penetrate deeply. For this purpose, ether is applied with small cotton pledgets starting at the proposed line of incision and working parallel to it, each stroke coming nearer the periphery. When the outer periphery is reached the pledget is discarded and a new one is used to repeat the process. This means that we are constantly working from the cleanest area toward the more contaminated surrounding area and never returning to the incision line with anything that has touched the periphery. When there is no longer evidence of fats or oils showing on the pledgets, the second step has been completed.

The application of a skin disinfectant to the operative area is the final step. Ethyl alcohol is a popular skin disinfectant and is very effective, except against spores, provided the concentration is kept at 70 per cent by weight. Its effectiveness is lost if the concentration changes appreciably. To improve its effectiveness it should be applied with rubbing, following the same pattern as used for defatting. Isopropyl alcohol, although not effective against spores, is an otherwise good germicide even in solutions as low as 30 per cent. Iodine, especially in aqueous solution (U.S.P. Aqueous Iodine 2 per cent), is a good germicide but may be somewhat irritating to the skin. Most of the dye-type antiseptics derive whatever germicidal power they may have from their alcoholic content.

After the patient is positioned on the table, it may be necessary to repeat the disinfecting procedure. It is a wise precaution and can do no harm, particularly in view of the fact that we cannot expect to sterilize the skin and are therefore simply attempting to reduce the number of organisms present at the incision site.

Because the positioning and draping of the patient in the usual positions are well known, we shall concern ourselves with procedures only insofar as they apply to surgery on the limbs. The position in most cases is lateral recumbency with the injured limb uppermost. Exceptions to this rule are the application of half pinning to the tibia and the medial approach to the hip joint. An attendant holds the limb in a vertical position by grasping the toes while the first drape is laid lengthwise covering the other limbs. The second drape, without being unfolded, is used to grasp the distal part of the limb as it is released by the attendant. The drape is then wrapped around the foot and lower limb up to the operative area, where it is fastened with towel clamps. This gives a much better protection from contamination than a

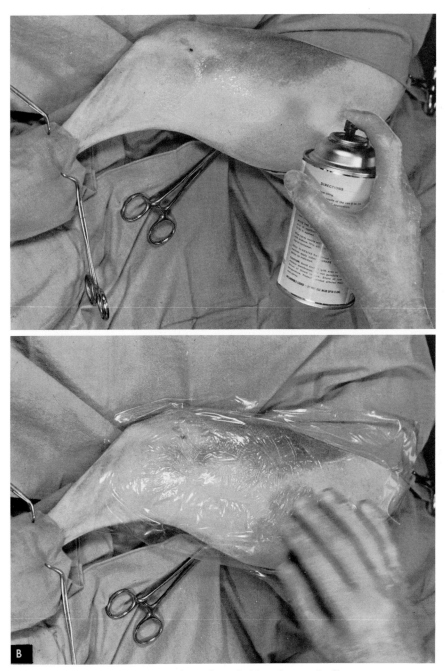

Figure 11. Using a plastic drape held in place with adhesive.

stockinette and still leaves the limb free above the first drape for easy manipulation. The third and fourth drapes are then placed crosswise over the patient so that they can be clamped above and beneath the injured limb (Fig. 10). Draping to the incision can be accomplished by using two muslin drapes, two small towels, or plastic draping material preceded by an adhesive spray. When this latter material is used (Fig. 11) the incision is made directly through it and the sutures for closure are also made without removing it. The plastic is finally removed along with the sutures. In order to apply this material, the hair must be clipped very close so that the plastic will adhere well.

PREPARATION OF THE SURGEON

The surgeon begins his preparation by changing his street clothes for appropriate clothing so that he can scrub to his elbows. He then should don cap and mask, which are clean but not sterile. The use of a mask might be questioned, but the cap is essential. The mask can do no harm, and may have some benefit, and for this reason it is usually recommended.

The scrubbing procedure consists of a preliminary washing of the hands and arms to remove debris. A sterile brush is then used to scrub thoroughly the fingers, the hands, and finally the arms, in that order. It is most important that the scrubbing proceed from the hands to the elbows so that the cleanest area will be the hands. Once the brush has been used on the arms, it should not be returned to the hands. Each finger should receive ten strokes on each surface, making a total of 40 strokes per finger. The fingernails and both surfaces of the hands should receive 20 strokes. The number of scrubbing strokes used is far more important than is the time spent in scrubbing. When the scrubbing has been completed, the hands and arms should be rinsed in warm water, allowing the water to drip from the elbows, thereby preventing contamination of the hands by drippings from the upper arms.

For the purpose of scrubbing, one may use a good soap or detergent. Many prefer to use hexachlorophene. If soap is used, alcohol may be used in the arm immersion. If, however, hexachlorophene is used, the arm immersion should contain a quaternary ammonium compound, such as Zephiran or Roccal (Winthrop). Eight ml. of a 12.8 per cent concentrate is used in 1000 ml. of distilled water. Soap and alcohol destroy some of the germicidal activity of the quaternary ammonium compounds. If the wet glove technique is used, the gloves may be placed directly in the arm immersion basin, and the gloves are donned at the end of the immersion. If the dry glove technique is used, the hands are dried on the sterile towel from the gown pack and the gown is put on before the gloves (Fig. 12). In most instances the gown and gloves can be put on without help, still maintaining sterility. To do this, grasp the gown by the ties at the back of the neckband and allow it to unfold. Toss it in the air and thrust the hands into the armholes,

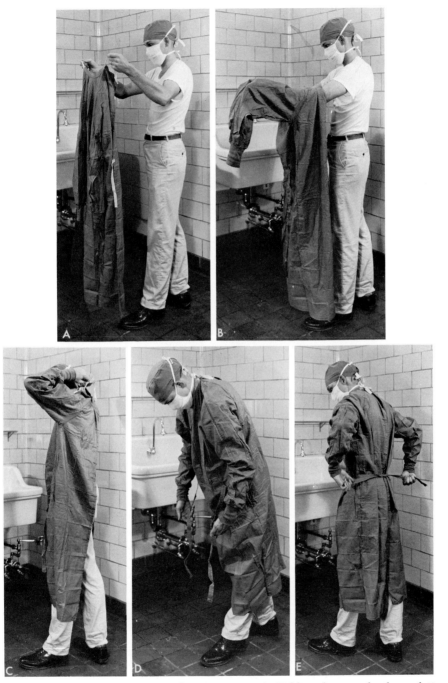

Figure 12. Donning the gown without assistance. A, Holding the gown by the neck ties. B, Hands in the armholes with neck band across the arms. C, Pulling gown into place by means of the neck ties. D, The operator leans forward to swing the belt ties away from the body before grasping them. E, Tying with hands away from body.

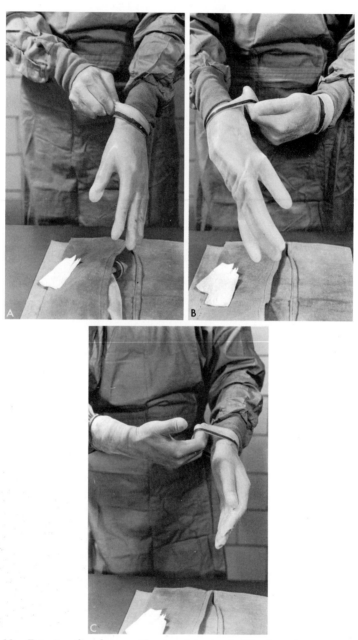

Figure 13.   Donning the gloves without assistance. A, The first glove is put on without covering the wrist. B, The second glove is completely donned. C, Wrist of first glove pulled into place.

allowing the neckband to fall across the arms at the elbow. The hands can then be worked out of the sleeves without touching the outside of the gown. When this has been accomplished, grasp the neck ties without allowing the hands to touch the body and pull the gown into place. The neck can then be tied, followed by the ties at the waist.

After the hands are powdered with the sterile powder from the glove pack, one glove is picked up and pulled on the opposite hand, care being taken not to touch the outside of the glove. The opposite glove is then lifted with the glove hand by holding the gloved fingers inside the wrist fold. When the glove is on, it is then turned over the wrist of the gown and the same operation is performed on the first glove (Fig. 13).

One person can follow an aseptic technique in surgery without extra help if he so desires by performing the several steps required in the following chronological order:

1. Anesthetize the patient.
2. Prepare the patient for surgery.
3. Position the patient on the table.
4. Open the instrument pack on the instrument tray.
5. Open the drapes and place them on the instrument tray with transfer forceps.
6. Using transfer forceps, place cutting instruments on the instrument tray.
7. Open bundles containing gown and gloves.
8. Don cap and mask.
9. Scrub and immerse hands and arms.
10. Don gown and gloves.
11. Drape the patient.

The foregoing illustrates the simplicity with which aseptic surgery may be carried out, but is not to be used as an excuse for skimping on help in the operating room. At least one good assistant seems quite necessary if one is to perform good orthopedic surgery.

REFERENCES

Armistead, W. W.: Aseptic veterinary surgery: Fact and fancy. Vet. Med., 52:79, 1957.
Leonard, E. P.: Fundamentals of Small Animal Surgery. Philadelphia, W. B. Saunders Co., 1968, Chap. 4.
Riser, W. H.: Canine Surgery. 4th ed. Evanston, Ill., American Veterinary Publications, 1957.
Walter, C. W.: The Aseptic Treatment of Wounds. New York, The Macmillan Co., 1948.
Walter, C. W., and Arlein, M. S.: Aseptic technique in veterinary surgery. J.A.V.M.A., 102:41, 1943.

Chapter 4

Methods and Materials

There are many methods and even more materials that can be used to assist in the repair of a fracture. The surgeon is fortunate to have such diversified ways and means at his disposal, but he must not lose himself in the forest of "gadgets." The use of mechanical appliances should be governed at all times by the cardinal principles of bone repair and the recognition that one is dealing with living tissue. The artisan's approach to a fracture problem is commendable to a point, but the final decision as to methods and materials must be controlled by the comfort of the patient, the simplicity of the method, and the effectiveness of the materials.

In this chapter we shall survey the possible methods of reduction and fixation as well as the materials that might be used to achieve proper and durable alignment. The reduction of a fracture can be classified as closed or open and its fixation as either external or internal.

CLOSED REDUCTION

Whenever a fracture is reduced without incising the skin or exposing the bone, it is known as a closed reduction. There are certain exceptions to this "rule of thumb" definition, for example, in the use of half pin splintage, full pin splintage with external traction, and some intramedullary splintage. Under these conditions, the skin has been incised in order to introduce the pin but the bone has not been exposed and reduction is carried out by external manipulation. On the other hand, a compound fracture frequently means the exposure of bone through a laceration in the skin. In such a case, if apposition of the fracture segment was brought about through external manipulation, this would still be a closed reduction.

In areas of the body where bone segments can be easily palpated (radius and ulna), it is common practice to use closed reduction. Fixation in such cases is usually of an external type. Perhaps the most common splintage is coaptation, although we shall see that other forms of external splintage with either skin or skeletal traction can be used following closed reduction. Much of the early work with intramedullary pins was done with closed reduction. Today, in the interest of more accurate reductions, most of this type of fixation is done with open reduction.

Closed reduction should always be carried out with as little injury to the surrounding tissues as possible. This frequently means that if the angle of the fracture is known and the position of the segments is taken into consideration, the fracture can be reduced by the use of simple mechanics rather than by the application of brute force.

This method is frequently referred to as "angulation" or "toggling" and works best when the segments are easily palpated, but may be employed wherever the bone segments can be manipulated. There are two types of fractures in which straight traction parallel to the long axis of the bone will not bring about reduction. One is the transverse fracture with overriding due to muscle spasm and the other is the short oblique fracture with the long sides overlapping. The latter cannot be extended enough because of the added length imposed by the two oblique ends (Fig. 14).

In both cases, if the limb is carefully bent at the fracture site until the two segments are at an angle to each other and then gently pushed away from the apex thus formed, the fractured surfaces will impinge. After the two segments have been "toggled" into position, the limb can be slowly straightened, thereby bringing about reduction. The angulation should be carried out in the direction of least resistance and with the welfare of surrounding soft tissues always in mind.

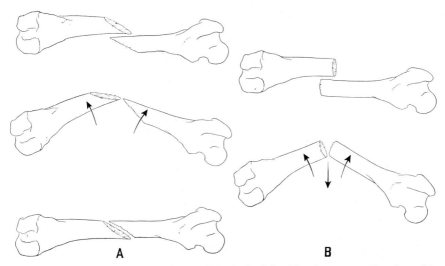

A   **B**

Figure 14. "Toggling" or "angulation" method of closed reduction. A, The short oblique fracture. B, The overriding transverse fracture.

OPEN REDUCTION

Open reduction can be defined as the proper alignment of a fracture through an incision which exposes the bone. This method of reduction is carried out in conjunction with internal fixation primarily, although there are times when external fixation is used following an open reduction. An example of this method would be the use of a half pin splint following an open reduction in repairing a non-union fracture of the radius.

EXTERNAL FIXATION

Immobilization of a fracture may be accomplished by external fixation through the use of coaptation, modified Thomas splints with either skin traction or skeletal traction, half pin splints, or full pins in combination with these three methods. A wide choice of methods is therefore available, but the best one in each instance is the simplest method that will achieve a comfortable fixation for the patient.

Coaptation

The oldest method of fracture fixation is coaptation, dating back some five thousand years. It still has its place in our modern orthopedic surgery because of its simplicity and effectiveness in certain types of fractures. It is frequently used in simple transverse fractures of the radius, ulna, tibia, and fibula as well as for distal fractures of these bones. It may also be applied to fractures of the scapula, ribs, and tail.

Coaptation should be durable yet as light as possible with a minimum of bulk to avoid being cumbersome. Materials should be carefully chosen with this in mind. Since there is no direct control of the bone segment with this method, it is extremely important that the fracture be carefully held in reduction throughout the application of the splintage (Fig. 15). In order to insure proper immobilization, it is generally agreed that the cast should include the joint above and the joint below the fracture whenever possible.

The cast must be snug enough so that apposition is maintained and yet must allow for ample circulation to the part. The amount of pressure to apply is learned only through experience. Until this has been established, frequent checks of the splint should be made. Even with the experienced operator, a weekly check should be made to ensure against loosening of the cast or development of spots of pressure necrosis. The cast may loosen as the edema recedes or uneven pressure may be applied by the cast because of inadequate padding. Care should also be taken in the case of certain materials that the cast is kept dry. Moisture will cause cotton bandage to shrink, thereby tightening the cast and causing necrosis.

If cotton is used for padding, it should be applied evenly (Fig. 16). This is best accomplished by using sheets or strips applied longitudinally. Spiral wrapping gives an uneven surface because there is either an overlap or a space left with each wrap. Cotton strips covered with gauze used in a longitudinal direction are the easiest to apply. Sheets of cotton can then be used to fill in the spaces between bony eminences so that an even pressure will result. Cotton should never be heavily applied over the prominences of the limb, but rather it should be used in the depressions, so that the bindings will give proper distribution of pressure. If the high points are excessively padded, the pressure at these points will be increased by the covering splintage.

Bandage can be wrapped over the padding, starting at the fracture site and continuing up and down the leg, making certain that even pressure is applied. In most instances, either one-inch or two-inch bandage will give the best results in evenness of application and pressure. If tongue depressors are to be used as splints (Fig. 17), they should be incorporated in the bandage as the wrapping proceeds. In case the cast is to be hardened with sodium silicate, the splinting material should be applied to the padding before the bandage is applied. When the bandaging has reached a point where the fracture site seems secure, cotton can be packed between the toes and the foot bandaged. Thin, flat pads of cotton should be laid carefully between the toes and the foot pads so that there is no bunching, which can cause excessive pressure when bandaged.

Basswood, aluminum sheeting, Alumafoam (aluminum backed with sponge rubber, Fig. 18), x-ray film, tongue depressors, and similar materials may be used for splinting. These should be applied to at least two and preferably three surfaces of the leg. Both the medial and lateral surfaces should be braced as well as the surface toward which the fracture angulates. Shaping of the splintage to conform with the leg is important. Wood can be shaped almost exactly with angles simulating normal posture. Basswood, when applied to the forelegs, should be extended to the shoulder on the lateral side so that the splint can be anchored to the body. A covering of heavy adhesive tape will complete this type of coaptation.

Plastic sheets for cutting and molding into splints are available. Isoprene (Johnson & Johnson) is manufactured primarily for human use, but it can be used on larger dogs successfully. These sheets are thick and extremely hard. They must be soaked in hot water in order to cut and shape them. Once the material is softened, it can be cut with bandage scissors. A cardboard pattern should first be made so that the Isoprene can be cut without waste, since it is very expensive. All the shaping must be done while it is warm and soft. As soon as it cools, it becomes hard and retains whatever shape it has been given. Because of its impervious nature, it should have holes bored through it before applying to the limb. This allows air circulation and prevents sweating.

The Mason meta splint (Fig. 19) is another form of coaptation in which a molded aluminum form is applied to the caudal, plantar, or palmar side of the limb over padding and then taped into place. This splint, as the name

(*Text continued on page 39.*)

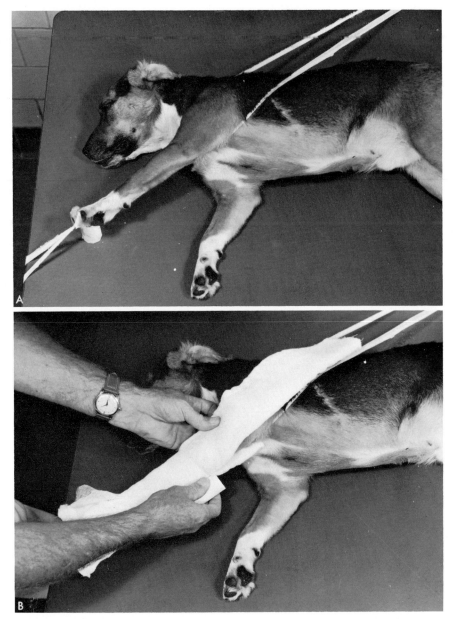

Figure 15.   Application of coaptation to the forelimb. A, Traction is applied to maintain reduction. B, Padding is used longitudinally. The padding is bandaged in place with even pressure.

(*Figure continued on opposite page.*)

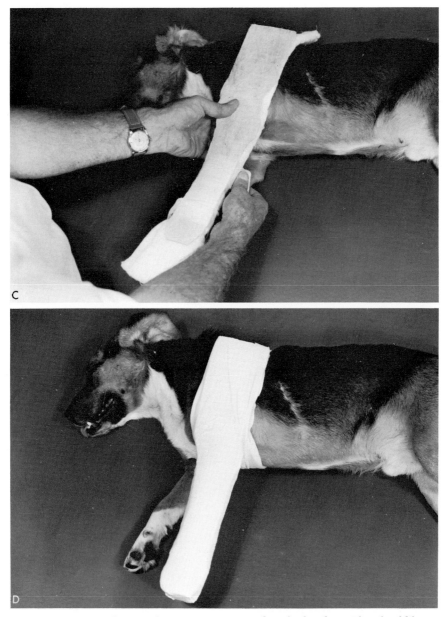

Figure 15 continued. C, Splintage is incorporated in the bandage. This should be cut to the shape of the leg. D, After padding between the toes with cotton, adhesive tape is used as covering.

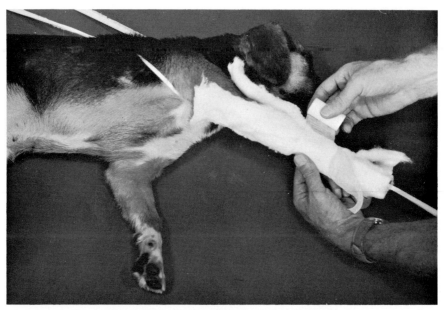

Figure 16.   Application of cotton to the limb.

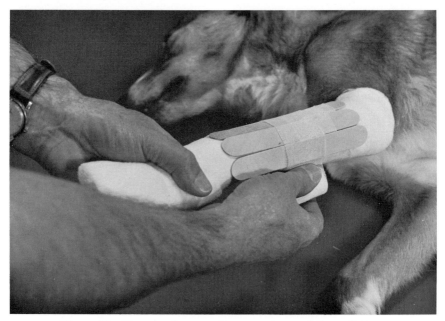

Figure 17.   The use of tongue depressors in coaptation splintage.

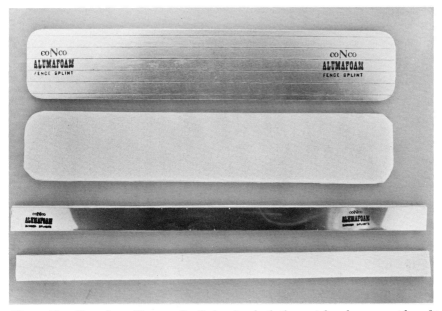

Figure 18. Alumafoam "fence splint" showing both the metal and sponge sides of two sizes.

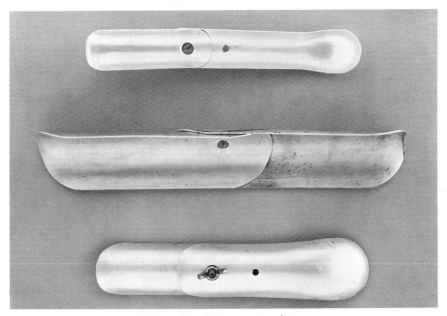

Figure 19. Mason meta splints.

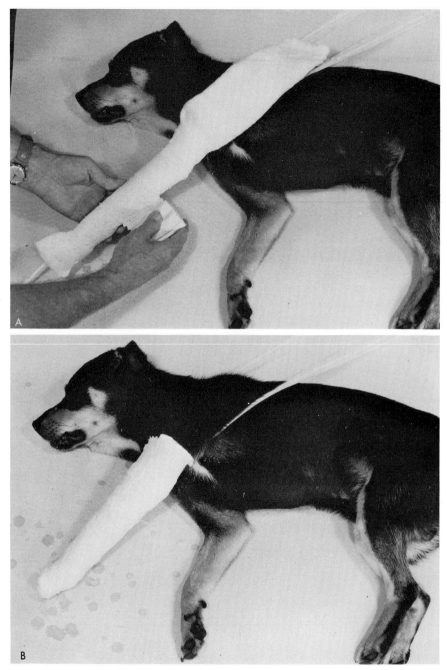

Figure 20. Application of plaster of Paris. A, The use of fast-setting plaster applied over padding. B, The completed cast with the foot padded and covered.

implies, is designed primarily for use on the metacarpals and metatarsals, as well as fractures distal to these bones. It is designed so that it can be lengthened or shortened and comes in a variety of sizes.

Plaster of Paris has gained popularity since it is now manufactured in a quick-setting formula which is extremely hard (Fig. 20). Because of these properties, it is possible to splint a dog's leg with two or three layers. This provides a relatively light splint which is quite durable. Plaster can be applied to the body or limbs without clipping the hair and need not be padded, except at the edges where excoriation can occur. Removal of a plaster cast can be simplified by imbedding a Fetatome wire after the first layer of plaster has been applied. Heavy scissors (Fig. 21) are also available for cutting plaster or other coaptation materials. Jenny applies plaster by molding the strips lengthwise over the leg so that each strip covers one half of the leg, either cranial or caudal. These two half shells are allowed to harden before they are bound to the limb. In this way the cast may easily be removed or adjusted as the leg swells or shrinks (Fig. 22).

Aire-Cast is the trade name for a plastic coarse woven cloth (Fig. 23) which hardens into a cast when soaked in a catalyst. This material is very porous and allows air to reach the skin easily. It is applied to a part in the same way as any bandage, after wetting with the catalyst. Because of the loose weave, it conforms to the contours without binding tightly. In fact, excessive pressure must be avoided because of slight shrinkage of the cast and possible swelling of the injured part. Undue tension is indicated by narrowing of the bandage and closing of the porous openings. The cast is

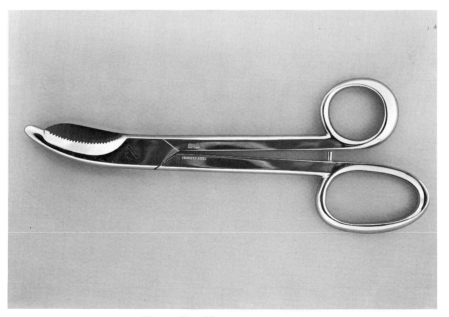

Figure 21.   Heavy cast scissors.

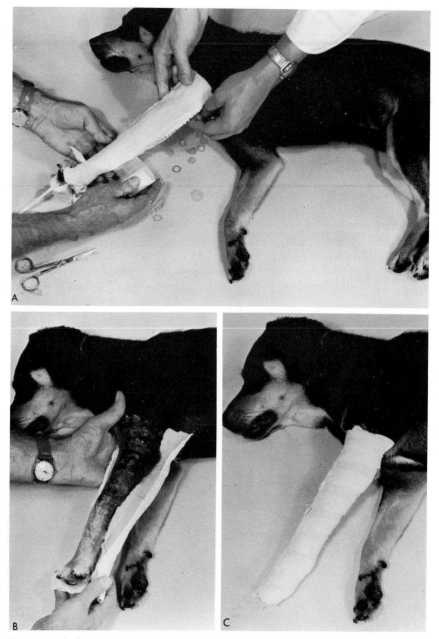

Figure 22. `The Jenny method of applying plaster. A, Wet plaster is held in place by bandage. B, The hardened shells. C, The cast taped in place.

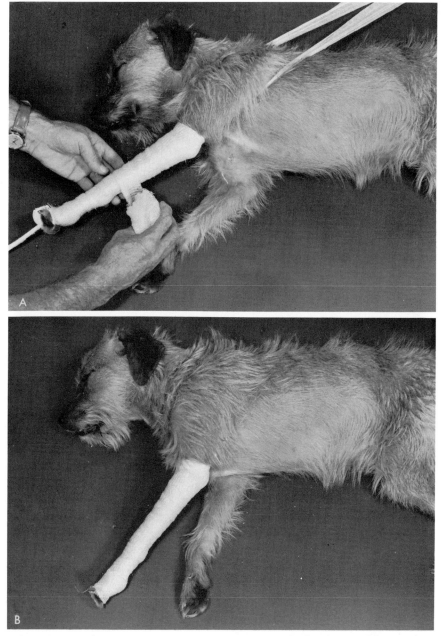

Figure 23. Application of Aire-Cast. A, Aire-Cast is applied without padding or clipping. B, Completed cast, which hardens in 30 minutes.

unaffected by water but may be softened for removal by applying some of the catalyst.

In most cases of cast destruction by the patient, either the reduction or the cast is at fault. The reduction should be inspected by roentgenogram and the cast should be checked to see that it is comfortable in all cases of chewing. If nothing is found amiss, then the cast can be protected by applying a layer of hardware cloth. It may also be necessary to maintain the patient on a tranquilizing drug until he becomes accustomed to the cast. If the cast is on a rear leg, a cradle (Fig. 24) may be used.

Modified Thomas Splint

Dr. E. F. Schroeder was largely responsible for the modification of the Thomas splint so that it could be used on small animals. This splint is still in popular use as a means of external fixation. When properly applied, it has many advantages. These splints are manufactured in several sizes and are adjustable in length. The author prefers, however, to use custom-built splints which can be made by anyone with a little mechanical ability.

Aluminum rod of various sizes can be used to make splints for dogs; an ordinary wire coat hanger is the best possible material from which to fashion one for a cat (Fig. 25). The rod should be an alloy, since tempered aluminum is too difficult to bend and has a tendency to crystallize and break when bent at a sharp angle. Hardness should be about 18 so that it molds well, yet holds

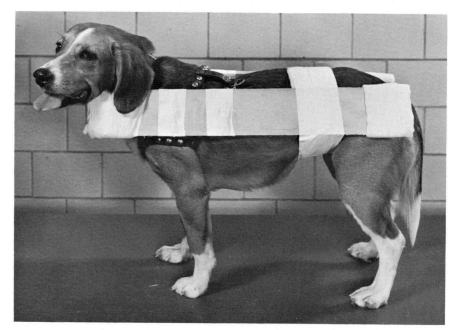

Figure 24. Cradle applied to a dog. This prevents the animal from reaching the rear parts with its mouth but allows freedom of movement in all other directions.

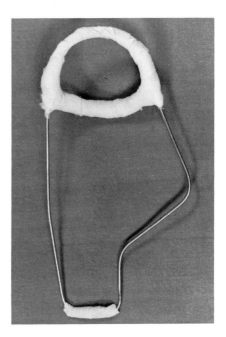

Figure 25. Thomas splint for a cat made from a wire coat hanger.

its shape when the splint is finished. Rods of three diameters ($^3/_{16}$ inch, $^1/_4$ inch, $^3/_8$ inch) are usually sufficient to make a wide variety of splints. This rod comes in 6 or 12 foot lengths.

In order to fashion the splint, two dimensions must be ascertained, i.e., the diameter of the ring and the length of the bars. Since the splint is used principally on the hindleg, we shall use this leg to illustrate our method of measuring. One can determine the ring diameter directly from the patient by using an x-ray caliper (Fig. 26) with the base along a line from the tuber ischii to the tuber coxae and the adjustable bar on the medial side of the thigh moderately snug to the flank. The splint bar length will then be the distance between the caliper bar and the tip of the toe when the leg is extended. With these two measurements, the total length of aluminum rod necessary for the splint can be calculated from the following formula: If D equals diameter of the ring and L equals length of the splint bar, then $2(3D + 1) + 2L + 8$ equals length of the rod (Fig. 27). $3D + 1$ would equal the circumference of the ring, and since the rod makes almost two complete circles, the rod required to form the ring would be $2(3D + 1)$. There are two bars, hence 2L with 8 inches added for overlap would constitute the amount of rod necessary to complete the splint. Calculations for the foreleg can be made in the same way, using the distance from the axilla to a midpoint on the scapula as the ring diameter. Since the leg does not vary in length whether flexed or extended, the amount of splint material required remains the same for all positions of fixation.

To fashion the ring, a splint mold is used (Fig. 28). After the rod is bent around the splint mold, the ring is taped wherever two pieces of rod are in

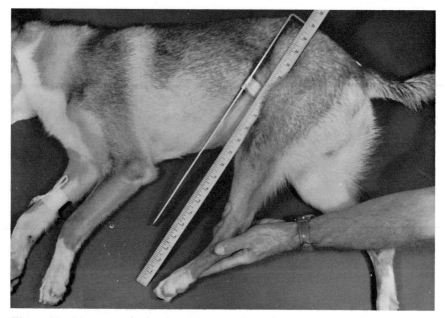

Figure 26. Measuring the leg for a Thomas splint. The measurements here would be ring diameter 5 inches and leg length 16 inches.

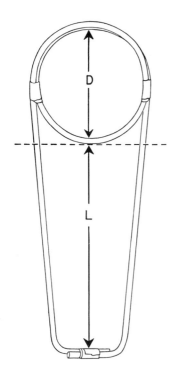

Figure 27. Diagram of Thomas splint, showing dimensions used in formula for determining rod length.

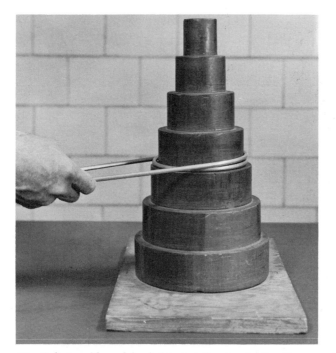

Figure 28. Splint mold used for fashioning the ring for the Thomas splint.

contact, making certain that there is reenforcement at the junction of the ring and bars. The bars are then shaped to meet the requirements of the case and the overlapping ends are firmly taped together. In general the splint should not be any longer than is absolutely necessary. The next step in shaping the splint (Fig. 29) is to bend the lower segment of the ring, which is between the bars, in a medial direction so that it will not put undue pressure on the medial side of the leg. Following this the padding is applied to the ring. It is quite unnecessary to use large amounts of padding; in fact, it is detrimental because of the excessive bulk it creates on the inner side of the leg. A double wrapping of orthopedic padding is quite sufficient; this can be tightly bound to the ring with one-inch bandage covering only that part of the ring which will be in contact with the body. Adaption of this splint will be discussed in conjunction with the various fractures.

Half Pin Splintage

Undoubtedly the name for this type of splintage arose from the fact that the pins are inserted through the bone but only part way through the limb. With this method there is direct skeletal control by means of pins, which are in turn controlled by an external apparatus. The splintage is applied to one aspect of the leg only and there is freedom of articular movement both above and below the fracture. This active motion improves the circulation, prevents atrophy of the muscles, and helps to avoid joint stiffness. Clayton

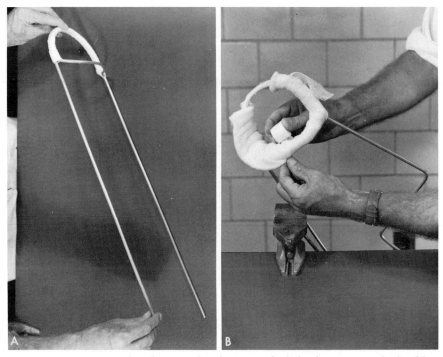

Figure 29. Preparing the Thomas splint for use with skeletal traction on the hind leg. A, The taped ring with inward contour of lower quadrant. B, Padding the ring with orthopedic padding and one-inch bandage.

Parkhill made the first attempt at rigid half pin splintage in 1897. He devised a splint with four screws which were seated in the bone at right angles to its long axis and controlled by a series of metal plates which could be bolted together with clamps (Fig. 30). Later Anderson devised a splint in which two pins were inserted at a 45° angle so that when clamped together they could not be pulled from the bone. After the segments had been thus anchored firmly, they could be manipulated into position and held by an extension bar fastened between the two pin bars. Further modifications of this idea were made by Schroeder, Stader, and Ehmer.

It cannot be overemphasized at this point that half pin splintage requires the same meticulous aseptic approach as does open bone surgery and that the danger of osteomyelitis is just as great if aseptic care is not used. Too often the disastrous results of poor preparation for this type of surgery are seen. This results in criticism of the method and, in some cases, of the profession itself. Osteomyelitis is not to be confused with pin seepage, which frequently occurs where pins protrude through the skin and is of little consequence except for the loosening of the pin.

APPLICATION.   A half pin splint (Fig. 31) consists of two half pin units connected by an extension unit. One half pin unit is anchored in the proximal segment and the other in the distal segment of the bone. It is important

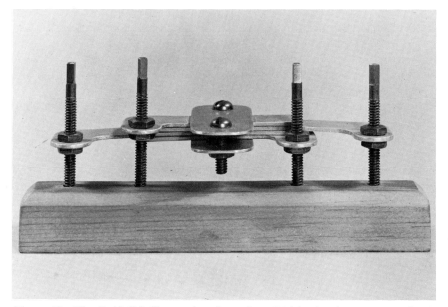

Figure 30. The Parkhill half pin splint devised in 1897 (replica by Dr. R. F. Olson).

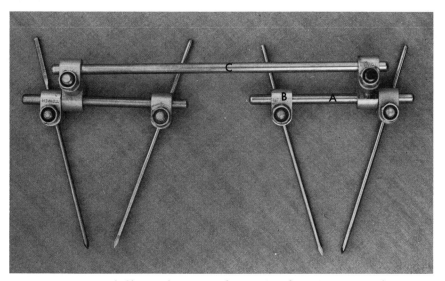

Figure 31. A half pin splint. A, Pin bar. B, Coupling. C, Extension bar.

to place the leg in a reasonably normal position with the fractured bone in at least a semi-reduced condition before beginning the pinning procedure. This allows introduction of the pins in the proper plane and without undue interference with muscular activity after complete reduction.

The pins are numbered from 1 to 4, starting at the proximal end. The number 1 pin is applied first and should be as near the proximal end of the bone as possible. After placing the pin in the chuck, a generous amount of skin is forced toward the fracture site so that there will be no binding when the fractured bone is extended to normal length. A small incision is then made in the skin with the point of the scalpel so that the pin will not carry infection from the skin into the deeper tissues.

The point of the pin should contact the bone at about a 45 to 50° angle. This will produce good holding power when the half pin unit is completed. It is important to insert the pin so that the pin bar will be parallel to the bone in both the dorsal and sagittal planes. The pin is driven through both cortices with a back-and-forth rotation of the wrist while moderate pressure is applied. A sharp pin does not require excessive pressure. Indeed, such pressure may cause the point to turn on small pins or misdirect larger pins. Forceful drilling also produces thermal necrosis of the bone and subsequent loosening of the pins. All pins should be hand-drilled. The use of electrically driven drills will cause thermal necrosis. Too much speed or force is therefore contra-indicated.

One can follow the progress of the pin as it penetrates each cortex by the grating sensation transmitted through the chuck handle as the point emerges from cortical bone, as well as from the ease with which it moves when it reaches softer tissue. The pin should be inserted far enough that the point is entirely free of the cortex but no farther (Fig. 32). When the pin is in this position, the forces exerted on it are in equilibrium and there is no tendency for the pin to back out. If the trochar point were still embedded in the cortex, the pressure against the point could force the pin outward, thereby causing it to loosen.

The number 2 pin is inserted at the same angle as number 1 and at a sufficient distance from it so that the point will emerge from the opposite cortex within a few centimeters of the number 1 point. As in the first instance, the skin is pushed toward the fracture site, a stab wound is made at the appropriate distance from number 1 pin, and the pin is inserted parallel to both the dorsal and sagittal planes of the bone.

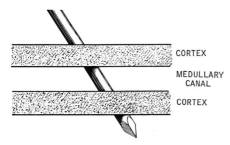

CORTEX

MEDULLARY
CANAL

CORTEX

Figure 32.   Diagrammatic sketch showing correct insertion of a half pin in a round bone.

When long segments are being pinned, the pins may be placed farther apart, while in pinning extremely short segments it may be necessary to change the angle of the pins so that the number 2 pin will not impinge on the fracture site.

Free skin is again pushed toward the fracture site before a skin incision is made for the number 4 pin. The distal pin unit is applied in the same manner as the proximal unit, starting with the number 4 pin as close to the distal end of the bone as possible.

The pin bars are now applied to the pins. One or two double couplings or clamps are placed on the pin bar or rod first. The number will depend upon the number of extension bars required to give rigid fixation. A single coupling is placed over each pin and the ends of the pin bar are inserted into these couplings. The pin bar is then held about a fingerbreadth above the skin and parallel to the bone while the single couplings are tightened.

When both pin assemblies have been readied, the pins are wrapped with sterile surgical sponges so that the area between the skin and the pin bar is covered and the puncture wounds protected. A pin cutter (Fig. 33) is used to cut the pins about ¼ inch above the pin bar. Each pin assembly can then be grasped and by careful manipulation the bone ends can be brought into apposition. If fine adjustment or retention is required, the Ehmer reduction gear is attached to the pin bars. This apparatus will hold the pin bars in position until the extension or fixation bars can be put in place and secured. The extension bars should reach from the number 1 pin to the number 4 pin and the double couplings should be fastened at a point that will produce maximum leverage.

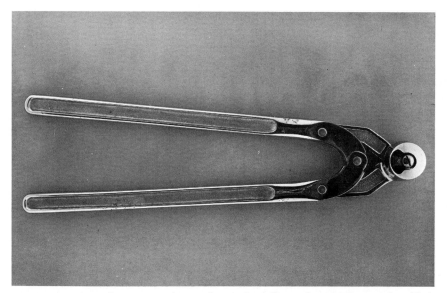

Figure 33. Type of pin cutters that can be used on all round pins. These are less likely to leave burrs.

It is well to cover the entire splint with adhesive tape to prevent projections of the splint from catching on surrounding objects. This covering should allow a small gap next to the skin to facilitate inspection of the pin holes and promote dryness in the area. At no time should antiseptics be applied around the pins. Such treatment stimulates granulation and promotes seepage. Where the skin movement is not great, a scab will form around the pin and the wound will remain dry.

Now that we have discussed the general application of half pin splintage, it might be well at this point to review the causes of failure when this type of splintage is used. In order to evaluate and visualize a fracture properly, it is necessary in most cases to radiograph the part. Whenever possible, this should be done in two planes, at right angles to each other. Once the fracture is clearly visualized, the mechanics of reduction and fixation can be carried out systematically. It seems very logical that overriding should be corrected first in a transverse fracture and that long axis rotation should be corrected first in an oblique fracture, but too often reductions with half pin splintage do not follow in such logical sequence simply because the fracture is not clearly visualized. If the reduction maneuvers are carried out in logical sequence in a recently acquired fracture, the fragments will come into apposition with comparative ease. It is only the fractures of long standing which may require some force to reduce. In these cases, the half pin assembly has the advantage of applying a small amount of force steadily until there is some stretching of the tissues and gradually the contracted muscles can be lengthened until the overriding bone segments are corrected.

In placing the pins, one should bear in mind that more bone control will be obtained if the pins are as near the ends of the bone as possible. Compromises are sometimes necessary, as in the proximal end of the radius, where pins placed too close to the end of the bone will interfere with flexion of the elbow joint.

If the reduction is carried out with too much force, there is excessive injury to soft tissues and interference with circulation. Care should be used in adjusting the extension bar so that the bone ends are not excessively distracted, thereby leading to non-union or delayed union. By the same token, the fractured ends should not impinge with excessive force, since this causes bone necrosis. In most cases in which satisfactory alignment is not forthcoming within a reasonable length of time, it is advisable to resort to open reduction.

The insertion of the pins is highly important. It should be emphasized that forceful or wobbly drilling will lead to loose pins. Too much force generates excessive heat, causing thermal necrosis of the bone. Wobbly drilling creates a hole larger than the pin. As previously indicated, failure to penetrate both cortices will also result in a loose pin. Whenever a pin is inserted so that the skin is under tension, a certain amount of skin necrosis and seepage will occur. Pushing the skin toward the fracture site is a good precaution against seepage and allows more maneuverability of the fracture as well. Fortunately, this oversight can be corrected by incising the skin on the side of the pin where tension exists.

Failure to penetrate both cortices, insertion of the pin into soft bone, joints, or tendons, infection of soft tissues, or improper preparation of the skin may lead to difficulty which should not reflect upon the method but rather upon the operator.

Finally, in young animals one should avoid placing pins directly into the epiphyses since this may interfere with or distort bone growth, especially in the long bones.

KIRSCHNER SPLINT. The Kirschner splint (Fig. 34) has been more widely used by veterinarians than any other form of half pin splintage. It is a modification made by Ehmer of the Anderson splint and is manufactured by Kirschner. This is strictly a fixation splint and requires a separate reduction apparatus (Fig. 35). The principal advantage of this splint is in its versatility. Pins can be inserted at any angle without regard to bone planes. It is possible to couple the pin assemblies together by means of the extension rods regardless of their position. While this has some advantages, it also has some disadvantages in that it allows the beginner to insert pins at incorrect angles and to couple splints together without regard to the natural lines of stress in a limb. To those acquainted with rules of half pin splintage, however, this splint has considerable merit. The pins as well as the extension rods may be used singly or doubly, depending on the stress at the fracture site and the location of the fracture. It can be used in conjunction with other types of splinting when additional pinning is required (anchoring an intramedullary pin) as well as in pelvic fractures and coxofemoral luxations. The

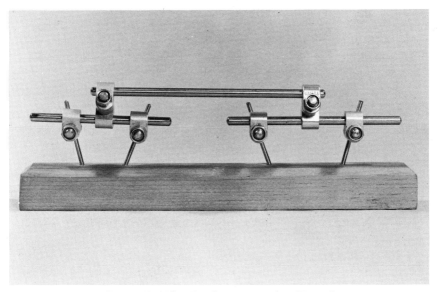

Figure 34. The Kirschner type splint (Tower).

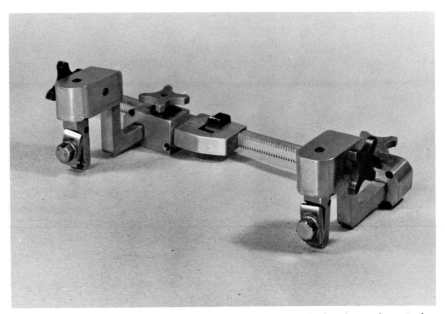

Figure 35. Ehmer reduction gear. The two clamps are attached to the pin bars. Reduction adjustments are then made by means of the thumb screws.

splint is light in weight but, because of the friction-type couplings made of relatively soft metal, it has not proved to be a very durable apparatus.

TOWER SPLINT. The Tower spint is almost identical to the Kirschner splint, but the couplings are stronger, making for a more rugged construction. In the hands of the author, this splint has seemed to be a little more satisfactory.

Full Pin Splintage

This form of external fixation is obtained by using pins which penetrate two surfaces of the skin as well as both bone cortices. It is employed in connection with some form of external splint which serves as a fixation point or anchorage. The pins used in most instances are in the form of wires which can be easily bent. Although the Steinmann pin is sometimes used along with coaptation, this is not as common in veterinary orthopedics as it is in the human field. Materials that are used in full pin splintage are the bicycle spoke, the Kirschner wire, and the Thomson beaded wire. The bone tong is not a form of full pin splintage, but since it is primarily employed in the same manner as the foregoing devices, it will be discussed in this category.

BICYCLE SPOKE. The bicycle spoke has been used by the author as a means of full pin splintage since 1935 with a high degree of success. It is important that this pin be properly prepared and that it be used only in those places where it can be removed after the fracture has stabilized. Figure 36

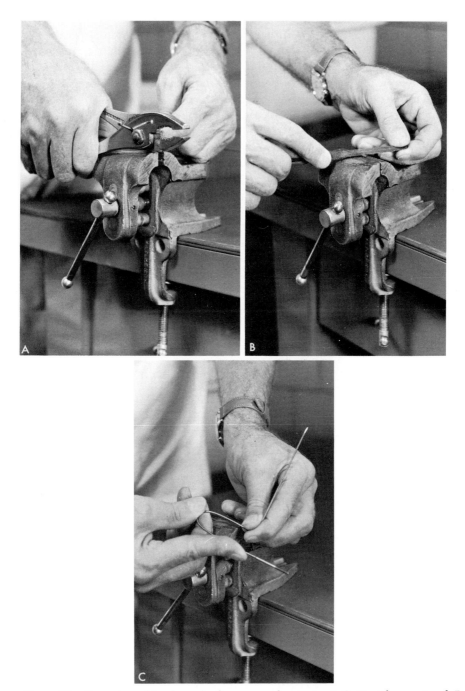

Figure 36. Preparing a bicycle spoke for use as a bone pin. A, Cutting the upset end. B, Filing a four-sided point. C, Bending the shaft to form a handle.

shows the preparation of a spoke. If possible, spokes should be selected that are not chromed or lacquered. Long sizes are usually required. The upset end is removed with wire cutters but the threaded end is left intact. The spoke is then placed in a vise and the cut end filed to a four-sided point. In order to assure a good cutting edge on the point, it should be filed in one direction only; a back-and-forth motion of the file will produce a rounded edge which will penetrate bone with difficulty. As soon as a good point is prepared, the spoke can be bent into a T-shape ready for hand drilling into any bone. The use of this pin will be described in conjunction with the Thomas splint and the Alumafoam splint, particularly as it relates to fixation of pelvic, femoral, and humeral fractures.

KIRSCHNER WIRE. This wire, introduced in 1909, is about the same diameter as a bicycle spoke and is pointed on one end and beveled at the other so that it can be fitted into a drill chuck. In its use in veterinary work, however, the wire is usually bent in the form of a T and hand-drilled into the bone. It can be used in the same manner as the bicycle spoke.

THOMSON BEADED WIRE. Similar in size and diameter to the Kirschner wire, the Thomson beaded wire has a metal bead about midway along its length, which makes it a decided adjunct to longitudinal traction when transverse traction is needed as well. It can be used wherever traction is needed in more than one direction. The pin is drilled through the bone and out through the skin. Traction is then applied until the bead is seated against the cortex. Two of these pins going in opposite directions can exert considerable force to bring opposing fragments together (Fig. 37).

BONE TONGS. Tongs are used for external fixation in the form of skeletal traction with the modified Thomas splint. Perhaps the most common

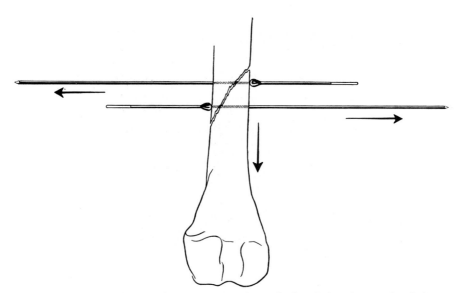

Figure 37. Diagram showing how traction can be applied with the Thomson beaded wire.

application is in cases of supracondylar fractures of the femur. Tongs are easily applied to the bone through small skin incisions, but have a tendency to slip unless the blades are set well into the cortex of the bone. Good control of the distal segment and the elimination of a spreader are their greatest advantages.

INTERNAL FIXATION

Internal fixation refers to the immobilization of bone fragments through the use of devices which exert a restraining force on the bone wholly from within the body itself. In most instances, these devices are completely buried in the tissue and are used in conjunction with open reduction. An exception is the installation of an intramedullary pin by closed reduction with the end protruding from the skin; this procedure is internal fixation, but the pin is not completely buried and the reduction is not open. The devices commonly used in internal fixation are intramedullary pins, bone plates and screws, wire, bone pegs, shuttle pins, and prostheses.

With the exception of bone pegs, these devices are made of metals which are relatively inert in the tissues. Galvanic activity is of less concern in those devices such as intramedullary pins, which will be extracted after the bone is healed, than it is in those which remain in the tissues indefinitely. Metals which differ in composition should not be used together for internal fixation because of the galvanic possibilities. This is particularly true of metals which are to be permanently embedded. If there is excessive pressure from metal, there may be rarefaction of the bone at the point of pressure. It is also true that metal may cause more inflammation if the soft parts are unduly traumatized during its application.

All metals will corrode under certain circumstances and for different reasons. Frequently, corrosion results from the galvanic action of two different metals, but at other times the corrosion can be produced by a difference in the oxygen potential at some point on the metal implant. One example would be the point at which a metal screw head contacts a metal plate.

Since corrosion usually is controlled by a time factor, the life expectancy of metals is better for small animals than for humans, since their life span is shorter. There is no perfect metal for orthopedic work, but any metal that can survive corrosion for 10 years (all other factors being equal) might be considered satisfactory for small animal orthopedics. Unfortunately, the fatigue factor is often more important than the corrosion factor, if the two can be separated for the purpose of discussion. A small amount of bending applied continuously will fracture metal. One might say then that bone is stronger than metal because it is rarely subject to fatigue fracture. It can reconstitute itself and maintain its strength, whereas metal cannot.

Sherman first proposed the use of vanadium steel, and this was widely used until the late 1930's. It had the toughness required but was not totally inactive in the tissues. This metal proved, however, to be quite satisfactory for purposes of half pinning and full pinning in those cases in which it was removed after a few weeks.

Vitallium, which is composed mainly of cobalt, chromium, and molybdenum, was proposed as the metal of choice for internal fixation by Venable in 1936. This cast metal, completely inert in the tissues, has found a place in veterinary orthopedics, particularly in the field of prosthetics.

Stainless steel, although it has a small amount of galvanic activity, has proved to be quite satisfactory in dogs and cats. Its principal ingredients are carbon, chromium, nickel, molybdenum, and manganese. Stainless steel will withstand strain during the healing period better than vitallium, but it tends to corrode at points where the surface is deeply scored. There are some 75 or 100 types of stainless steel with a wide variety of physical and chemical properties commercially available. Bone plates and screws made of vitallium are available and are commonly used in skeletal repair of dogs and cats.

The American Iron and Steel Institute (A.I.S.I.) type 316 and 317 stainless steels are produced by adding 2 and 3.5 per cent molybdenum respectively to 18.8 stainless steel. These two stainless steels give superior performance in the body because of the presence of the molybdenum. They both possess good strength, but type 317 is slightly more resistant to corrosion, according to Laing. Since stainless steel is an alloy, the chemical composition may vary slightly from batch to batch. It is important, therefore, not to use implants from different manufacturers for the same repair. Such materials will be of different composition and will increase the galvanic potentiality even though they are both classified as the same type of stainless steel.

Intramedullary Pins

Intramedullary pinning is probably the most popular form of internal fixation used by veterinarians today. Most of the pins are applied in conjunction with open reduction, but occasionally an application may be made with closed reduction. A wide variety of devices are available, and each will be discussed here as well as under the various fractures for which they are applicable (Fig. 38).

As in all forms of fixation, it is of great importance to select those cases in which intramedullary fixation will be the most effective. Transverse fractures, particularly in young patients, are ideal; some oblique fractures in which the fracture line is sufficiently irregular so as to prevent overriding also will respond well to intramedullary treatment. Generally speaking, with the exception of the Kuentscher nail, intramedullary pins are contraindicated in comminuted or oblique fractures. Figure 39 shows clearly what usually happens when a round pin of a diameter much smaller than the medullary canal is applied to an oblique fracture of a long bone. The tendency is for the short sides of the fracture to impinge on the pin, thereby allowing the fragments to override, so that a large irregular callus is formed and the limb is shortened. It can easily be seen that a transverse fracture or an oblique

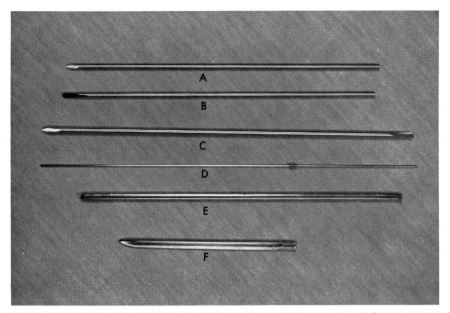

Figure 38. Various types of intramedullary pins and Thomson beaded wire. A, Single point (trocar). B, Single point (chisel). C, Double point. D, Thomson beaded wire. E, Kuentscher nail "cloverleaf." F, Kuentscher nail "V."

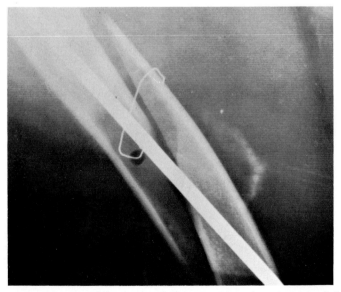

Figure 39. Incorrect use of the intramedullary pin. Note the migration of the short sides of the oblique fracture toward the pin, resulting in overriding and angulation. The feeble attempt to correct this by wiring has aborted.

fracture with sufficient gripping power due to irregularities in the fracture line would not produce such a result with the conventional round intramedullary pin.

KIRSCHNER INTRAMEDULLARY PIN. This pin is used more than any other for intramedullary fixation. It can be obtained in diameters ranging from $\frac{1}{16}$ inch to $\frac{1}{4}$ inch and lengths from 7 inches to 12 inches. The points may be trochar, chisel, or screw types (Fig. 40), and the pins are sold as single-pointed or double-pointed with various combinations of points. The trochar point has three faces and works well in cortical bone most of the time. However, bone dust can "build up" on the faces of the point and interfere with effectiveness of the cutting edges. The chisel point, on the other hand, has a beveled cutting edge which is almost at right angles to the two faces of the point and is less likely to be impeded by bone dust "build-up." Either the trochar or the chisel point is satisfactory for most intramedullary work in small animals.

The screw point on an intramedullary pin is of little or no value for two reasons: (1) The cutting edge of the point is the same width as the thread. This means that the hole that is cut in the bone is the same diameter as the thread portion of the pin, leaving no solid bone to engage the thread. In such a case, the thread has added no value to the pin. (2) The threads are coarse and therefore much too "fast" for the cutting edge. This means that if the threads did engage solid bone, they would strip out of the bone, because the pin would not be moving forward rapidly enough. Such a situation could be corrected by increasing the number of threads per inch or by first drilling a hole slightly smaller than the threaded end. This is done when screws are used with bone plates, but it probably would prove to be a considerable task in intramedullary pinning. If such a method is attempted, the intramedullary pin should have a self-tapping end. Figure 41 illustrates the futility of a threaded point.

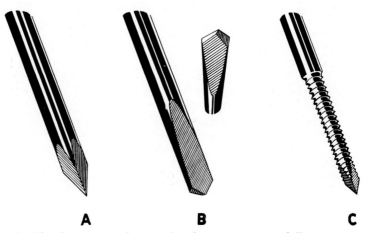

A   B   C

Figure 40. The three types of points found on most intramedullary pins. A, Trocar. B, Chisel. C, Screw.

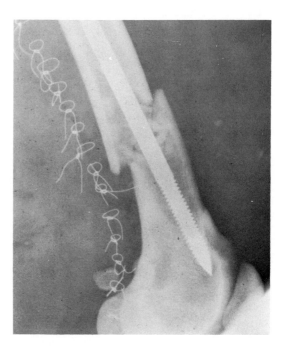

Figure 41. A threaded pin placed in a femoral fracture. Here the thread is embedded in cancellous bone and adds nothing to the support of the distal fragment. Note also the tendency for the short sides of an oblique fracture to migrate toward the pin.

Since the Kirschner intramedullary pin is round, the problem of long axis rotation should always be considered. This does not occur when the line of cleavage is irregular enough for the fragments to enmesh, but it is likely to occur in smooth transverse fractures. A good example of this type of case is the transverse fracture of the midshaft of the femur. With a round pin, this is quite likely to heal with the stifle adducted and the hock abducted, creating a "pigeon-toed" effect. Longitudinal rotation can be avoided by using a pin such as the Kuentscher nail. It can also be controlled by applying some sort of external splintage for about one week in addition to the round intramedullary pin. Fortunately, most fracture lines are sufficiently irregular to minimize this type of rotation. Contrary to popular belief, muscle pull will not correct this kind of rotation because it is the force applied to the bone by the contracted muscles which brings about rotation in the first place. It is true, however, that once the proper extension of the fractured bone has been achieved, the muscles have a tendency to press any free fragments toward the fracture site, thereby helping to promote a proper reduction.

Insertion of the Kirschner intramedullary pin is best accomplished with a Jacobs type chuck having a hollow handle and a hollow safety extension which can be attached (Fig. 42). Since more experience is required to place the pin properly with closed reduction, it is usually recommended that an open reduction be performed. Nevertheless, in some instances open reduction is not feasible. Since it is easier to align a short segment with a longer one, the closed operation is facilitated by placing the pin in the short segment first. An exception to this rule is a supracondylar fracture of the

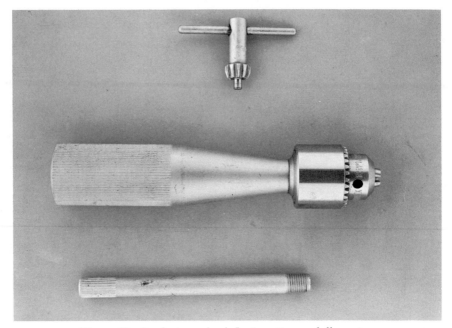

Figure 42. Jacobs-type chuck for inserting medullary pins.

humerus, in which the elbow joint interferes with pin placement from the distal end. This obstacle may be overcome by inserting two small pins or two screws in the epicondyles at such an angle that they penetrate the opposite cortex at a point proximal to the fracture line. The fixation pins or screws thus form an X across the fracture line.

The pin should be inserted the full length of the bone (Fig. 43) so that the proper leverage is obtained and migration is minimized. We speak of the pin movement as migration and not gravitation because it frequently does not gravitate, but rather follows a path of migration brought about by muscle action. An anchor pin placed at right angles to the intramedullary pin will control this tendency. Migration can be controlled in open reduction by inserting a single-pointed pin into the proximal segment and out through the skin (retrograde). The procedure is then reversed and the blunt end inserted as far as possible into the distal segment. The excess pin, along with the point, is then cut off, leaving a pin with both ends blunt.

Finally, pins of small diameter should be used wherever the medullary canal of the bone has sufficient curvature to require a pin to bend in order to remain in the canal and not penetrate the cortex. It is quite possible to insert several small pins if more strength is required, but a pin of large diameter is unyielding and therefore will not follow the contour of the bone.

KUENTSCHER NAIL. The Kuentscher nail is designed for proximal and midshaft fractures of the femur and is of particular value if the fracture is oblique or if half pin splintage or the conventional intramedullary pin is not

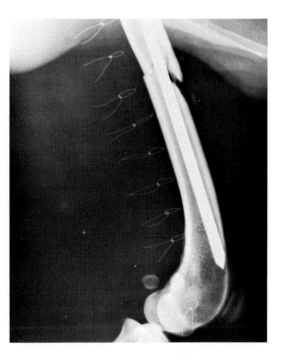

Figure 43. An intramedullary pin correctly inserted in a femoral shaft fracture. Note the stainless steel sutures in the skin.

feasible. The equipment necessary for the application of this nail is shown in Figure 44.

The size of the nail is extremely important. The femur can easily be shattered by a nail that is too large, since it is driven through the medullary canal with some force. The variations and curvature of the canal should be considered in selecting the proper size. The simplest method of determining diameter is by measuring the roentgenogram at the narrowest point and subtracting at least $1/16$ of an inch for magnification. Length is estimated by measuring from the proximal border of the patella to the base of the trochanter major. The nail should be cut to the proper length before driving and any rough edges should be filed smooth to avoid irritation to the tissues. It goes without saying that at least one hole should remain in the nail so that it can be extracted.

Application is best accomplished by open reduction so that all parts are exposed and under control. With this method, no guide pins are necessary. The trochanteric fossa is exposed, and with the reamer an opening is made in the cortex large enough to accommodate the nail. The mallet and punch are then used to drive the nail into position. When it reaches the distal end of the proximal segment, driving is halted long enough to reduce the fracture manually, after which the nail is driven into the distal segment. After healing is completed, the trochanteric fossa is again exposed and the nail withdrawn. The hook of the extractor is placed in the hole in the pin and the weight driven against the heavy end of the extractor.

RUSH PIN. The Rush pin has never had wide acceptance by veterinar-

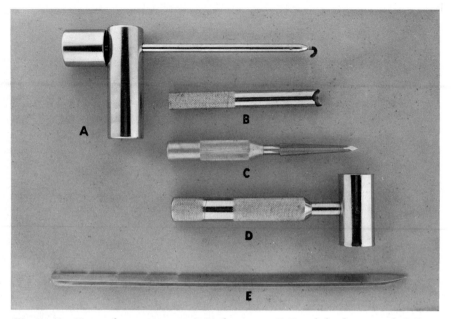

Figure 44. Kuentscher equipment. A, Nail extractor. B, Punch for driving nail. C, Reamer. D, Mallet. E, Large size nail.

ians. Its principal use has been in fractures of the radius and supracondylar fractures of the humerus in smaller dogs and cats. It is usually employed in connection with closed reduction. The pin has a hooked end so that it will anchor outside the bone and will not migrate. It is driven through a hole drilled near the proximal end of the bone. Because of its flexibility, it follows the medullary canal and bridges the reduced fracture. When the fracture is healed, the pin is removed (Fig. 45).

Jonas Splint

The use of this splint was first reported in 1953 by the inventor, Dr. Jonas. It consists of three parts which are assembled into a permanent unit. A cylindrical sleeve containing a spring and pin is manufactured in several diameters and lengths. It is made of "non-magnetic surgical stainless steel" for a permanent insertion into the medullary canal. The apparatus is "cocked" before use and is held in this position by a small pin until it has been placed within the bone. The "firing pin" is then released so that the splint extends itself along the medullary canal. Figure 46 shows the splint in place and extended.

This device has been recommended for fractures of the radius, ulna, and tibia, or for situations in which the short segment has insufficient length for plating. The splint is introduced through open reduction, the sleeve being placed in the longer segment of the bone which has been reamed out to accommodate it. After reduction, the released pin extends into the shorter

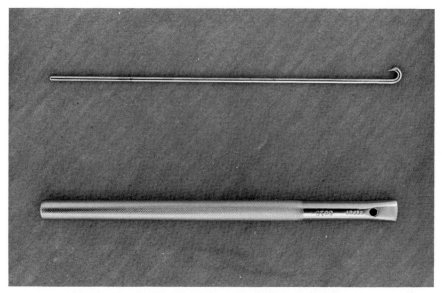

Figure 45. Rush pin and special punch used for driving it.

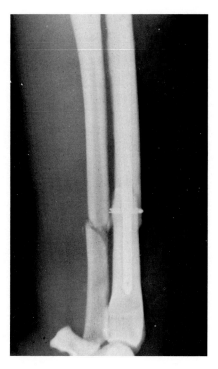

Figure 46. The Jonas splint applied to a fractured radius. Additional support has been added by wiring.

segment. The pin end can be cut and sharpened to whatever length is needed, but the splint should not be allowed to overextend, since this will impair its effectiveness. The Thomas splint is frequently used for additional support. Holes are provided in either end of the splint to permit withdrawal if necessary at some subsequent time. It is suggested that the extended splint be ½ inch longer than the entire medullary canal.

We have been called upon from time to time to remove this splint from a patient because a fistula has developed. It usually requires considerable bone destruction in order to retrieve the splint.

Leighton Shuttle Pin

This is a modified form of intramedullary pinning proposed by Leighton in 1950. The method consists of embedding a short shuttle-type pin at the site of the fracture. Successful use of this pin has been reported in the radius, the ulna, the tibia, and the femur. Some form of external splintage must be applied in order to support the repair, since the short loose-fitting pin merely holds the fracture ends in mild apposition. It eliminates the need for traction and provides prolonged support when the distal fragment is short.

Figure 47 illustrates the equipment needed for installing the pin, which is made of 18-8 SMo type 304 stainless steel so that it can remain in the bone indefinitely. Open reduction is performed and the medullary cavity of the bone ends is reamed with a simple hand drill to facilitate introduction of the

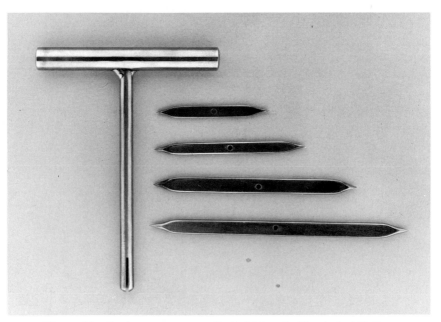

Figure 47. Equipment necessary for Leighton shuttle pin installation.

pin. A long heavy silk or wire suture is threaded through the hole in the middle of the pin, after which it is inserted into the long segment of the fractured bone until only a tiny portion of the distal end protrudes. The fracture is then reduced with the suture emerging from between the fractured ends. The twisting rod or tightener is then brought into play by twisting on the suture so that the pin will be pulled into position across the fracture line. This method should work well in selected fractures of the radius and ulna, but external support in the form of coaptation should always be used to avoid angulation and excessive movement at the fracture site.

Bone Plates and Screws

The use of steel plates with screws for the fixation of fractures was popularized by Lane in 1910. Since that time, the Sherman type plate (Fig. 48) has come into wide use and seems to be most acceptable. This plate is made of vitallium or type 316 or 317 stainless steel. The vitallium plate, since it is cast, is x-rayed for flaws and the screws are tested for strength by torsion before it is offered for sale. It is widely used in veterinary orthopedics at the present time. Archibald and Chappel have written about the use of vitallium bone plates in dogs; these men report favorably and it is reasonable to assume that vitallium plates should work well because of their lack of galvanic activity. Stainless steel has had a slightly wider acceptance, but vitallium is gradually replacing it in the veterinary field.

The steel formula was developed with the cooperation of the Bureau of Standards of the American Academy of Orthopaedic Surgeons and Military Surgeons. Some manufacturers make their own alloys and by very exact processing they are able to produce batches that are very similar in composition. Since manufacturers now use a standard grade of material, selection of plates can be narrowed to type and thickness. The Sherman type plate has all the mechanical advantages for firm fixation, yet it is light in weight. In spite of the lightness it has proved to be a strong, durable plate. For the best immobilization, a plate should have at least three screw holes, and preferably more. The length should be five times the diameter of the bone at the fracture site. Because scratches cause increased corrosion, the plate should be marred as little as possible during installation. Sizes commonly used are 4 to 11, 4 being the large size and 11 being the small.

The screws should be of a machine type with self-tapping ends (Fig. 49). Tapering screws are inadvisable. Inasmuch as the screw length should be exactly right it is advisable to have on hand all of the lengths from $3/8$ inch to $1\frac{1}{2}$ inches. Both coarse-threaded and fine-threaded screws are available; in general, the fine thread is preferable because of its greater contact surface.

Bone plating in dogs requires even more care and attention to details than bone pinning, for two reasons. First, there is little muscular covering in most instances, so that the plate is near the surface and more likely to loosen. Every care must be taken, therefore, that the plate is properly seated and that the screws maintain maximum holding power. This means that the plate must be bent to conform to the shape of the bone and there should be no

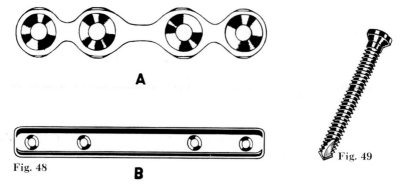

Fig. 48

A

B

Fig. 49

Figure 48.   A, Sherman type bone plate. B, Lane type bone plate.

Figure 49.   A machine type screw with self-tapping end.

points of excessive pressure to cause decalcification (Fig. 50). It also implies that the screw holes be exactly the right diameter and drilled without "wobbling" so that the threads will contact as much cortical bone as possible. Second, the periosteum is thin and does not easily separate from the bone. The periosteum is especially difficult to handle in areas near the ends of long bones where plating is sometimes mechanically advisable. On the other hand, these are the very areas where a covering of periosteum over the plate would be most helpful because of the proximity to the skin.

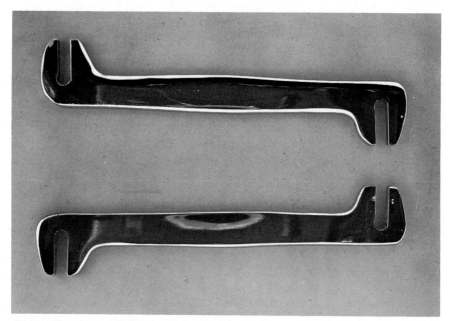

Figure 50.   A pair of plate benders. The plate can be molded to fit the bone by applying leverage with these instruments.

To install a plate, a generous incision is made so that the fractured ends are well exposed. Where possible, the periosteum is loosened so that the plate will be directly in contact with the bone. The fracture is reduced and the plate held in position with bone-holding clamps. Care is taken to see that the plate is correctly bent in easy curves and without sharp angles. At least two holes in the plate should appear on either side of the fracture line whenever practicable (Fig. 51). A bit with a slightly smaller diameter than that of the screws should be selected for boring the holes. Some have recommended a bit seven sizes smaller than the screw. In general, however, Sherman screws require a Number 32 drill for the coarse thread and a Number 30 drill for the fine. A "starter" bit with a sharp point is excellent for centering before drilling the hole. Both cortices should be penetrated with the bit without undue side motion. The screws should be set with an orthopedic type screw driver which grasps the screw head so that it can not slip (Fig. 52). The screw should be started slowly until the thread is well engaged. The final turn should be sufficient to hold the plate firmly but not exceedingly tight.

When the work of attaching the plate has been completed, and before the bone clamps are removed, a transfixion screw should be placed across the fracture line at right angles to the screws holding the plate. If the fracture is oblique, the screw hole can be bored directly across the bone. However, should the fracture line be transverse, the screw hole should be

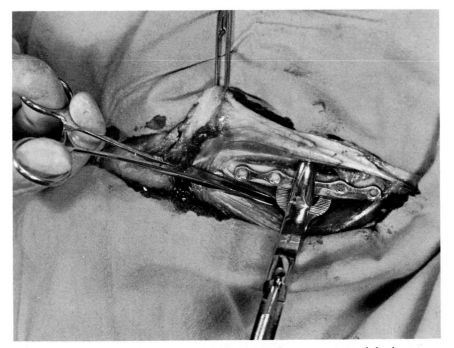

Figure 51. Bone clamp applied to hold the bone plate in position while the screws are inserted.

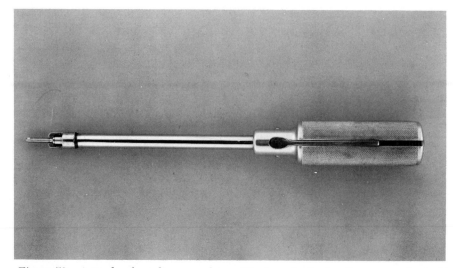

Figure 52. A good orthopedic screw driver. The lever in the handle operates the locking and releasing device holding the screw.

made obliquely. This transfixion screw does much to overcome torsion of the bone segments and reduces cortical absorption due to pressure on the plate and screws. Figure 53 illustrates the use of a transfixion screw.

Screws do not hold well in cancellous bone. They also have a tendency to loosen if placed too near the skin surface or if subjected to excessive pressure.

According to most human orthopedic texts, a periosteal flap should cover the plate, but it is well known that the dog and cat have a very thin friable periosteum which, in most cases, is virtually impossible to manipulate in such a manner. As much tissue as is available should be used to fill the incision and to pad the area between the plate and the skin. External support is generally required during the clinical healing period. It is not necessary to remove plates unless they cause trouble by loosening.

In 1958, a group of Swiss orthopedic surgeons began an evaluation of fracture treatment in humans. This group was known as "Arbeitsgemein-schaft für Osteosynthesefragen" and later referred to as "AO." As a result of these studies, a new method of bone plating, known as compression plating, evolved. Davis was of the opinion that axial compression promoted osteo-genesis. On this premise the AO group developed a plating method using the principle of impaction and rigid fixation. The purpose of the method is to stimulate first intention bone healing without callus formation and at the same time to allow the muscles and joints to be mobilized.

Plates and screws for this method of fixation are made of A.I.S.I. type 316 stainless steel. This steel is practically inert in the tissues and ranks close to vitallium. It is an austenitic steel which is non-magnetic and highly resistant to corrosion. The screws have an extremely coarse thread which is also cut deep with a sharp right angle toward the head and a sloping angle

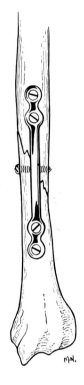

Figure 53. Drawing to illustrate method of applying transfixion screw.

away from the head. This produces greater holding power with less possibility of stripping. They are not self-tapping, and therefore the cortex holes must be tapped before inserting the screws (Fig. 54).

Since this method was developed for human orthopedics, it was necessary to adapt it to smaller animals. Smaller screws and plates have been made by Richards Manufacturing Company of Memphis, Tennessee, along with some modification of the plates to meet the needs of fractured bones in dogs and cats. Hirschhorn has developed some modifications of the compression system manufactured by Richards which are said to have some advantage over the original AO system.

The instruments, plates, and screws developed by AO are referred to as AOI. More recently, in the United States, the Smith, Kline, and French Laboratories has provided this type of equipment under the name of ASIF (Association for the Study of Internal Fixation).

Compression plating requires a very exacting technique and should not be attempted unless the operator is prepared to use the specified equipment and method of application. The method is built primarily around the type of screw that is used. These screws are deep threaded with the upper surface of the thread almost at a right angle to the axis of the screw. The threads are extremely coarse, so that maximum holding power is produced.

This technique requires a good exposure of the bone and a plate that is long enough for at least two screws on either side of the fracture. The plate

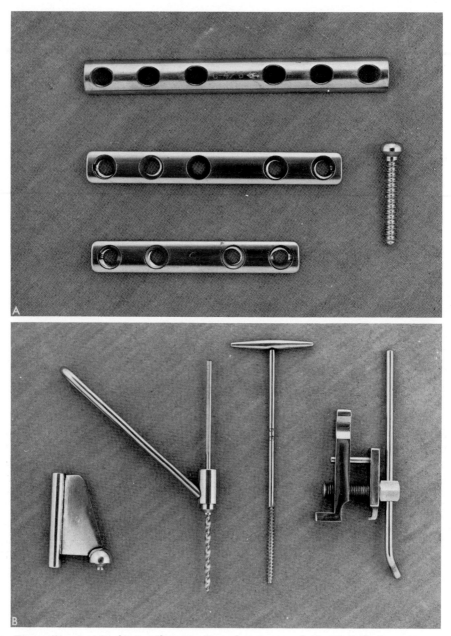

Figure 54. A, AO plates and screw. Top plate is curved. B, AO drill sleeves, tap, and compression instrument.

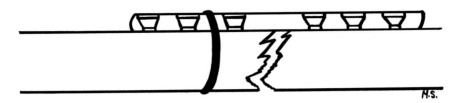

Figure 55. Bone plate placed over fracture.

should be centered over the fracture site and held in place by clamping or cerclage wires until the fragments are firmly fixed with screws (Fig. 55). After the bone segments have been properly aligned, a hole is drilled through both cortices of the short segment with a 3.2 mm. drill bit. A drill sleeve should be used to ensure that the hole is drilled exactly in the center of the hole in the plate as well as to keep the bit and the plate separated from each other (Fig. 56).

Once the cortices have been drilled, a thread is cut with a special tap (Fig. 57). No downward force should be applied to the tap, but rather gentle turning with the fingers to avoid stripping of the bone threads. Complete tapping of the distal cortex is extremely important, since any binding of the screw at this point will cause it to strip the bone. A 6 mm. nipple on the end of the tap serves as an indicator when the threading is completed. A screw is then inserted and tightened enough to hold the plate in position. This process is repeated until all screws in the short segment are in place and firmly tightened (Fig. 58).

The original AOI method of compression began the next step by applying a special drill sleeve to the end hole of the plate on the long bone segment (Fig. 59). This places the bit beyond the end of the plate, where a

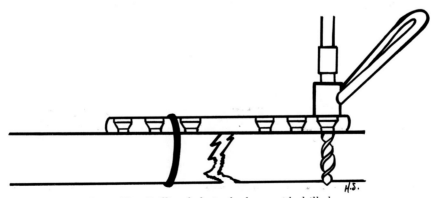

Figure 56. Drilling hole in the bone with drill sleeve.

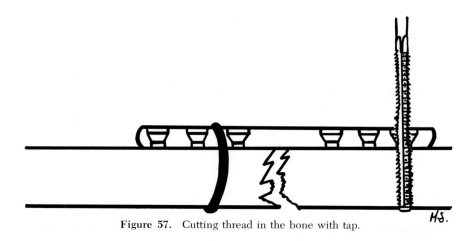

Figure 57.   Cutting thread in the bone with tap.

hole is drilled and tapped through the proximal cortex. The compression
instrument is hooked in the end hole of the plate and screwed to the bone at
the previously prepared point (Fig. 60). By tightening the compression
instrument, the bone segments are apposed, and the screws nearest the
fracture are applied. The last screw is applied after the compression instrument is removed (Fig. 61).

If the Hirschhorn modification of the Richards plating technique is
used, a slightly different approach is made to the compression of the fracture. The Richards plate has a slot in place of one of the center screw holes
(Fig. 62). The plate is placed on the bone so that the near end of the slot is at
least 10 mm. from the fracture site. Screws are inserted into the short
segment as usual. A screw hole is then prepared in the long segment by
drilling in the center of the slot. The screw used in this hole should be about
3/4 inch longer than is required to penetrate both cortices and should be left

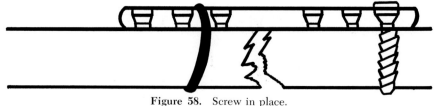

Figure 58.   Screw in place.

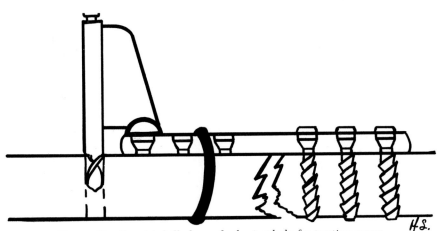

Figure 59. Special drill sleeve for boring hole for traction screw.

protruding above the plate (Fig. 63). The compression device is fastened to this screw and hooked into the nearest screw hole in the plate (Fig. 64). The compression of the fracture is accomplished by tightening the compression device and the remaining screws are inserted in the usual manner. After the compression device is removed, the long screw is replaced by one of proper length (Fig. 65).

The advantage claimed for this method is more direct leverage at the fracture site with less bowing and displacement. This eliminates the need for cerclage or clamps. A shorter incision is required, since the compression device operates in the middle of the plate instead of from the end.

The compression plating technique has been recommended primarily for the repair of non-union fractures of long bones, although it has been used with success on some fresh fractures. The use of this method in dogs has met

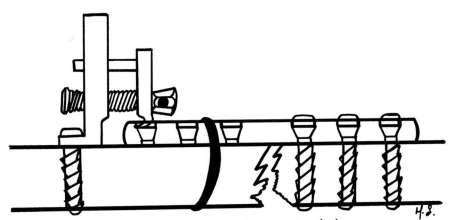

Figure 60. Compression instrument applied.

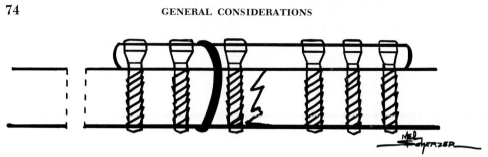

Figure 61. Completed application.

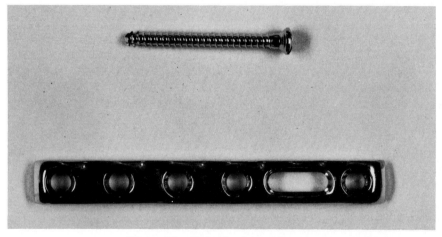

Figure 62. Richards plate and screw.

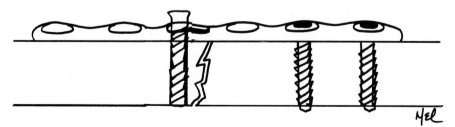

Figure 63. Long traction screw applied.

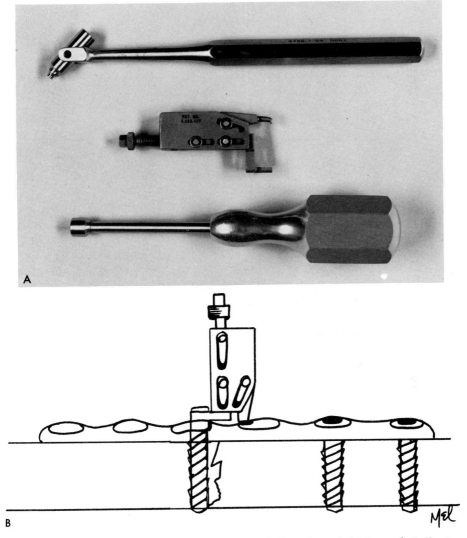

Figure 64. A, Hirschhorn compression device, drill guide, and driving tool. B, Fracture compressed.

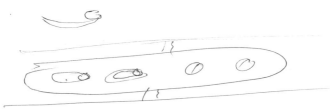

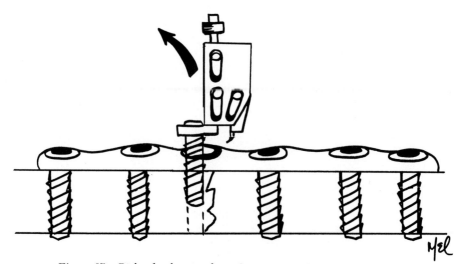

Figure 65.   Richards plate in place. Compression device being removed.

with varying degrees of success. There have been reported failures due to screws backing out or stripping. In all probability the thin cortex found in the dog has some bearing on this result, since better success has been reported where the method has been used on old non-unions where the cortex has been thickened by callus formation. It has also met with success in horses, in which the cortex is considerably thicker than it is in dogs.

The method has been recommended in fractures of femur, tibia, and humerus in dogs, but the human equipment is too large for smaller bones. The Richards equipment is also adapted from human equipment and therefore has some of the same drawbacks.

Femoral Head Prostheses

Four types of prostheses have been proposed for use in dogs. Brown designed one of stainless steel which consisted of a three-quarter sphere with a simple stem. Archibald fashioned one of the same shape from plastic resins (methyl methacrylate or Vibrin 108) with a stainless steel stem. Gay's prostheses consists of a stainless steel head piece rounded on one end to fit the acetabulum and attached at an angle to an intramedullary pin on the other. The intramedullary pin is designed to fit into the medullary canal of the shaft and a smaller pin acts as an anchor (Fig. 66).

The Gorman prosthesis (Fig. 67) is a ball and socket arrangement designed to replace both the femur head and the articular cartilage of the acetabulum. It attaches to the pelvis with three toggle bolts and to the femur with an intramedullary pin. The recommended approach for installation is through a dorsal paramedian skin incision which transverses the hip just ventral to the trochanter. The superficial muscles are separated and the joint is exposed by osteotomy of the trochanter. The designer recommends the

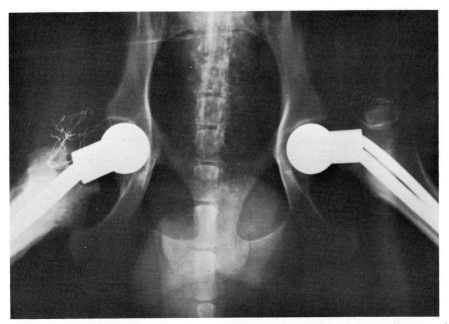

Figure 66. The Gay femoral head prosthesis installed in both hips. The installation on the right shows both the intramedullary pin and the anchor pin. (Courtesy of Dr. W. I. Gay, National Institutes of Health, Department of Health, Education, and Welfare.)

use of this prosthesis in the following conditions: "(1) Osteoarthritis of the joint; (2) aseptic necrosis of the head and neck; (3) congenital luxations and subluxations; (4) intracapsular fractures; (5) separation of femoral epiphysis; (6) fracture of the acetabulum; (7) dysplasia of the head; (8) chronic luxations; (9) coxa plana, coxa vara, or coxa magna; (10) tumors of the head and neck."

It might be well at this point to say a word about the use of plastics in hip prostheses or about their use as implants in general, since there is no doubt that synthetic materials will be tried more frequently in the future. Most plastic resins contain additives such as catalysts, plasticizers, pigments, stabilizers, fillers, and stripping agents, which may cause tissue reaction. The acrylic resins have been used as implants but with questionable results. Scales lists the qualifications of synthetic materials to be used as implants as follows: The implant (1) must not be physically modified by tissue fluids; (2) must be chemically inert; (3) must not incite an inflammatory or foreign cell response in the tissues; (4) must be non-carcinogenic; (5) must not produce a state of allergy or hypersensitivity; (6) must be capable of standing mechanical strain; (7) must be capable of being fabricated in the form required with reasonable ease and at relatively low cost; and (8) must be capable of being sterilized.

Since the Brown type of prosthesis has come into more common use than the others, the installation of this device will be described in detail.

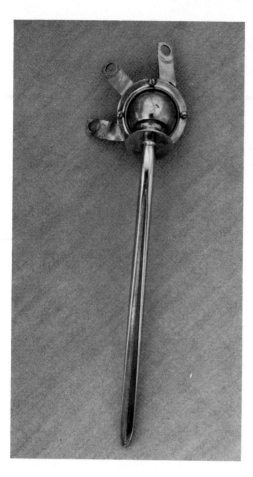

Figure 67.   Gorman hip prosthesis.

The original prosthesis was made of 18-8 SMo, type 303, stainless steel rod turned down on a lathe, polished, and passivated with nitric acid for twenty minutes. This prosthesis can also be made of vitallium as well as the stainless steels previously mentioned as being inert in the tissues (see page 56). Some have been fabricated in two pieces with the stems screwed into the head instead of from a single piece of metal. Either type seems to work well. The sizes usually available are Number 5 through Number 16, each number representing $1/16$ of an inch in head diameter. The head size is determined by measuring the diameter of the normal femur head on the roentgenogram and subtracting one size to allow for magnification. The stem varies in diameter and length with the head size, but must be long enough to penetrate the lateral cortex of the femoral shaft. The head should be protected before use, since small scratches in the surface will have an abrasive action on the joint cartilage whenever the leg is moved.

The instruments required for installation are shown in Figure 68. The procedure for wide exposure of the hip joint. The skin incision should extend from the dorsal midline over the trochanter major to midthigh. The

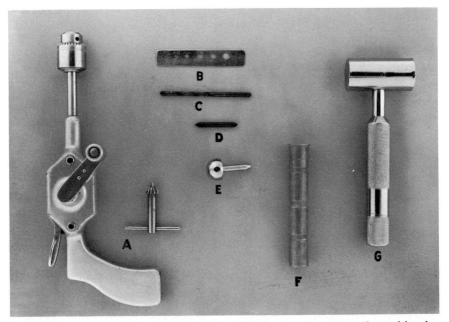

Figure 68. Equipment necessary for the installation of a Brown type femoral head prosthesis. A, Drill with chuck that can be sterilized. B, Gauge for comparing the bit size with the size of the stem of the prosthetic head. C, Bone bit slightly smaller than the prosthetic stem. D, "Starter" bit. This is a sharpened bit to be used for starting the drill hole. E, Prosthetic head. F, Punch used for setting the head. This is a piece of soft aluminum tubing. G, Soft metal mallet.

fascia lata and the tensor fascia lata are divided, exposing the gluteal muscles (Fig. 69). These attach on the cranial and dorsal sides of the trochanter and should be severed close to their attachment, leaving sufficient tendinous tissue for suturing. The capsule lies beneath the muscles and usually needs no incision, since it is already badly mutilated. As soon as the joint has been opened, the femur can be lifted and rotated so that the cranial and medial surfaces are exposed. Cutting or putting excessive pressure on the caudal side of the joint should be avoided, since the sciatic nerve lies in this area.

Frequently the ligamentum teres is still intact with the femur head attached. If such is the case, the head is lifted with a pair of Backaus towel clamps so that the ligament can be easily cut with a pair of scissors. The acetabulum is cleared of any debris and the femur neck shaped to accommodate the prosthesis (Fig. 70).

A bit is then selected which is just a trifle narrower than the prosthetic stem and a hole is drilled so that one end lies in the center of the neck and the other end just distal to the base of the trochanter major (Fig. 71). This hole can be started from whichever side seems most acceptable to the operator so long as the result is accurate. The stem is started by hand and then firmly seated by driving with a mallet and soft aluminum punch (Fig. 72). When the prosthesis is in place, the stem should protrude slightly from the opening in the lateral cortex of the femur.

(*Text continued on page 83.*)

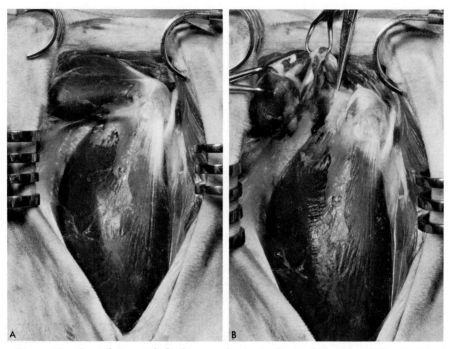

Figure 69. Cranial approach for hip prosthesis. A, Exposed gluteal muscles. B, Divided gluteals exposing the joint capsule at the tip of the hemostat.

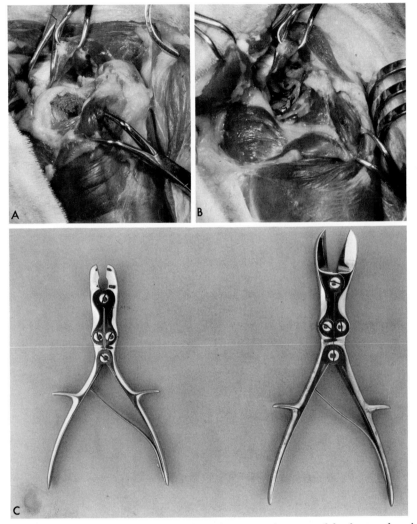

Figure 70. Removal of the femur head. A, The proximal portion of the fractured neck with the femur head still retained within the torn capsule. B, The femur head removed, exposing the acetabulum. C, Instruments used to shape and smooth the femoral neck. Bone rongeurs (left) and bone cutters (right).

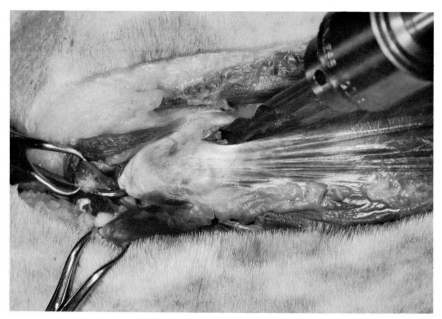

Figure 71.   Drilling the femur to accommodate the stem.

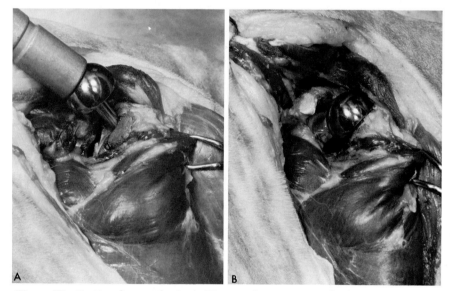

Figure 72.   Seating the prosthesis. A, The punch is a section of soft aluminum tubing. B, The head in place ready for seating in the acetabulum, which can be seen in the background.

After the acetabulum is cleared, the head is replaced and the capsule sutured if possible. If the capsule is so badly lacerated that suturing is impossible, the tissues surrounding it are secured with a few sutures and the capsule will reestablish itself. Synovial fluid will be secreted to lubricate the joint following closure of the capsule. If the fluid is not confined, a large bursa may form. The gluteal muscles are now brought into place and sutured with a suture material that will retain its strength for some time. Size 000 multifilament wire is recommended. If the muscles have been divided too close to the trochanter, small holes may be drilled into the bone and the sutures secured in this manner. It is important that this part of the closure be done well so that there is sufficient support for the joint. The fascia and skin are closed in the usual manner (Fig. 73).

Other Prostheses

Whittick describes a prosthesis used to rebuild the elbow joint in a cat after the natural joint had been totally destroyed. Intramedullary pins were placed in the ulna and humerus. These were coupled to form a joint and a projection was added for the attachment of the triceps tendon.

A mandibular prosthesis was also described. In this case there was bone loss in the body of both mandibles in a whippet. A U-shaped prosthesis was fashioned of steel and fastened to the remaining mandible by means of screws.

Description of prostheses in more common use will be found in the discussion of treatment of the specific orthopedic problem.

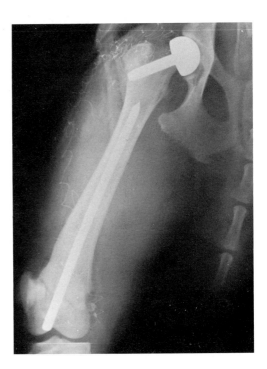

Figure 73. Roentgenogram showing Brown prosthesis in place. This also shows the repair of a distal epiphyseal fracture with an intramedullary pin.

Bone Grafts

The use of bone grafts has not been as common in veterinary surgery as it has been in human surgery. This method of repairing non-union fractures has been referred to by both Brinker and Coleman but to date has not been widely used in our profession. Although there are numerous types of grafts in use in orthopedic surgery, only about four are of interest to the orthopedist working with dogs or cats. These are the *onlay graft*, the *inlay graft*, the *intramedullary bone peg*, and *bone "seeding"* or *"packing"* with bone chips.

Inasmuch as non-union fractures require rigid immobilization in the form of skeletal fixation, and since the bones are relatively small in many cases, packing the freshened fracture site with bone chips seems to be the most logical procedure. This is easily accomplished by cutting autogenous cancellous bone into small pieces and filling the fracture space after the bone ends have been cut with a bone saw or cutters and properly immobilized.

In other cases it may be advisable to cut cortical bone into the form of a peg that can be inserted into the medullary canal. The bone peg has some splintage value as well as furnishing a transplant, but it must definitely be reinforced. One of the most easily obtained pegs is a section from the patient's rib. There is an added advantage here in that the rib curves and therefore fits into the medullary canal under a slight spring tension.

The onlay and inlay grafts differ only in the fact that the onlay is fastened on the outside of the cortex and the inlay is countersunk. These are made from cortical bone and require at least four screws to hold them in place.

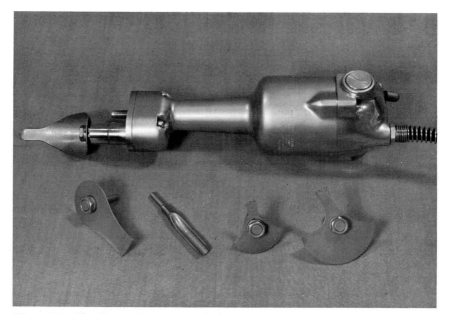

Figure 74. The Stryker bone saw with various types of blades. This equipment can be completely sterilized by autoclaving.

The fracture is freshened, apposed, and the graft is then laid in place and held with bone clamps. The drilling and screwing are done after the graft is in place. In the case of the inlay, the bed is prepared in advance with the use of a Stryker saw (Fig. 74) or a bone chisel. It can be readily seen that such a procedure is applicable only to the larger bones.

REFERENCES

Anderson, R.: Fractures of the radius and ulna. A new anatomical treatment. J. Bone Joint Surg., 16:379-393, 1934.

Anderson, R.: The Anderson splint. Surg. Gynec. Obstet., 62:865, 1936.

Anderson, R.: Ambulatory method of treating femoral shaft fractures, utilizing fracture table for reduction. Am. J. Surg., 29:538-551, 1938.

Baker, J., and Braken, F. K.: Plastic fracture sleeve. Vet. Med., 48:28, 1953.

Bjorck, G.: A transfixation plaster cast in the treatment of small animals. Nord. Vet. Med., 4:89, 1952.

Brinker, W. O.: Use of intramedullary pins in small animal fractures. N. Am. Vet., 29:292, 1948.

Brown, R. E.: A surgical approach to the coxofemoral joint in dogs. N. Am. Vet., 34:420, 1953.

Carney, J. P.: Rush intramedullary fixation of long bones as applied to veterinary surgery. Vet. Med., 47:43, 1952.

Charnley, J.: The Closed Treatment of Common Fractures. 2nd ed. Baltimore, Williams & Wilkins Co., 1957.

Cofield, R. B.: Technique in handling simple and compound fractures. N. Am. Vet., 15:32, 1934.

Coleman, D.: Bone transplant of femur in dog. J.A.V.M.A., 129:143, 1956.

Danis, R.: Theory and Practice of Internal Fixation. Paris. Masson et Cie, 1947.

Dibbell, E. B.: Splints for fixation of fractures and dislocations in small animals. N. Am. Vet., 11:29, 1930.

Dibbell, E. B.: Lower third femoral fractures in dogs. N. Am. Vet., 12:37, 1931.

Eastman, D. A.: Kirschner wires in femoral fractures. N. Am. Vet., 16:43, 1935.

Ehmer, E. A.: Bone pinning in fractures of small animals. J.A.V.M.A., 110:14, 1947.

Elmer, E. A.: Traumatic injuries in small animals. J.A.V.M.A., 112:246, 1948.

Freeman, L.: The application of extension to overlapping fractures. Ann. Surg., 70:231, 1919.

Frick, E. J., Witter, R. E., and Mosier, J. E.: Treatment of fractures by intramedullary pinning. N. Am. Vet., 29:95, 1948.

Gay, W. I.: Preliminary evaluation of a femoral head prosthesis in the presence of coxitis. J.A.V.M.A., 126:85, 1955.

Gay, W. I.: A method for surgical lengthening of the femur of the dog. Military Med., 123:282, 1958.

Gorman, H. A.: Master's Thesis, Ohio State University, 1955.

Green, J. E., Hoerlein, B. F., Konde, W. N., and McBee, J. A.: The indications and limitations of the medullary nail in small animals. Cornell Vet., 40:331, 1950.

Hickcox, J. P.: Treatment of fractures with Hirschhorn compression plates. J.A.V.M.A., 156:187-196, 1970.

Jacobs, P. A., and Guten, G. N.: Compression fixations of bone. Wisconsin Med. Jour., 66:412-417, 1967.

Jenny, J.: Kuentscher's medullary nailing in femur fractures of the dog. J.A.V.M.A., 117:381, 1950.

Jenny, J.: Today's standard of fracture treatment in small animals. Proc. 89th Ann. Meet., A.V.M.A., 1952; 187, 1953.

Knight, G. C.: A report on the use of stainless steel intramedullary pins and Sherman-type vitallium bone plates in the treatment of small animal fractures. Brit. Vet. J., 105:294, 1949.

Knowles, A. T., Knowles, J. O., and Knowles, R. P.: Clinical application of pinning in fracture reduction. Vet. Med., 44:259, 1949.

Knowles, A. T., Knowles, J. O., and Knowles, R. P.: Clinical application of splints in fractures of the pelvis. Vet. Med., 44:308, 1949.

Laing, P. C.: Available metals. In Metals and Engineering in Bone and Joint Surgery. Baltimore, Williams & Wilkins Co., 1959.

Lambotte, A.: Evaluation of fractures. Brit. Med. J., 2:1530, 1950.

Lauder, J. S. J.: Fracture repair by bone pinning. Brit. Vet. Rec., 61:866, 1949.

Lawson, D. D.: The use of Rush pins in management of fractures in the dog and cat. Vet. Rec., 70:760, 1958.

Lawson, D. D.: Toggle fixation for recurrent dislocation of the hip in the dog. J. Small Animal Pract., 6:57-59, 1965.

Leighton, R. L.: A new method of permanent intramedullary pinning. J.A.V.M.A., 117:202, 1950.

Leighton, R. L.: Further reports of new method of permanent intramedullary pinning. J.A.V.M.A., 120:189, 1952.

Lyon, W. F.: The technique of plating long bone fractures. Surg. Clin. North America, 25:99, 1945.

MacAusland, W., and Russell, W.: Medullary nailing of fractures of the long bones. Surg. Gynec. Obstet., 84:85, 1947.

Mason, C. T.: Useful appliance for fractures of the extremities of dogs. N. Am. Vet., 29:360, 1948.

Mason, C. T.: A new appliance for metacarpal and metatarsal surgery. Auburn Vet., 4:91, Spring, 1948.

McCarroll, H. R.: Use of small threaded wires in the treatment of fractures. Arch. Surg., 54:138, 1947.

Muller, H.: Anatomische grundlagen und klinik der stabilen osteosynthese (marknagelung nach kuntscher) bei Hund und Katze. Zentralbl. Veter., 2:105, 1955.

Müller, M. E.: Internal fixation for fresh fractures and for non-union. Proc. Roy. Soc. Med., 56:455-460, 1963.

Müller, M. E., Allgöwer, M., and Willenegger, H.: Technique of Internal Fixation of Fractures (G. Segmüller, ed.). English edition. Springer-Verlag, New York, 1965.

Nichols, R. E.: Mechanics of fracture therapy in small animals. N. Am. Vet., 23:325, 1942.

Nichols, R. E.: Mechanical principles in fracture diagnosis and therapy. Cornell Vet., 32:37, 1942.

Obel, N.: Intramedullary fixation of diaphyseal fracture of the femur in dogs by stainless steel pins. Nord. Vet. Med., 3:723, 1951.

Olson, R.: External fixation of fractures in small animals. Student thesis No. 05737, N.Y.S. Vet. Lib.

Parkhill, C.: A new apparatus for the fixation of bones after resection and in fractures with a tendency to displacement. Tr. Am. Surg. A., 15:251, 1897.

Pease, C. H.: Beaded wires in treatment of fractures of the leg. Surg. Clin. N. Am., 25:174, 1945.

Ross, G. E., Jr.: Personal communication.

Ryerson, E. F.: Modern methods in treatment of fractures. Surg. Gynec. Obstet., 84:562, 1947.

Scales, J. T.: Tissue reaction to synthetic materials. Proc. Roy. Soc. Med., 46:647, 1953.

Schroeder, E. F.: The traction principle in treating fractures and dislocation in the dog and cat. N. Am. Vet., 14:32, 1933.

Shaar, C. M., and Kreug, F. P., Jr.: Manual of Fractures. Philadelphia, W. B. Saunders Co., 1943.

Stader, O.: A method of treating femoral fractures in dogs. N. Am. Vet., 15:25, 1934.

Stader, O.: Treating fractures of long bones, Part II. N. Am. Vet., 20:54, 1939.

Stader, O.: Treating fractures of long bones, Part III. N. Am. Vet., 20:62, 1939.

Stader, O.: Some Pertinent Notes about Fractures and Treatment with Stader Reduction Splints. Monograph (private publication), 1943.

Street, D. M., Hansen, H. H., and Brewer, B. J.: The medullary nail. Arch. Surg., 55:423, 1947.

Turnbull, N. R.: Fractures of humerus and femur repaired by intramedullary pins. Brit. Vet. Record, 61:476, 1949.

Venable, C. S., and Stuck, W. G.: Internal Fixations of Fractures. Springfield, Ill., Charles C Thomas, 1947.

Whittick, W., Bonar, C., and Reeve-Newson, J.: Two unusual orthopaedic prostheses. Canad. Vet. J., 5:56-60, 1964.

Wickstrom, J., Hamilton, L., and Rodriguez, R. P.: Evaluation of the AO compression apparatus. J. Trauma, 7:210-227, 1967.

PART TWO

Fractures

Distribution of Fractures in the Body (Based on 4146 cases)				
	Location	Frequency Per cent	Location	Frequency Per cent
The Pelvic Limb	Femur	25.8	Tibia and Fibula	10.2
	Shaft & Condyles	19.0	Tarsus	0.6
	Neck & Head	6.8	Metatarsus	1.4
	Patella	0.1	Phalanges	0.9
The Pectoral Limb	Scapula	1.3	Radius	5.1
	Humerus	6.9	Ulna	3.7
	Shaft	5.7	Olecranon	0.4
	Condyles	1.2	Carpus	0.5
	Radius & Ulna	9.8	Metacarpus	1.8
The Skull, Spine and Pelvis	Calvarium	1.4	Pelvis	22.6
	Maxilla	0.7	Ischium	1.7
	Mandible	6.3	Acetabulum	1.4
	Spine	5.7	Pubis	1.4
	Ribs	1.6	Ilium	18.1

Figure 75.

The chart shown in Figure 75 is derived from 4146 fracture cases admitted to the Small Animal Clinic, New York State Veterinary College. It represents the fractures seen in dogs and cats only. Because of the location of the college, it probably would be safe to say that this chart roughly represents the distribution of fractures seen in the average practice in the northeastern United States, exclusive of those practicing in large cities. It is interesting to note that fractures of the femur are first in frequency, followed closely by fractures of the pelvis. The two combined comprise nearly half of all fractures seen.

A fracture of bone or cartilage can be described as a disruption of the continuity of living connective tissue. It has been defined as the breaking of bone or cartilage resulting from external force or disease. The latter condition is usually referred to as a pathological fracture. The force causing a fracture may be direct or indirect. Fractures resulting from direct force occur at or near the point of violent impact and seldom follow any definite pattern of cleavage. Those occurring as a result of indirect force are usually typical because the force is transmitted through a bone or bones to a vulnerable spot where the pattern of the fracture can be predicted with fair accuracy. Fracture of the medial or lateral condyle of the humerus furnishes a good example of fracture by indirect force. Whenever a dog jumps from a high place or from a moving car, a fracture of the lateral condyle is likely to occur because the force is transmitted from the forefoot through the radius and ulna to the trochlea of the humerus, shearing off the lateral condyle and epicondyle (Fig. 76). On the other hand, if the dog is hit by a vehicle so that the force is applied just below the elbow joint, the olecranon transmits this force to the medial condyle of the humerus, thereby causing a break through the condylar shaft on the medial side (Fig. 77). In the latter case the force is moving in a horizontal direction; in the former it is travelling in a vertical direction.

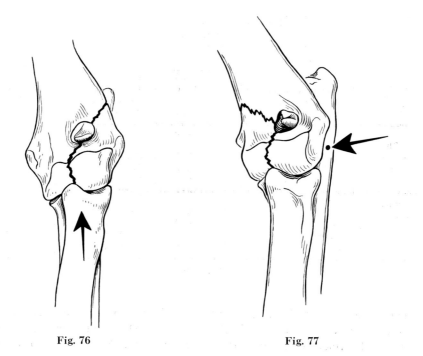

Fig. 76   Fig. 77

Figure 76. Diagrammatic drawing showing forces responsible for cleavage of the lateral condylar shaft of the humerus.

Figure 77. Diagrammatic drawing showing forces responsible for cleavage of the medial condylar shaft of the humerus.

CLASSIFICATION OF FRACTURES

Fractures may be classified as *simple* or *closed* when there is no communicating wound to the outside, or as *compound*, sometimes called *open*, when the fracture is exposed. From a clinical standpoint, if a wound exists in the region of the fracture it is considered compound whether there is absolute communication or not. Often in such cases the fracture becomes compound due to necrosis of badly traumatized tissues overlying it. When an open reduction is attempted, it is important to remember that a simple fracture has been converted into a compound fracture with all the attending dangers.

When classified according to extent of bone damage, a fracture may be called complete or incomplete. A *complete* fracture is one in which there is total disruption of the continuity of bone. The fracture line in this instance may be single or multiple. If it is multiple, it is designated as a *comminuted* fracture. Single fracture lines are named according to their direction in relation to the bone, i.e., *transverse, oblique, spiral,* or *longitudinal* (Fig. 78).

Complete fractures may also be classified according to displacement.

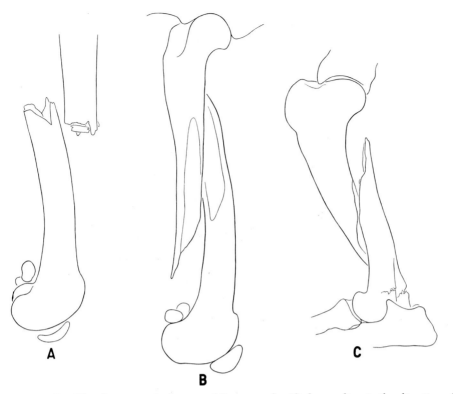

Figure 78. The three principal types of fractures classified according to the direction of the fracture line. Longitudinal fractures seldom occur except in the carpals and tarsals. A, Transverse. B, Oblique. C, Spiral.

Common types seen in this category are impaction and distraction. An *impacted* fracture is one in which the fractured ends are driven into each other or one bone is driven into the fracture site of another (femur head into a fractured acetabulum, Figure 79). When bone ends are not impacted by muscular contraction but simply lie side by side with shortening of the limb, this is called *overriding*. A *distracted* fracture occurs when there is sufficient muscle pull to separate the fracture segments (fracture of the olecranon, Figure 80). *Compression* fractures occur in cancellous bone, such as the vertebrae, with an apparent reduction in size of the bone due to pressure. Occasionally a compression fracture may occur in the bones of the skull, but more frequently skull fractures are *depression* fractures, meaning that they are displaced inward, causing a concavity in the vault of the calvarium.

The *incomplete* fracture is characterized by partial loss of continuity and only slight displacement. Two types of incomplete fractures are commonly seen in dogs. The *fissure* fracture (Fig. 81) is one in which a fine, hairlike crack penetrates the cortex for a short distance, usually in a transverse direction but at times longitudinally. In the *green stick* fracture (Fig. 82) there is usually some angulation of the bone with separation on the convex

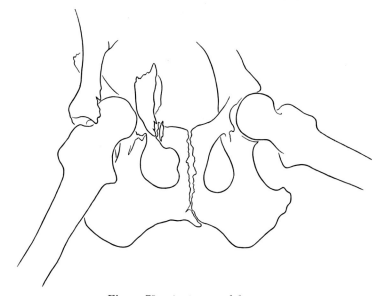

Figure 79. An impacted fracture.

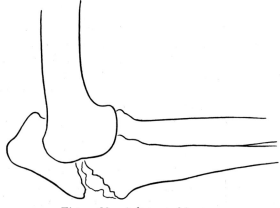

Figure 80. A distracted fracture.

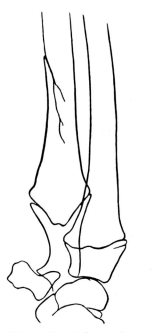

Figure 81. A fissure fracture.

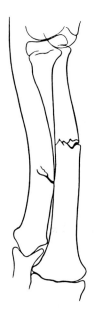

Figure 82. A green stick fracture.

side and with impacted cortex and periosteum on the concave side. The fracture derives its name from its resemblance to a broken live tree branch. This type of fracture usually occurs in dogs with soft bones, such as pups or those suffering from rachitis.

Fractures can be further classified according to their anatomical location in specific bones, an example of which is the supramalleolar fracture of the tibia. These will be discussed under their appropriate headings.

It has been suggested by Charnley that fractures should be classified from a practical clinical point of view according to their physical suitability to fixation. This would divide fractures into three main groups according to their stability against a telescoping force applied after reduction. Group I would be those fractures having no stability against shortening. This would include oblique, spiral, and comminuted fractures, all of which require some traction or skeletal fixation against overriding. Group II would be those fractures with complete stability against shortening. This would refer to the transverse fracture in which a splintage or fixation is used only to control angular deformity. Group III would consist of those fractures which have some potential against shortening, such as the jagged oblique fracture whose fracture line is less than 45° from the transverse. These are probably the commonest fractures and sometimes require close inspection in order to determine whether they belong in Group III or Group I.

DIAGNOSIS

Ordinarily the diagnosis of a fracture requires very little skill, since the signs are obvious and striking. On the other hand, the signs may be quite obscure, as in the case of a fractured fibula or tuber ischii. At other times it may be perplexing to differentiate between a fracture, a dislocation, and a sprain. Even when the presence of a fracture is quite evident, one must be careful not to overlook the possibility of multiple injuries: for example, fracture of the femoral shaft with luxation of the coxofemoral joint. An accurate diagnosis requires a systematic examination of the patient, using the five cardinal signs laid down by Schroeder 35 years ago: deformity, abnormal mobility, crepitus, loss of function, and pain.

Whenever the patient is ambulant, the first observations should be made from a point a few feet distant and before undertaking to palpate the injured parts. These preliminary observations may help to establish some of the signs such as deformity, mobility, and function. After the patient has been placed on the examining table, other signs such as pain and crepitus may be sought by gentle palpation. The approach should be gentle and gradual so as to cause as little discomfort as possible. If sedation is necessary for the comfort of the patient and can be given with comparative safety, it will simplify the examination, particularly the roentgenographic survey.

Deformity will be manifest by swelling, angulation, rotation, shortening, abduction, adduction, or any deviation from the normal posture or position. Certain deformities are pathognomonic, such as the abduction of the paw in Colles' fracture of the radius and ulna and supination of the paw in fracture of the lateral condyle of the humerus.

Abnormal mobility or immobility is seen when bones exerting leverage or acting as anchors are broken. Fractures in the pelvic region often cause the leg to deviate from its normal pattern of movement. This would be an example of abnormal mobility. When there is nerve injury, motor paralysis may cause immobility of a part. This then would not be a sign of fracture but rather of nerve injury. An example of immobility caused by fracture can be seen in such instances as fracture of the shaft of the femur.

Crepitus is a common sign in fractures and is essentially reliable, but occasionally a luxation will produce crepitus. There are also times when the fractured ends are distracted or muscles intervene so that crepitus cannot be produced.

Loss of function is a less reliable sign, since it may be seen with injuries to muscle, ligaments, tendons, nerves, bone, or cartilage, and the degree of injury may vary from a bruise to complete disruption. This sign is usually considered as part of the fracture picture but is not particularly diagnostic in itself.

Pain may be self-evident or may be elicited on palpation. Diffuse pain is quite likely to indicate a sprain or bruise. This calls for some interpretation in dogs that are highly sensitive, unless they have been tranquilized. Incomplete fractures with no displacement frequently can be located by palpation because the patient will flinch when the exact spot is touched. Pain seems to be more localized in the case of fracture than it does in other tissue injuries.

Verification of all fractures should be made by roentgenography. This will give the operator an exact picture of the injury and will help to locate any complicating factors. Views in two planes should be taken in areas such as the elbow. It is advisable to have the patient under sedation so that reliable roentgenograms can be taken, except on those rare occasions when sedation seems too hazardous.

TREATMENT

Since treatment will be discussed in detail under the heading for each type of fracture, it is necessary here only to remind the reader of the general requirements of good treatment for all fractures. Open reductions being in such common use, along with the various external pinning methods, a word of warning concerning the surgical techniques seems justified. Venable states, "Bone normally possesses less power of resistance to infection than soft tissues and traumatized bone as well as soft tissues at a fracture site are even less resistant to infection." From experience, we know this to be true and therefore recommend that the first rule of treatment of any open fracture be a strict aseptic approach.

Fractures should be properly reduced with a minimum of trauma. Excessive trauma cannot be excused as necessary to exact reduction. Good alignment is, nevertheless, important so long as it does not have to be achieved through the use of excessive force. Good length is of less consequence in the dog than in man because of the angulation in a dog's leg, but it should be accomplished as frequently as possible. One should endeavor to produce an end-to-end reduction but never at the expense of surrounding tissues through excessive trauma.

Proper immobilization is probably the most important factor in fracture treatment. Motion must be minimized if good healing is to be expected. In selecting a method of fixation, the first question should be, "Will it immobilize the fracture?" Naturally, the simplest method of fixation which will produce rigid immobility is usually the method of choice, all other things being equal.

The most valuable treatment after a fracture has been immobilized is that which will improve circulation. The cast or bandage should not be unduly tight. In case of swelling, steps should be taken to reduce the edema. Passive methods such as massage will help, but active motion performed by the patient himself is far superior. If massage is used, it should be gentle and the stroking should be in the direction of venous flow. Active exercise of a limb will usually be encouraged by the use of splintage which leaves the joints free. When the leg is constantly held in flexion, the application of a small amount of sheet lead to the foot will usually bring about active exercise of the leg. The weight of the lead will extend the leg and the dog will then flex it, thereby setting up an active exercise.

REFERENCES

Charnley, J.: The Closed Treatment of Common Fractures. 2nd ed. Baltimore, Williams & Wilkins Co., 1957.

Jenny, J.: Proc. 89th Ann. Meet., A.V.M.A., 1952.

McCunn, J.: Fractures and dislocations in small animals. Vet. Record, 47:1236–1254, 1933.

Perkins, G.: Rest versus activity in the treatment of a fracture. Lancet, 252:49–54, 1947.

Schroeder, E. F.: The use of traction in the treatment of fractures. Cornell Vet., 25:111–131, 1935.

Schroeder, E. F.: Diagnostic methods in small animal practice. Vet. Med., 30:323–330, 1935.

Venable, C. S., and Stuck, W. G.: Internal Fixations of Fractures. Springfield, Ill., Charles C Thomas, 1947.

Wright, J. G.: Some observations on the incidence, causes and treatment of bone fractures in the dog. Vet. Record, 49:2–16, 1937.

Chapter 5

Fractures in the Pelvic Limb

FRACTURES OF THE FEMUR

It is readily apparent from Figure 75 (p. 89) that fractures of the femur in the dog and cat occur more frequently than fractures of any other bone in the body. They constitute 25 per cent of all fractures seen in our clinic in the past 20 years.

Fractures of the Femoral Head and Neck

Definition

These fractures may be classified as *capital* (fractures of the head), *epiphyseal* (fracture through the epiphyseal line), or *neck* fractures. Depending on the location of the fracture line, they may be classified as *intracapsular* or *extracapsular.*

Incidence

Fractures in the region of the femur head and neck constitute 6.8 per cent of all fractures. The incidence is much higher in dogs under one year old than in old dogs, thereby increasing the incidence of epiphyseal separations over neck fractures.

Etiology

As a result of an indirect force transmitted through the femur, either the head or neck is fractured, provided that it is well seated in the acetabulum. If for some reason the head is not well seated, it may be forced out of its socket, resulting in a luxation.

Pathology

Blood circulation is an extremely important factor in intracapsular fractures. Although the vascular system for the hip joint in the dog has not been thoroughly investigated, enough work has been done so that we know there is some slight difference between this animal and the horse or man. Miller has described the gross arterial supply as follows:

"The obturator branch of the deep femoral artery branches to supply the neck of the femur and the caudal part of the hip joint capsule. The cranial femoral artery bifurcates at the neck of the femur and the ascending branch sends many twigs to the cranial part of the hip joint capsule."

It is doubtful that the blood vessels in the ligamentum teres supply any great amount of blood to the femur head. Notice how many times a dislocated femur with rupture of the ligamentum teres has been replaced without subsequent necrosis of the femur head. On the other hand, it is not uncommon in epiphyseal fractures in which the ligamentum teres remains intact to find the head still normal but the neck undergoing aseptic necrosis* (Fig. 83). This would indicate that at least some circulation is obtained through the ligament.

---

*The terms "aseptic necrosis" and "avascular necrosis" of bone have been used in veterinary literature to describe a condition which is actually a decalcification in the presence of hyperemia. Bone that is undergoing necrosis because of ischemia appears denser by comparison with the decalcified bone because there is retention of calcium. "Aseptic necrosis" or "avascular necrosis" should therefore not be applied to areas of bone showing rarefaction.

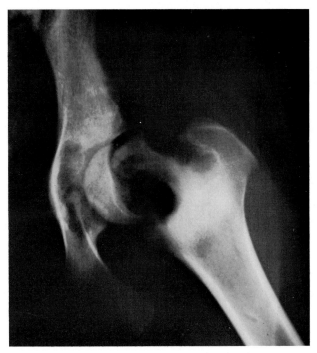

Figure 83. Epiphyseal separation of the femur head with subsequent necrosis of the neck. Note that the head is still intact, probably because it still receives some slight blood supply through the ligament.

There is much disagreement as to what actually takes place to bring about aseptic necrosis. It seems logical to assume that, inasmuch as necrosis is directly related to circulation, extensive damage to the capsule would cause neck necrosis and probably head necrosis if the ligamentum teres is also severed (Fig. 84). When circulation of the capsule is preserved, necrosis is not likely to occur. There is certainly some circulation through the cancellous bone in the area, but this can be effective only when the fractured ends are apposed. It has been thought by some that accurate reduction and fixation is the answer to proper healing of these fractures. It seems more logical to assume that those successfully treated by this approach still maintain good capsular circulation and that the failures are due to inadequate capsular circulation.

There is no doubt that some of the blood supply arrives through the periosteum, but since this is from one direction only, disruption of the periosteum curtails further blood supply to the proximal segment.

If the fracture is extracapsular, the circulation remains established on either side of the fracture line and there is much more likelihood of uncomplicated healing (Fig. 85).

A puzzling phenomenon frequently occurs in connection with aseptic necrosis of the neck. If the injury is several weeks old, necrosis may involve the trochanter major and even a small portion of the proximal shaft. Since this statement is based only on radiographic observations, it is quite possible that this is a decalcification rather than a necrosis. Nevertheless, it can

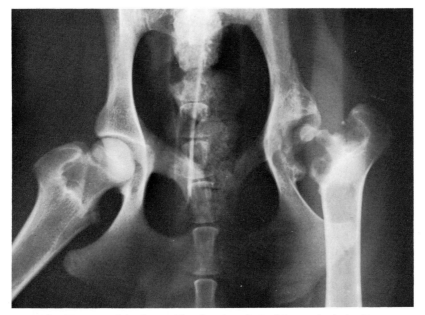

Figure 84.   Necrosis of the femoral head and neck. In this case both the ligamentum teres and the joint capsule were ruptured.

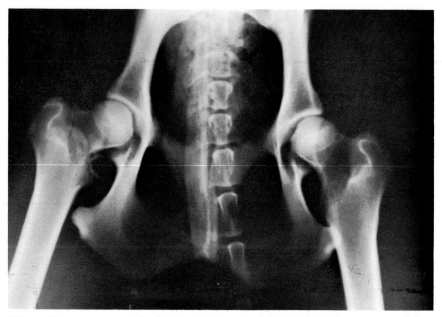

Figure 85. An extracapsular fracture of the neck of the femur. With proper immobilization this should heal.

readily be seen that these bone changes have a very direct bearing on the treatment and prognosis.

Signs

Older dogs with fractures of the femoral neck tend to show more pronounced signs than young dogs with capital or epiphyseal fractures. The limb is usually carried adducted and flexed at the stifle and tarsal joints. There is outward rotation of the thigh with the femur pointing downward. The trochanter major is elevated and surrounded by diffuse swelling. Severe pain can be elicited when the limb is manipulated, although there is usually a lack of resistance to such handling. Crepitation can be produced by extending and rotating the limb. Lack of resistance to abduction is a good differentiating sign when dislocation is suspected.

If the dog is anesthetized and placed on a table in dorsal recumbency, the leg length can be compared with that of its mate. If the legs are held in the perpendicular position, the injured one should be shorter. If they are held in horizontal position, both should be the same length. This is also true in the case of a dorso-lateral luxation and therefore this possibility should be kept in mind.

The femoral neck can be tested further by placing the dog on its side so that the femur can be maneuvered from this position. Digital pressure on the femur will often produce crepitus and a feeling of instability in the joint. Deep palpation with the thumb between the trochanter major and the tuber ischii will reveal that the femur does not pivot at the hip joint when abducted, adducted, rotated on its long axis, or flexed and extended.

Complications which can occur and which may confuse the typical signs are other fractures in the region of the trochanter major, the upper femoral shaft, or the acetabulum (Fig. 86).

Diagnosis

Before making the diagnosis it is important that a roentgenogram be made to substantiate the physical evidence and rule out or confirm any complicating factor. The patient should be anesthetized and placed on the x-ray table in dorsal recumbency. The hindlimbs should be extended in the horizontal plane and the feet should be elevated to the level of the hip. The limbs should be held so that the lateral edge of the patella is in the same vertical plane as the lateral edge of the femur. The cone should be centered over the injured hip. One good roentgenogram in this position should confirm the diagnosis. If there is doubt, a second exposure can be made, but usually the error in diagnosis is in fractures without gross displacement that are dismissed as sprains or bruises without benefit of a radiograph.

Prognosis

Without some surgical interference these fractures do not heal. Poor healing and necrosis are often encountered even when attempts are made to hold the segments in good apposition. The prognosis will depend to a large

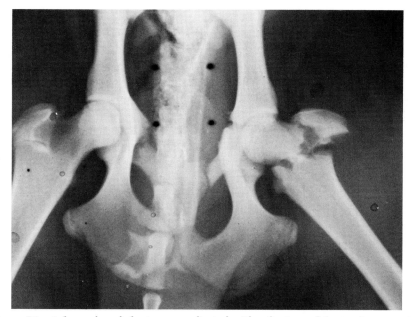

Figure 86. A femoral neck fracture complicated with a fracture of the trochanter major.

extent on the location of the fracture. Intracapsular fractures are less likely to heal than extracapsular. On the whole, the prognosis should be guarded.

Treatment

A good treatment for fractures of the femoral neck has long been sought, with the result that many methods have been proposed. As pointed out previously, the success of each treatment seeems to depend largely on the location of the fracture and the patency of the circulation to both segments. The accuracy of reduction may have some bearing on the results, since most of the bone at the fracture site is cancellous and therefore requires some direct contact. Schroeder, Ehmer, and others first recommended closed reduction in extracapsular fractures with the use of the Thomas splint or "figure eight" bandage as a means of fixation. Even with flexion of the thigh to compensate for rotation of the head (a common occurrence in these fractures), good apposition was largely a matter of good fortune.

Later, Schroeder described a method of fixation in which he employed two pins inserted at a slight angle through the femur, the neck, and into the head. This was further supported by a Thomas splint. Anderson et al. reported on the experimental use of pins in four dogs, but the results of this type of repair seem inconclusive in the light of clinical experience with this type of reduction.

Cawley et al., using pins in femoral neck fractures, found that fixation must be accomplished very early (less than a week after the fracture occurs), that apposition must be perfect, that pins must be small, and that even then some necrosis will occur. Their work was done primarily on intracapsular fractures.

Nilsson described the use of a screw for the repair of the fractured neck, but here again the problem of the intracapsular fracture was not solved. Furthermore, the holding power of the screw is slight in cancellous bone.

Brinker has described the use of a screw as being a successful method of femoral neck repair in several cases. He attributes his success to the fact that the fracture is reduced early and that apposition is as nearly perfect as possible. After the hip area is opened by the cranial approach, a tract *slightly smaller than the screw* is drilled through the center of the femoral neck so that it emerges just below the trochanter major. The screw point is flattened with a file. It is then inserted through the neck and into the head as far as possible without damaging the articular surface of the joint.

Tovee and Gendron, reporting on a series of 150 experimental dogs, found that after they had produced subcapital fractures of the femur, the head died in nine days. They also found that the fracture would heal and the head revascularize in from three to six months. Clinical healing of the fracture was complete in four weeks provided that there was perfect reduction and good fixation with a screw. Blood supply to the head and neck was evaluated by use of radioactive phosphorus. These authors are of the opinion that aseptic necrosis in fractures of the neck of the femur is due to inaccurate reduction, poor nailing, or premature weight bearing.

In 1944, reference was made to the use of a prosthetic femur head in a dog. Since that time Jenny has recorded the use of a "plastic femur head and neck fastened to the shaft with screws and a Sherman plate." The first extensive work done on femoral head prostheses in dogs was by Brown in 1953. Later Archibald and Ballantyne, Gay, and Gorman also investigated the use of hip prostheses, each using a different design.

Prostheses offer a method of treatment for intracapsular fractures of the femoral head and neck regardless of age so long as the acetabulum is normal and necrosis of the neck has not progressed to the point where it encroaches on the proximal shaft. The stem of the prosthesis will not hold if the bone is decalcified. It is expected that there will be growth of the skeleton in young animals, and therefore concern has been expressed over the installation of a prosthesis in these patients. We have found that although there is growth of bones of the hip joint after prosthetic repair, the acetabular cup remains the same size. This is probably due to the fixed size of the femur head and the lack of growth pressure which serves to enlarge the socket. In those cases in which the femur head was installed during the growing period we have found the results to be quite satisfactory. Gay, on the other hand, feels that a prosthesis should only be used in fractures of the femoral head or neck after other means of repair have failed and that a prosthesis is contraindicated in recently acquired fractures.

We have used the Brown type of prosthesis made from stainless steel type 316 by the Ludwig Products Company, Cortland, New York, or vitallium made by Austenal of New York City. Some of these prostheses have been in place as long as 15 years, with every clinical evidence of good function. We have not had experience with either the Gay or the Gorman types of prostheses. They require a more radical type of surgery.

The use of prostheses, however, as a means of repair for fractures of the femoral head and neck has never been widely accepted by veterinary orthopedists. More recently, a cementing substance known as methyl methacrylate has been used in conjunction with prostheses to prevent loosening (the most common cause of failure).

The use of intramedullary pins has met with some success, particularly in extracapsular fractures that were pinned early. It is well to perform an open reduction with the skin incision starting close to the dorsal midline, crossing the trochanter major, and ending near the middle of the thigh. The incision is continued as described for hip prosthesis (p. 79). The capsule usually does not need to be opened, since the fracture should be exposed by the time the capsule is reached. An intramedullary pin is then inserted through the lateral cortex of the femur just below the trochanter major at an angle which will bring the point into contact with the femur neck in a reduced position. The pin is then forced through the neck to the head, making sure that it does not penetrate the metaphysis. Another pin is then placed through the same structures, but at an angle to the first pin. After closure of the incision the two pins should be anchored to each other with a Kirschner bar.

Small diameter threaded wires (0.050 inches) have been used with success in smaller breeds of dogs and in cats. Two converging holes are first drilled with a smooth Kirschner wire through the distal neck and trochanter in a retrograde direction so that they will be properly centered at the fracture site. The threaded wires are then placed with a hand drill at slow speed. When the points reach the fracture site, a very accurate reduction is made. The threaded wires are screwed into the head by turning the hand drill slowly until they reach subchondral bone. The depth of penetration of the wire should be carefully ascertained before drilling so that the joint cartilage will not be broken.

It is important that the wires be set in the head in divergent directions to enhance their holding power.

They are cut close to the lateral cortex of the femur and allowed to remain in the bone unless otherwise indicated at a later time.

As a last resort, when other methods have failed and there is non-union, an excision arthroplasty may be performed. There are a number of choices open to the surgeon as to the avenue of approach to the hip joint. It may depend to some degree on the amount and type of surgery already performed on the hip and the recency of such surgery. The most common approach is the dorsal approach of Brown, but the cranial (anterior) approach is quite effective in dogs with smaller muscle masses over the hip joint. The ventral approach is used successfully by some surgeons, but the caudal (posterior) approach is seldom used.

The skin incision for the cranial approach (Fig. 87–1) begins at the cranioventral edge of the wing of the ilium and procedes in an arc over the trochanter major and two-thirds the length of the femur. This will expose the tensor fascia lata, gluteus medius, and biceps femoris muscles. The fascia lata is incised along the border of the biceps femoris and over the trochanter major. The gluteus medius and the tensor fascia are bluntly separated. This will lead to exposure of the rectus femoris. By separating the vastus lateralis and the rectus femoris, the joint capsule will be uncovered. However, this separation should be done with caution in order to avoid injury to the lateral circumflex artery and vein or the cranial branch of the femoral artery and vein.

Probably the most common approach to the hip is the dorsal approach of Brown (Fig. 87–2). The skin incision begins near the dorsal midline and extends over the trochanter major to about midthigh. Transection of the fascia lata will expose the gluteal muscles and the vastus lateralis. One at a time, the gluteals are bluntly separated and the tendon of insertion transected about 1 cm. from the trochanter. This provides enough stump for rejoining when the incision is closed. When the gluteals are reflected, the joint capsule will be exposed. Since the sciatic nerve passes just caudal to the joint and trochanter major, it is necessary to be exceedingly careful not to injure it.

The dorsal approach of Gorman (Fig. 87–3) requires a skin incision in the craniocaudal direction. It begins midway between the trochanter major and the wing of the ilium and passes caudoventrally in an arc below the

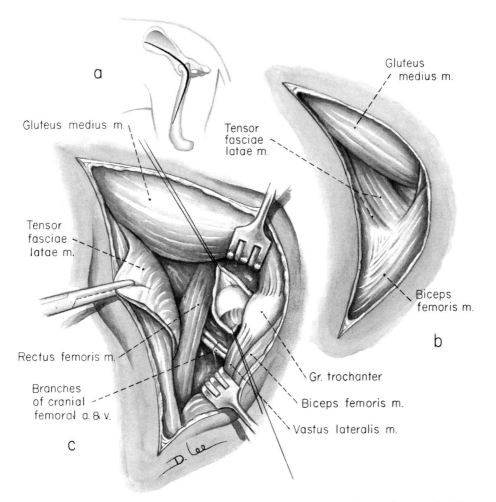

Gluteus medius m.

a

Gluteus medius m.

Tensor fasciae latae m.

Tensor fasciae latae m.

Biceps femoris m.

b

Rectus femoris m.

Branches of cranial femoral a. & v.

Gr. trochanter

Biceps femoris m.

Vastus lateralis m.

c

D. Lee

Figure 87–1. Cranial approach to the hip joint. (By permission of *Animal Hospital* and Dr. R. B. Hohn.) a, Outline of skin incision. b, Superficial field. c, Deep field.

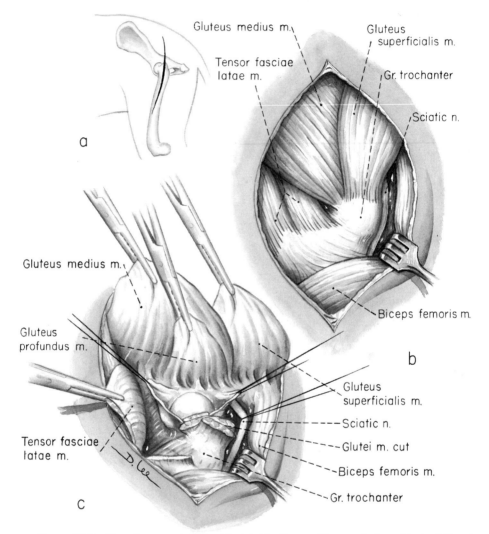

Figure 87-2. Dorsal approach to the hip joint by Brown. (By permission of *Animal Hospital* and Dr. R. B. Hohn.) a, Outline of skin incision. b, Superficial field. c, Deep field.

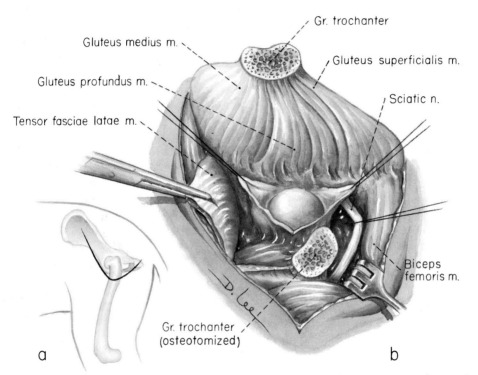

Gr. trochanter

Gluteus medius m.

Gluteus superficialis m.

Gluteus profundus m.

Sciatic n.

Tensor fasciae latae m.

Biceps femoris m.

Gr. trochanter (osteotomized)

a

b

Figure 87-3. Dorsal approach to the hip joint by Gorman. (By permission of *Animal Hospital* and Dr. R. B. Hohn.) a, Outline of skin incision. b, Deep field.

trochanter major to the ischial tuberosity. The fascia is transected and re-flected to expose the trochanter. The trochanter is separated from the femur with an osteotome and the gluteal muscles reflected dorsally. This exposes the joint capsule and affords rather free access to the joint. On closure the trochanter must be held in place by pins, a screw, or wires.

The caudal approach (Fig. 87–4) requires an incision which begins on the dorsal midline at a point that is caudomedial to the trochanter. It should pass caudal to the trochanter and end at midthigh over the femur. The cranial edge of the biceps femoris is separated and reflected caudally. In-ward rotation of the limb, after reflecting the superficial gluteal, brings the muscle mass that inserts on the trochanteric fossa into position for transec-tion. These muscles are the external and internal obturators and the gemelli. The tendons of insertion are divided so that a reasonable stump is left for reattachment. The quadratus femoris attaches immediately distal to the fossa and this too must be detached. Care should be taken not to disturb the artery which supplies this area. It arises at the obturator branch of the deep femoral artery and supplies the structures of the trochanteric fossa and the caudal joint capsule as well as the neck of the femur. Care must also be exercised in moving the sciatic nerve out of the field. While this approach is slightly more difficult, it gives a satisfactory exposure of the hip joint.

The patient must be placed in dorsal recumbency for the ventral or medial approach to the hip joint (Fig. 87–5). The body is rotated toward the injured side so that the limb will lie flat on the table. The skin incision begins toward the body midline and continues over the medial side of the hip joint to the middle of the femur. The femoral artery and vein lie fairly close to the surface at the distal end of the incision. The pectineus muscle is carefully separated and divided near its origin on the pubis. This exposes the deep femoral artery and vein which lie on the surface of the iliopsoas muscle. By blunt dissection, the iliopsoas and adduction muscles are sepa-rated and reflected to expose the joint capsule. Severe damage and hemor-rhage will result if the femoral vessels are not retracted from the area with great care.

Exposure of the hip joint by the dorsal approach (Brown) gives an adequate exposure of the femur head and neck but care must be taken not to injure the sciatic nerve. It lies just caudad to the acetabulum and is quite vulnerable. Injury to this nerve can be disastrous.

If the fracture is extracapsular, it is sometimes easier to trim and smooth the stump with rongeurs before proceding with the removal of the proximal segment. This is done by rotating the femur outward until the fractured neck is accessible. On the other hand, if the fracture is intracapsular, it may require removal of the proximal segment first.

Since a variety of conditions may exist in the proximal segment, it may be necessary to separate it from the capsule or the ligamentum teres or it may be free except for a few fibrous attachments. Once it is removed, the capsule and ligament are trimmed as close to the acetabulum as possible before the closure begins.

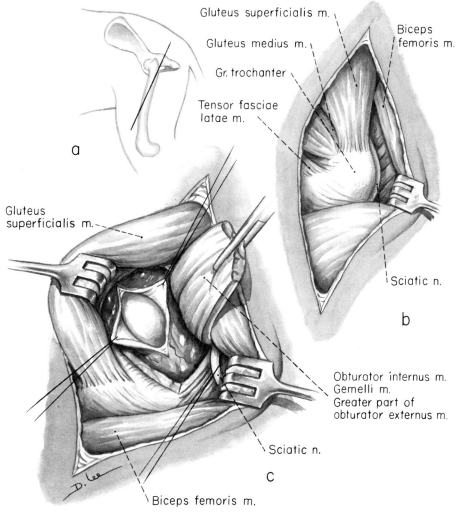

Figure 87-4. Caudal approach to the hip joint. (By permission of *Animal Hospital* and Dr. R. B. Hohn.) a, Outline of skin incision. b, Superficial field. c, Deep field.

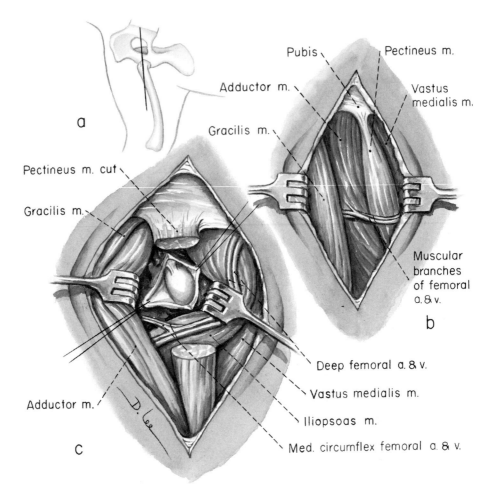

Figure 87-5. Ventral or medial approach to the hip joint. (By permission of *Animal Hospital* and Dr. R. B. Hohn.) a, Outline of skin incision. b, Superficial field. c, Deep field.

In the case of capital fractures, the neck must be transected lateral to the capsule. This may be done with a Gigli saw or with a simple bone saw after the capsule has been excised and the femur rotated outward to fully expose the head. The line of excision should be close to the shaft of the femur so that the stump will be smooth (Fig. 88). Bleeding of the medullary stump can usually be controlled with bone wax or Gelfoam (Upjohn).

Closure following the dorsal (Brown) approach requires more care than the cranial (anterior) approach because of the transected gluteal muscles. These muscles should be securely anchored to the trochanter major with a few well-placed stitches. Excessive suturing may weaken the closure. Mattress stitches of small gauge wire work well. These may pass through previously drilled holes in the bone or they may be anchored in the fibrous muscle attachment.

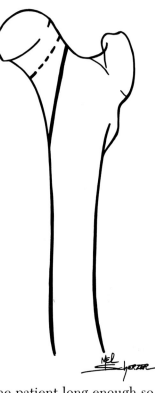

Figure 88. Line of excision arthroplasty of the femoral head. Dotted line indicates improper excision.

Usually weight bearing will be curtailed by the patient long enough so that immobilization of the leg is not necessary. Freedom from external bandages and splints has the advantage of full circulation to the leg as well as the elimination of the danger of torsion due to unwieldy splintage.

Fractures of the Proximal Segment

Definition

These are fractures of the femur occurring in the upper third of the shaft, usually in the region of the lesser trochanter. In some cases fractures occur through the trochanter major and in others there is an epiphyseal separation.

Incidence

While fractures of the femoral shaft comprise over one-fifth of the total fractures occurring in the dog and cat, fractures of the proximal segment constitute the smallest proportion of shaft fractures (see Fig. 75).

Etiology

Fractures in this area usually occur as a result of direct violence, the most common, of course, being collision with moving vehicles.

Pathology

Comminuted fractures are common, but compound fractures are seldom seen in the proximal segment probably because the upper segment is short and the musculature is heavy. Trauma to the muscles is usually extensive, although hemorrhage is less profuse than in lower shaft fractures. The upper segment is rotated due to muscle spasm. Overriding is variable.

Signs

The signs may be similar in many respects to luxation of the coxofemoral joint or fracture of the neck. The leg hangs limp with the appearance of dangling. There is an incoordinated swinging of the member when the animal moves. The leg is shortened in the standing position. The upper fragment is flexed, abducted and rotated due to the pull of the gluteal muscles. The lower segment is displaced upward and forward. Pain is not usually an outstanding sign, and the ease of manipulation of the leg depends on the degree of displacement of the distal segment and length of time the condition has existed. For a short time after the fracture has occurred the distal segment is movable, but after muscular contraction begins, movement becomes more difficult.

Diagnosis

The final diagnosis should be made by roentgenogram, the signs being used in making a provisional diagnosis.

Prognosis

Prognosis is good in uncomplicated cases but should be guarded if there are also fractures of the neck, trochanter major, or pelvis.

Treatment

Fractures of the trochanter major may be repaired by drilling and wiring with a No. 30 monofilament wire. Usually two well-placed sutures will fix it in position.

When the proximal shaft is fractured, fixation can be accomplished with the Kuentscher nail following open reduction (Fig. 89). Most often the proximal segment is too short for half pin splintage, although in certain instances a bicycle spoke or Kirschner wire can be drilled through the trochanter major and then bent to fit in a Stader pin bar. The wire is best drilled from the medial side of the trochanter through the lateral cortex in a ventral direction so that a good purchase of the segment is obtained. A single half pin can be inserted alongside the pin bar and taped to it to control long axis rotation.

If the fracture does not involve the femoral neck, it may be possible to insert two Kirschner half pins to form the upper assembly by inserting one pin in the trochanter at a sharp downward angle and one through the upper shaft and into the neck at a slight upward angle.

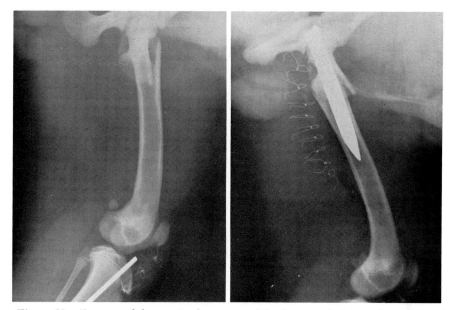

Figure 89. Fracture of the proximal segment of the femur with fixation by a Kuentscher nail.

On occasion when there has been both a neck fracture and a proximal shaft fracture, the author has repaired the shaft fracture by inserting an autogenous rib through a previously prepared hole in the trochanteric fossa and driving it into position as an intramedullary pin. Following this open reduction procedure the neck fracture is repaired by a Brown prosthesis. It is quite possible that the same repair could be accomplished with the Gorman prosthesis.

Fractures of the Middle Segment

Definition

Mid-shaft fractures of the femur are arbitrarily classified as those fractures occurring in the middle third of the femur.

Incidence

Seen in dogs and cats of all ages, fractures in this location are the most common and probably account for half the femur fractures that occur.

Etiology

Direct violence is the cause, in spite of the fact that this part of this particular bone is afforded the best protection of any bone in the body.

Pathology

Extensive tissue damage and hemorrhage is prevalent, resulting in swelling at the fracture site and edema of the distal parts of the leg. Usually these fractures are transverse, oblique, or comminuted. Only occasionally are they compound. There is gross displacement and overriding which tends to aggravate the soft tissue, thereby stimulating excessive granulation in the area. In some cases fascia or muscle may be interposed between the fractured ends.

Signs

Swelling is a frequent sign, along with pain and crepitus. The dog lies on the injured member, a common sign in most fractures. The proximal segment of the femur is in semiflexion, abducted, and slightly rotated. The distal segment is retracted toward the thigh with a caudal displacement.

Diagnosis

A lateral roentgenogram should be taken in order to confirm the diagnosis. Too often the exposure is made with the patient in a dorsal position. This leaves much to be desired in the resulting roentgenogram, since it is difficult to extend the injured leg fully. Foreshortening in the roentgenogram is a consequence. If pelvic complications are suspected, two exposures should be made, one in the ventro-dorsal position for the pelvis and one in the lateral position for the leg.

Prognosis

A good prognosis can usually be given because this area of the femur usually heals well. Complications in the middle segment are usually man-made and can be avoided by using correct methods coupled with aseptic surgery.

Treatment

Correction and fixation of midshaft fractures can be accomplished in a number of ways, depending on the type of fracture and the size of the patient. Seldom is it possible, however, to reduce and fix them by coaptation. In transverse fractures an intramedullary pin of the Kirschner variety serves very well. This type of fracture does not override after reduction and seldom gives cause for concern about long axis rotation because the fractured ends impact readily (Fig. 90).

Although it is quite possible to repair this type of fracture by closed reduction and the insertion of a single pointed pin through the trochanteric fossa and thence along the medullary canal to the condyles, it is much simpler to do an open reduction and to insert the pin retrograde. After the skin is incised directly over the femur and for approximately its entire

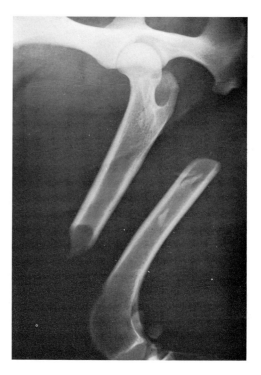

Figure 90. A midshaft fracture of the femur.

length, the fascia lata is divided so that the biceps femoris can be reflected caudally and the vastus lateralis cranially to expose the fracture site (Fig. 91). The pin is started in the medullary canal at the distal end of the proximal fragment and emerges at the trochanteric fossa. After the skin is incised at this point, the pin is retracted until the blunt end is flush with the fracture. After reduction has been accomplished, the blunt end of the pin is thrust into the distal medullary canal until it contacts the condyles. It is then withdrawn slightly and cut off, whereupon it is driven into place with a punch. Both ends of the pin being blunt, there is very little likelihood of migration. When healing is complete, the pin is removed by incising the skin over the trochanteric fossa and extracting it with sterile pliers (Fig. 92).

When the fracture line is more than 45° off the transverse, the method of treatment must be changed to meet the needs of an oblique fracture unless the line is jagged enough to restrain rotational movement when the two segments are impinged. Overriding is a major problem in oblique fractures. This can be overcome by using the Kuentscher nail or half pin splintage.

The principal landmarks for half pinning the femur are the trochanter major and the patella. Having located these two parts, orientation for all other areas of the femur becomes simple. The No. 1 pin is inserted just distal to the crest of the trochanter and the No. 2 pin in the shaft. A point opposite the middle of the patella and on the longitudinal midline of the femur is the site of insertion of the No. 4 pin, and the No. 3 pin is inserted just proximal to it. General rules concerning the use of half pin splintage will be found in

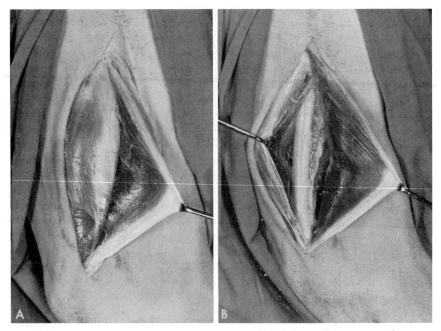

Figure 91. Incision site for open reduction of mid-shaft femur fractures. A, Skin incision from the trochanter major to the stifle. The fascia lata is incised along the cranial border of the biceps femoris and this muscle is reflected caudally. B, When the vastus lateralis is reflected the femur shaft is exposed.

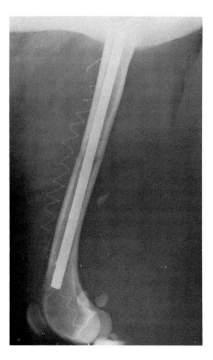

Figure 92. Open reduction of fracture shown in Figure 90 with intramedullary fixation. Note that a single pointed pin was used retrograde.

the chapter on Methods and Materials. In dogs under 40 pounds, as well as in cats, the Thomas splint with skeletal traction may be employed (Figs. 93 and 94).

The landmark for inserting the full pin used with the Thomas splint is found by locating the patella. The approximate location for the pin is a point on the lateral condyle where a line through the center of the patella intersects the midline of the femoral shaft. If there is considerable caudal displacement of the distal segment, it may be necessary to insert the pin just cranial to this point in order to bring about the proper rotation of the distal segment (Fig. 95).

After insertion, the pin is bent at right angles on both the medial and lateral aspects of the leg and the ends are put through a spreader and clenched. The spreader can be made from a piece of aluminum rod about 3 inches long with holes bored near each extremity to accommodate the pin ends. Traction can then be applied by heavy rubber bands running from the spreader to the extension bar of the splint. Another way to obtain traction is through the use of No. 19 soft steel bundle wire which can be tightened by twisting (Fig. 96).

The splint should be fashioned (Fig. 97) so that the gastrocnemius

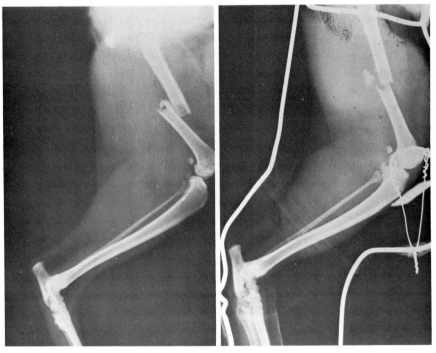

Fig. 93   Fig. 94

Figure 93. Midshaft fracture of the femur in a cat.

Figure 94. Repair of the fracture shown in Figure 93. The splint is fashioned from a coat hanger. A bicycle spoke has been drilled through the femoral condyles and traction applied with No. 19 soft steel bundle wire. Note the spreader which keeps the traction wires from pressing on the stifle.

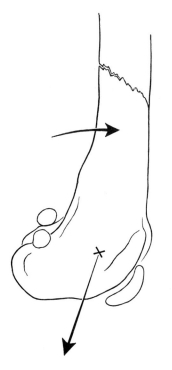

Figure 95. Diagram showing rotation of distal femoral segment into place following skeletal traction with a full pin.

muscle is relaxed, thereby releasing the distal femoral segment so that it will rotate into place. This is accomplished by flexing the stifle and moderately extending the hock.

Extensive comminution is best handled with the half pin splint. Open reduction may be employed and large bone fragments replaced after reduction and fixation of the two principal segments. Bone should not be removed from the fracture site unless contaminated. In some cases, if the periosteum has been stripped from a fragment, it may be chopped into small pieces with bone cutters and used to seed the fracture site. Comminuted fractures usually heal more rapidly than transverse fractures because of the more extensive bone surface exposed. The callus is larger and the bone reaction greater during the healing process.

In recent years, compression plating has become quite popular as a method of repairing femoral shaft fractures. A description of this method will be found on page 68. Considerable special equipment as well as special training is required to use this method, especially in dogs. Its use in humans and in horses has met with considerable success, possibly because of the comparatively thick cortex of the bones. In the dog the cortex is relatively thin. Some workers have claimed a high degree of success with this method in dogs, but others have found that it works best in cases of non-union in which there is a large callus and thickening of the cortex. In fact, some maintain that the method should not be used in fresh fractures. Great care

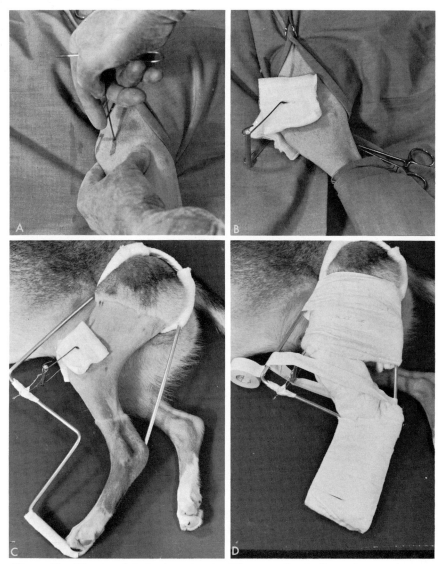

Figure 96. The use of skeletal traction in a Thomas splint for femur fractures by means of a bicycle spoke. A, Insertion of the pin. Note the landmark laid out on the skin. The semicircle at the edge of the stifle represents the patella. The horizontal line indicates a plane through the center of the patella. The vertical line runs parallel to the central axis of the femur. B, The pin has been inserted, bent at right angles, and the spreader has been attached. C, How traction is applied with the use of No. 19 soft steel bundle wire. D, Applying the padding and tape. This should be carefully applied on the medial side of the thigh so that no skin is left uncovered ventral to the ring of the splint.

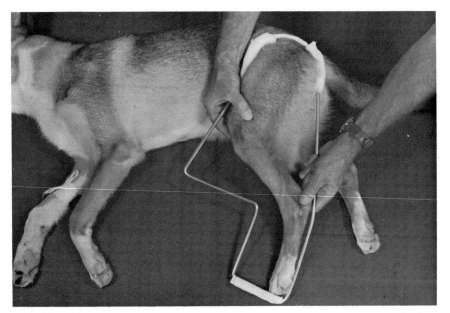

Figure 97.   The Thomas splint applied to the hindleg showing the position of the leg so that the gastrocnemius is relaxed.

must be taken to place the proper amount of torque on the screws, since those that are not tightened enough will back out and those that are set with too much pressure will strip the cortex.

Compression plating produces a very precise reduction of the fracture and minimizes callus formation.

Fractures of the Distal Segment

Definition

These fractures may be supracondylar, intracondylar, or epiphyseal (Fig. 98). The former two conditons occur mostly in mature dogs and the latter is seen in young animals. Infrequently there may be a single condyle split from the femur, and sometimes T fractures are seen, but these are not nearly as common in the femur as in the humerus. Most of the supracondylar fractures are transverse, although occasionally one may be oblique.

Incidence

Fractures involving the distal end of the femur constitute about one-quarter of all fractures seen in the femur. They occur in dogs of all ages but seem to be a little more prevalent in young dogs in which the fracture is in the form of an epiphyseal separation.

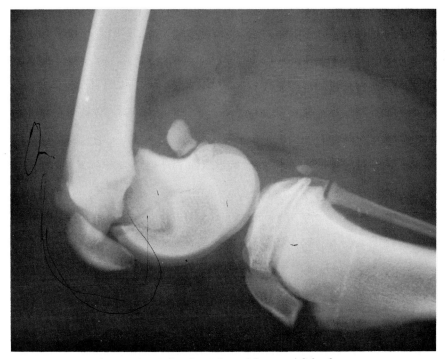

Figure 98. A distal epiphyseal fracture of the femur.

Etiology

Fractures of the distal segment are caused by both direct and indirect force. Direct violence brought about by moving vehicles is usually the cause, although in farm dogs this injury may be the result of a kick from a horse or cow. Falling from high places and jumping are usually the forms of indirect violence involved.

Pathology

Soft tissue trauma is usually severe, with associated joint damage in many cases. Compound fractures are not unusual, the distal end of the proximal segment piercing the skin on the medial or dorsal aspect of the stifle in most cases. Grossly, these fractures do not look as severe as midshaft fractures, but the short distal segment and the possibility of joint involvement may cause serious pathologic changes. In cases of long standing the callus overgrows the joint, causing stiffness, and in compound fractures the infection may spread to the joint, thereby setting up arthritic changes.

Signs

The limb is not in a fixed position but there is a definite change in the contour of the stifle. There is a double convexity, the second convexity being at the distal end of the upper segment. When the patient moves, the limb is carried with the metatarsus parallel to the thigh. Because of a spasm of the gastrocnemius, the tarsus is overextended. Swelling is moderate in the immediate area of the fracture. Crepitus is usually difficult to obtain because of the separation of the fragments, the upper fragment being slightly flexed, abducted and rotated inward while the lower fragment is displaced backward and flexed on the stifle joint. This is due to tension from the gastrocnemius. Frequently there is some lateral displacement of the distal segment. Digital pressure over the area of the fracture causes great pain but the surrounding areas seem much less sensitive.

Diagnosis

Any abnormal mobility in the region of the stifle should lead one to suspect a supracondylar fracture in an old dog and an epiphyseal separation in a young dog. The contour of the joint and localized pain are diagnostic. Torn ligaments do not usually give such well-defined signs. A roentgenogram must be made in these cases to evaluate the damage accurately.

Prognosis

If the injury is more than one week old, the prognosis is poor to guarded. Granulation is well under way and in all probability involves the joint, particularly in the region of the patella. This usually means ankylosis of the joint, or at least limited movement. In cases that are repaired early the prognosis is quite good and the limb usually is restored to normal function, provided that the fracture is properly reduced.

Treatment

Epiphyseal fractures may be repaired by inserting a Kirschner-type intramedullary pin, by applying a Thomas splint using skeletal traction in dogs under 40 pounds, or by bridging the stifle with a half pin assembly (Kirschner). Use of the intramedullary pin as described by Armistead and Lumb is the most satisfactory method.

The pin is inserted by open reduction (Fig. 99). A skin incision is made on the cranio-medial side of the stifle and usually traverses the groove made by the separation of the two segments. The fascial insertions are cut longitudinally and the two bellies of the sartorius muscle are separated. The rectus femoris and the vastus medialis are also separated in a like manner, and the incision is carried downward beyond the head of the tibia. By reflecting the rectus laterally, the joint will be exposed, and then by flexing the stifle the condyles will be brought into position for the first stage of the operation.

A single-pointed intramedullary pin is started in the intercondylar space at the point where the caudal cruciate ligament attaches. This is easily located as a small, flesh-colored, crescent-shaped area surrounded by the whitish appearance of bone and cartilage. After the pin has penetrated the distal segment, it should be gently lifted until the point of the pin is

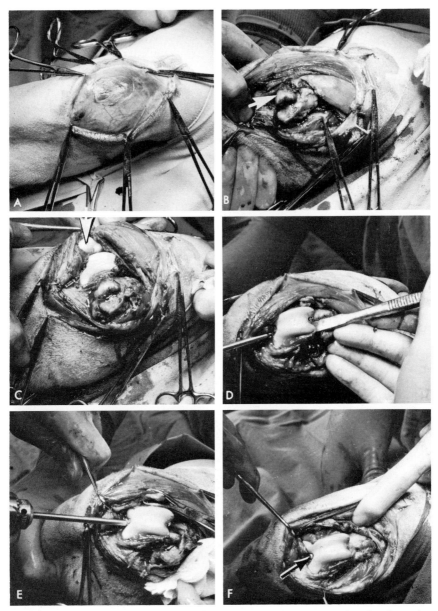

Figure 99. The method of Armistead and Lumb for the repair of a distal epiphyseal fracture of the femur. A, The skin incision. B, Exposure of the distal end of the proximal segment. C, The distal segment. Note the patella directly above the condyles. D, The intramedullary pin is inserted in the distal segment, which is being elevated to the level of the proximal segment. E, The pin being driven into the proximal segment with the distal segment over-reduced. F, Fixation completed. Note the end of the pin between the condyles.

centered in the medullary canal of the proximal segment. This should be done cautiously since the distal fragment is soft and fragile. Sometimes it is necessary to insert a flat chisel between the two segments and, using the distal end of the proximal segment as a fulcrum, to lift the distal segment by prying with the chisel and lifting with the intramedullary pin. Never pry with the intramedullary pin, as this is quite likely to split the condyles.

The pin is drilled through the proximal segment until it emerges through the skin at the trochanteric fossa. The chuck is then changed to the pointed end of the pin, and with a careful rotary motion the pin is withdrawn until the blunt end is flush with the intracondylar fossa.

It will be quite evident that the fracture has been overreduced, but this is as it should be. The overreduction will allow callus to form away from the patella and stifle joint, thereby avoiding ankylosis (Fig. 100). Supracondylar fractures should be either very accurately reduced (Fig. 101) or overreduced, never underreduced. In epiphyseal fractures overreduction is safer and easier.

Closure is carried out starting with the joint capsule, then the fascial layers, and finally the skin. The pin is cut so that it can be covered with skin,

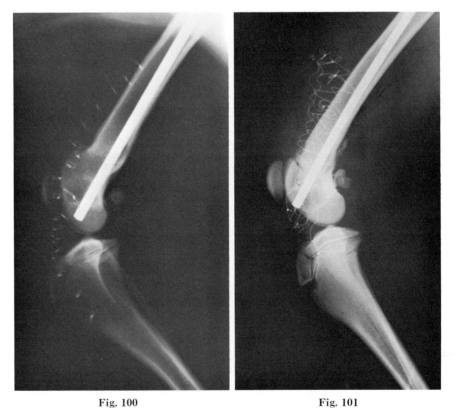

Fig. 100   Fig. 101

Figure 100.   An overreduced bone after healing. Note that the patella is free.
Figure 101.   An accurately reduced epiphyseal fracture.

and a gauze pad held in place with liquid adhesive is used to cover the incisions. Ordinarily no supporting splintage is used unless there are complicating injuries which might require extra support.

If the Thomas splint is used for epiphyseal fractures, some form of skeletal traction must be applied. Since epiphyseal fractures occur in young dogs, it must be borne in mind that the distal segment is soft and therefore likely to tear when force is applied to the full pin or tongs. This type of splintage may be used in some of the small breeds where rigorous traction is not required or when the patient is approaching maturity. Detailed instructions for application will be found under the treatment for supracondylar fractures.

Brinker has described a method of fixation whereby the stifle joint is bridged with a Kirschner splint. This method depends on the accurate reduction and impaction of segments to immobilize the fracture, since only the tibia and the proximal segment are immobilized by the splint, thereby leaving the distal segment free of splint control. If this method is used, two extension bars should be applied to the splint so that both pin assemblies are well anchored (Fig. 102).

Supracondylar fractures in older dogs are usually characterized by a larger distal segment than is seen in the epiphyseal fracture. This allows more latitude in the choice of splintage. If the distal segment is long enough a half pin splint may be applied. If the segment is short the Thomas splint with skeletal traction can be used. In either case an intramedullary pin can

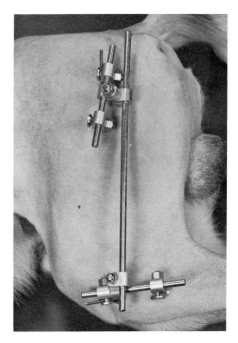

Figure 102. Bridging the stifle joint with a Kirschner splint. A method of fixation for distal epiphyseal fractures.

be used so long as there is a reasonable amount of bone to engage the distal end of the pin.

Application of the half pin splint in supracondylar fractures may require that the pins in the distal assembly be placed closer together because of the short bone segment. The distance between pins can be reduced until their points converge just as they emerge from the medial cortex. Pins can be inserted so that they cross each other, but the correct angle of insertion should be observed if they are to maintain their holding power. A complete description of the application of half pin splintage to the femur will be found under Fractures of the Middle Segment.

When the patient is under 40 pounds in body weight, a simple and effective fixation may be accomplished by using a Thomas splint, made as described in the chapter on Methods and Materials, and applying skeletal traction to the distal segment. To overcome the rotation caused by the gastrocnemius, the bicycle spoke or pin should be inserted slightly cranial to the center of the condyle and about opposite the upper border of the patella. When traction is applied, there will be sufficient counterrotation to bring about alignment of the segment. In recent fractures complete reduction can be obtained when the splint is applied. Older cases may require heavy rubber bands in order to maintain traction for long periods of time until overriding has been eliminated. Control of the upper segment is brought about by wrapping the upper leg with padding and taping it to the caudal bar of the splint.

Supracondylar fractures repaired with intramedullary pins are handled best by open reduction. Using a double-pointed pin or a single-pointed pin, drilling is begun at the open end of the proximal segment. The pin is thrust through the skin over the trochanteric fossa after traversing the medullary canal. The chuck is then changed to the upper end of the pin so that the distal end can be "backed off" flush with the fractured end of the bone. After the fracture is reduced, the pin is drilled into the distal segment until it is in contact with the cortex beneath the patellar surface of the femur. A blunt end will seat just as well as a pointed end and probably has a more stabilizing influence.

In all supracondylar fractures of the femur in which the fracture line is in close proximity to the patella, it is especially important to avoid under-reduction because callus formation is likely to involve the patella, thereby causing a stiff joint.

Fractures of a single condyle are frequently repaired by the use of screws. These screws must be long enough to penetrate both cortices and should be inserted according to the rules laid down under Methods and Materials.

The Rush pin has been recommended for the repair of condylar fractures of the femur, but it is doubtful that this method will produce the desired result in the hands of the average surgeon. This method seems better adapted to the condyles of the humerus and is particularly more suitable in the smaller breeds.

There are two main features in the treatment of distal fractures of the femur which must be constantly kept in mind during the selection of splintage for fixation. The first is to use a method which will absolutely immobilize the distal segment. The second is to make certain that callus formation will not involve the patella and the stifle joint.

FRACTURE OF THE PATELLA

Although fracture of the patella occurs with relative frequency in humans, it is rather rare in dogs and cats. In every one thousand fractures, one would be likely to encounter this fracture about once. The usual cause is direct force from some sharp or semi-sharp object. Unless the patella is weakened by disease or congenitally malformed, it does not fracture by indirect force. The cause being an outside force, the nature of the fracture is not predictable, although the patella is usually separated into a proximal and a distal segment.

Most frequently the injury is compound, with edema and hemorrhage around the stifle but with very little bleeding from the bone fragments. The area is moderately painful and the leg is held in complete flexion, thereby causing a gross distraction of the segments. There is always grave danger of infection with severe arthritic changes.

Diagnosis is usually obvious, but a lateral roentgenogram is extremely helpful as confirming evidence.

The prognosis should be guarded because of the nature of the wound and its proximity to the joint.

Wiring of the segments seems to give satisfactory results and should be done whenever possible. In most cases two strands of wire will be required in order to immobilize properly. Using a fine drill or a very small intramedullary pin, drill two holes from the fracture site to the cranial surface in each segment. An attempt should be made to align the starting points so that the two segments will approximate properly when the wire is drawn taut. Using a single strand of fairly heavy monofilament stainless steel wire and starting on the cranial side of one segment, thread one end through each hole. Then thread the ends through the matching holes in the other segment, starting at the fracture site. When the wire is twisted tight, there will be two strands holding the segments so that the wire has no contact with the joint surface (Fig. 103). The twisted end is then cut off and flattened to the surface of the patella so that it will not cause undue irritation. Support in the form of extension in a Thomas splint should be given this type of fracture until healing seems reasonably advanced.

Since this is usually a compound fracture, antibiotics are recommended during the aftercare. Some decalcification may be noticed during the healing process. This is due to pressure and will gradually correct as healing proceeds.

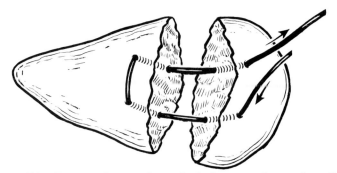

Figure 103.   Diagram showing the method of wiring a fractured patella.

FRACTURES OF THE TIBIA AND FIBULA

Although fractures may occur in one of these bones without necessarily involving the other, it seems advisable to consider the two together. The fibula may fracture without damage to the tibia but seldom is the reverse true. Most tibial fractures involve the fibula. According to Miller, the fibula is probably undergoing phylogenetic reduction and its importance as a separate bony structure is diminishing. We shall discuss fractures of the tibia, in the main, supplementing information about the fibula where it seems pertinent.

Considered together, fractures in these bones represent 10.2 per cent of the total fractures seen at our clinic.

Fractures of the Proximal Segment

Definition

Fractures occurring in the proximal segment of the tibia usually take the form of epiphyseal separations (Fig. 104), separation of the tibial tuberosity (Fig. 105), or transverse diaphyseal fractures.

Etiology

Separation of the tibial tuberosity and, occasionally, separation of the proximal epiphysis are brought about by indirect force such as might be applied if the animal is dropped so that it alights on one hind foot. The quadriceps can exert great force through the patellar ligament. Contraction of this group of muscles can cause avulsion of the tibial tuberosity in young dogs. Other fractures of the proximal segment are usually caused by direct force.

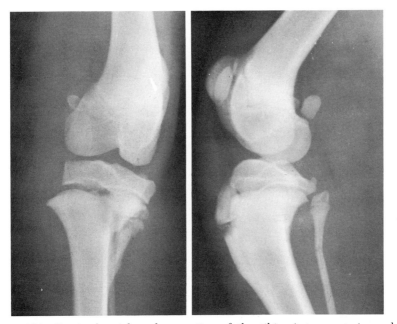

Figure 104. Proximal epiphyseal separation of the tibia. Antero-posterior and lateral views.

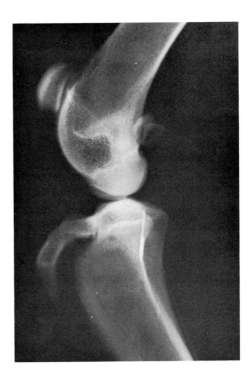

Figure 105. Separation of the tibial tuberosity.

Pathology

These fractures are simple, seldom compound, and produce little swelling. Hemorrhage is often very moderate, although this area of the bone and adjacent tissues are more vascular than the distal areas. Displacement of the fractured ends is ordinarily not great, although there is always distraction when the tibial tuberosity is fractured.

Signs

The leg is carried in flexion in both the moving and standing positions. In the case of fracture of the fibula, the dog carries the leg when moving but will extend it in the standing position. Pain is a constant sign whenever the leg is manipulated. The toes are rotated inward and there is a slight adduction of the lower limb. Fractures in this part of the tibia, because of slight displacement, are not likely to show gross distortion of the leg, and some may even be difficult to discern on palpation.

Diagnosis

A roentgenogram is essential for diagnosis both from the standpoint of the original fracture and to detect any complicating factors which might be present.

Prognosis

Aside from the fact that tibial fractures heal slowly, the prognosis can usually be considered good.

Treatment

It is quite possible that either an epiphyseal separation or a high transverse fracture will respond to simple coaptation. A little experimenting by slightly flexing the limb to see if the segments will appose is worthwhile. If the fracture does reduce with some manipulating, coaptation can be applied with the leg held in slight flexion. The cast should include the stifle joint and all parts distal to it. For most dogs, except very large ones, something lighter than plaster of Paris should be used. Aire-Cast may be applied directly to the leg or the leg may be padded with cotton pads and taped, using tongue depressors or basswood for splintage. The angulation of the leg will prevent the cast from slipping, so that excessive pressure is not required to hold it in place. Since there is some shrinkage with Aire-Cast, care must be exercised that is not applied too tightly. Whatever the cast material used, the toes should be padded with cotton and even pressure should be applied to the limb so that pressure spots can be avoided.

A very firm fixation can be achieved by inserting a Kirschner-type intramedullary pin. The medullary canal of the tibia is not straight, so that when the pin is inserted it will contact the cortex at two places as it traverses the distal segment. The pin should therefore be slightly flexible and not too heavy.

Fixation can be accomplished under closed reduction. The stifle is flexed and a small stab incision made in the skin just medial to the patellar ligament. The pin is inserted close to the ligament, slightly medial and anterior to the medial meniscus. It is drilled along the medullary canal until cortical bone is contacted at the distal end of the tibia. It is then withdrawn about one-quarter of an inch, cut level with the skin, and buried by driving it into place with a punch. These fractures are usually uneven enough so that long axis rotation is controlled. If there is rotation, characterized by abduction of the hock and inward rotation of the foot, some external splintage is indicated. This may take the form of coaptation or a Thomas splint.

Separation of the tibial tuberosity may be handled by placing the leg in a Thomas splint so that it is extended, thereby taking much of the tension off the patellar ligament. In addition to the external support, an open reduction may be performed and the fracture segment screwed into place.

Fractures of the Middle Segment

Definition

These fractures occur in the middle third of the diaphysis and are usually oblique, spiral, or comminuted. A few will be transverse. It is not at all uncommon to encounter compound fractures in this region. Middle segment fractures are the commonest tibial fractures and almost always involve the fibula.

Etiology

These fractures are the result of a direct force such as a kick, a blow, or, not infrequently, a bullet.

Pathology

So far as tissue damage is concerned, some of the most severe fractures of the body occur in the middle of the tibia. Many are comminuted and compound with grossly lacerated tissues surrounding the bone. They are attended by considerable edema and swelling but relatively little hemorrhage. Circulation is usually poor and healing is slow.

Signs

The patient presents a rather helpless-looking leg with the stifle flexed and those parts distal to the fracture partially extended, distorted, sometimes swinging, and seldom rigid. Angulation and rotation vary with the degree of injury. Pain can be elicited but ordinarily is not excessive. The foot and lower part of the appendage are swollen.

Diagnosis

The diagnosis is evident and requires a roentgenogram only to indicate the extent of bone damage.

Prognosis

Most tibial fractures of the middle segment heal well if properly immobilized for a long enough period. Tibial fractures heal slowly and usually require from four to eight weeks to produce a callus strong enough to support the leg without mechanical assistance. The tibia is one of the slowest-healing bones in the body, probably because it seldom has a good hematoma from which to form a callus, or perhaps because the blood circulation to this part of the bone is scanty.

Treatment

Coaptation can be used to immobilize fractures in this area of the tibia and is applied as directed on page 32. Ordinarily, coaptation leaves much to be desired in oblique, spiral, or comminuted fractures. Once in a while, spiral and oblique fractures can be brought into apposition by mild flexion of the leg. In such a case, coaptation will be ideal.

The Thomas splint works well when the fracture is not badly comminuted. By placing a pin through the femur and attaching to the front bar of the splint and another pin through the tuber calcis and fastening to the back bar, traction can be applied to the tibia to overcome any overriding. The fracture area can then be covered with coapting material or supported by wooden splints laid across the bars. If necessary, Thomson beaded wires can be inserted into the bone fragments and anchored to the bars of the splint (Fig. 106).

Becker and Henschel have suggested the use of full pins which are inserted into each segment (at least two to a segment). The fracture is then reduced and the pin ends are embedded in polyethylene. When the plastic has hardened the pins become firmly fixed. Padding is placed between the plastic and the skin.

Perhaps the best way of reducing and fixing middle tibial fractures, even though comminuted, is the use of half pin splintage (Fig. 107). The splint should be applied to the medial aspect of the leg, since this offers a flat surface of the bone on which to pin, and it is close to the surface, so that little soft tissue damage is inflicted. Application of the splint does not vary from the instructions given under Methods and Materials except that the patient should be placed in lateral recumbency with the injured leg down. In preparing for surgery, the dog is placed on its back and a sterile drape is laid lengthwise on the table alongside the fractured leg. The leg is then wrapped and the dog is rolled so that the prepared leg comes to rest on the sterile drape. Further preparation is carried out as usual. The half pin splint allows free use of the leg immediately after surgery, thereby improving circulation, reducing swelling, and preventing muscle atrophy.

Intramedullary pinning is seldom indicated except in the occasional fracture that is transverse (Figs. 108, 109, and 110).

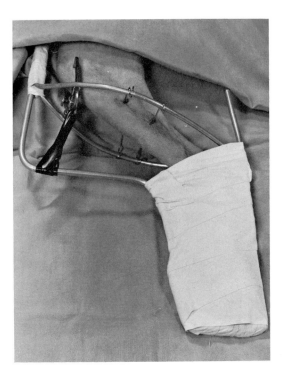

Figure 106. Fixation of a tibial fracture with Thomas splint and Thomson beaded wires.

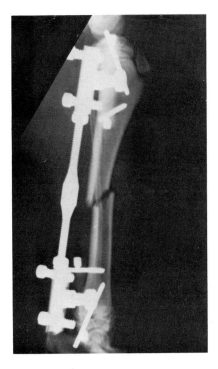

Figure 107. Fixation of a tibial fracture with half pin splintage.

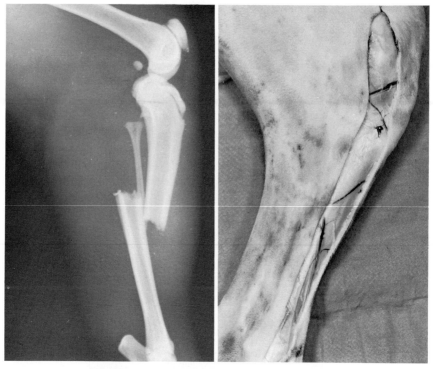

Fig. 108   Fig. 109

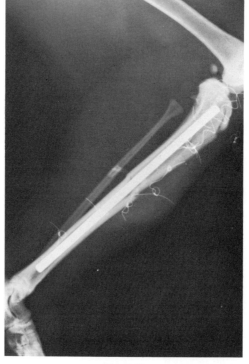

Fig. 110

134   *(See legends on opposite page.)*

Fractures of the Distal Segment

Definition

Fractures involving the distal tibia are usually spoken of as distal epiphyseal, supramalleolar, or malleolar. Strictly speaking, the lateral malleolus is part of the fibula. Since both bones are being considered together, and especially in view of the fact that the two bones are sometimes fused at this point, malleolar fractures, whether medial or lateral, will be discussed as one.

Incidence

It is estimated that fractures in this region of the tibia comprise less than one-fourth of the total tibial fractures.

Etiology

Supramalleolar fractures (Fig. 111) result from direct force. Malleolar fractures (Fig. 112) may arise from the application of either direct or indirect force. The indirect force is brought about by turning or twisting of the hind foot so that excessive pressure is put on the lateral or medial side of the hock.

Pathology

The supramalleolar fracture is usually transverse, although occasionally one sees a short oblique separation. Mild displacement is the rule, the long proximal segment being forced forward and overriding the length of the distal segment. Ordinarily, swelling and hemorrhage are not great. Simple fractures are most common.

Signs

The leg is held in a flexed position with a distortion at the hock joint. The Achilles tendon is relaxed, but the limb below the hock seems somewhat

---

Figure 108. Transverse fracture of the middle segment of the tibia with separation of the fibula.

Figure 109. A skin incision on the medial side of the tibia. The entire tibia can be exposed in this way. Care must be exercised in working around the blood vessels shown in the illustration. The tibia lies beneath this fascial layer.

Figure 110. Fixation of the tibial fracture shown in Figure 108 with an intramedullary pin. This is an open reduction using a single-pointed intramedullary pin which is inserted at the fracture site and drilled through the proximal segment, emerging at the stifle. After reduction, the blunt end of the pin is thrust deep into the distal medullary canal. The pointed end of the pin is then cut short enough so that the buried pin can be driven beneath the surface.

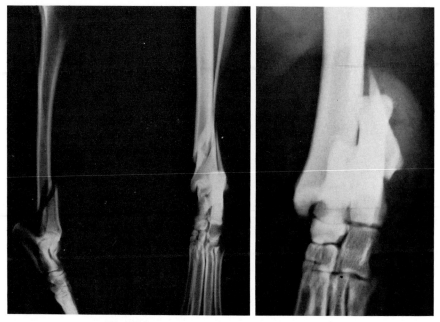

Fig. 111   Fig. 112

Figure 111.   A supramalleolar fracture of the tibia.
Figure 112.   A malleolar fracture of the tibia.

fixed. The patient will not bear weight on the limb, but shows only mild
pain except when palpated over the fracture area. The foot is held in a
downward position but seldom shows any other positional deviation except
in the malleolar fracture, when there is a tendency for the foot to rotate in
the direction of the bone separation.

Diagnosis

A tentative diagnosis can usually be made by palpation because of the
meager covering of the skeleton, but this should always be followed by a
roentgenogram.

Prognosis

With reasonable reduction and fixation, fractures of the distal end of the
tibia should heal, but they usually require a somewhat extended healing
time. One exception is distal epiphyseal separation, which seems to heal
quite rapidly, probably because of the age of the animal.

Treatment

The most satisfactory method of repairing supramalleolar and distal
epiphyseal fractures of the tibia is with the Kirschner-type intramedullary
pin. While the leg is held in mild flexion (about the normal standing angle),

a stab incision is made in the skin on the plantar surface of the hock directly opposite the distal end of the tibia. The intramedullary pin is then drilled through the tibial and fibular tarsal bones and into the distal segment of the tibia. The fracture is reduced by angulation (toggling) and the pin threaded up the medullary canal of the proximal segment. The initial insertion of the pin must be done carefully so as to avoid the plantar branch of the saphenous artery and the lateral plantar nerve, both of which pass close to the insertion point and sometimes must be pushed aside to avoid injury (Fig. 113).

During the time the pin is in place, the joint will be immobilized, but since the angle of this joint changes very little in ordinary locomotion, this will cause the patient slight inconvenience. When the pin is removed, full movement will return to the joint.

External support is frequently required in these cases to prevent rotation. Usually coaptation is sufficient.

The treatment of choice for a malleolar fracture is the vitallium or stainless steel screw. Open reduction is performed and the fracture fragment is drilled to accommodate a screw long enough to engage the opposite malleolus. The screw should be set with an orthopedic screw driver so that there is no wobbling or slipping during its insertion. It should be set deep to

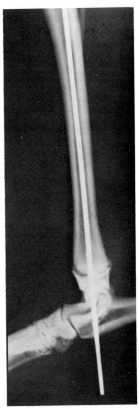

Figure 113. Fixation of a distal epiphyseal fracture of the tibia with an intramedullary pin.

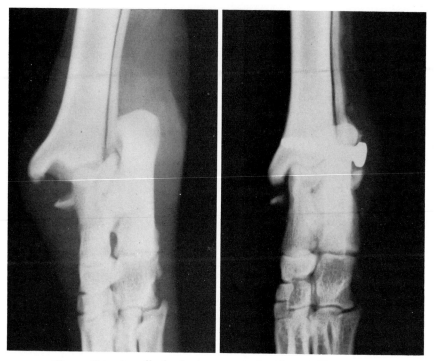

Figure 114. A malleolar fracture repaired with a vitallium screw.

avoid pressure on the overlying skin. Some decalcification will result, but recalcification occurs after about three months. The screw is allowed to remain indefinitely (Fig. 114).

It is important that coaptation be applied so that there is firm support during healing. A light material should be applied with the hock in slight flexion.

FRACTURES OF THE TARSUS, METATARSUS, AND PHALANGES

Definition

These bones are grouped together because they constitute the bones of the true foot, although the dog walks digitigrade and therefore uses only the phalanges to perform the duty of a foot.

Incidence

Of the total fractures in the dog, this group constitutes 2.9 per cent, and of these, tarsal fractures occur least frequently. Most of the tarsal fractures occur in the three proximal bones, and a great majority of these are seen in racing greyhounds. Fracture of the distal tarsal bones is seldom encountered.

Fracture of the tuber calcis and the central tarsus (scaphoid) are the most common tarsal fractures. Metatarsal and phalangeal fractures are not uncommon and are seen in all breeds.

Etiology

In racing greyhounds, an indirect force is responsible for the fracture of the central tarsus (scaphoid), and this in turn is responsible for fracture of the tuber calcis. All this is brought about by overextension during the strain of hard racing. Fracture of the tuber calcis is frequently seen in farm dogs as a result of mowing machine injuries. It is not uncommon to find tarsal fractures in conjunction with tibial fractures, particularly if the causative force is severe (Fig. 115). Fractures of the metatarsus and phalanges are usually the result of direct crushing injuries and are frequently compound.

Pathology

These fractures follow no set pattern, except possibly those of the central tarsus and the tuber calcis. The central tarsus (scaphoid) commonly splits longitudinally in a frontal plane, and the tuber calcis usually fractures transversely. Scaphoid fractures are never compound, but they are often comminuted. In the tarsal region, there is separation and tearing of the interosseous ligaments (Fig. 116). Since other fractures in the region are frequently

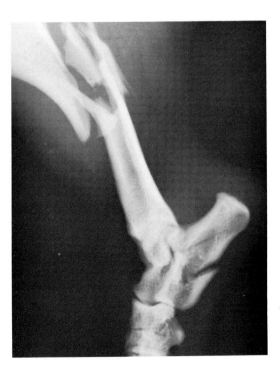

Figure 115. Fracture of the fibular tarsal along with fracture of the tibia.

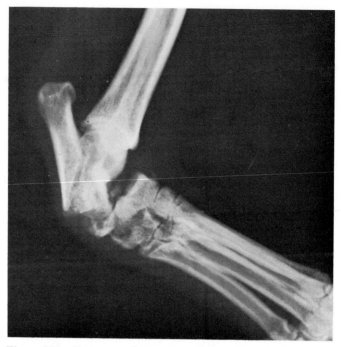

Figure 116. Fracture and separation of the proximal tarsal bones.

caused by a crushing injury, it is not unusual to see lacerations, contusions, swelling, hemorrhage, and gross contamination. Many times irreparable soft tissue damage has been done so that circulation to the foot is hopelessly interrupted. The appendage is cold, discolored, and lifeless. Needless to say, fractures of the metatarsal and phalangeal bones may be single or multiple regardless of whether the injury is simple or compound.

Signs

Fractures of the lower extremity are usually self-evident, especially those that are compound. The usual signs are crepitus, swelling, pain, inability to bear weight, and sometimes distortion of the foot. When the tuber calcis is fractured, the Achilles tendon is relaxed and the animal walks plantigrade. Fracture of the scaphoid produces a circumscribed swelling on the dorsal side of the hock which is painful on palpation. Bowing at the hock is common because of the displaced bone.

Diagnosis

The diagnosis should always be confirmed with a roentgenogram, using both the lateral and A-P views. Luxations and fractures can easily be confused because of the small size and location of the bones. It is also important to know whether the injury is single or multiple.

Prognosis

Only in case of extensive soft tissue damage would the prognosis be considered poor. Most of these fractures heal well, even those that are compounded and grossly contaminated. A fractured scaphoid will heal in about three months. A grave prognosis should be given, however, when there is serious interruption to circulation of the foot as indicated by coldness, discoloration, and swelling.

Treatment

FRACTURE OF THE TUBER CALCIS. A simple and effective repair can usually be made with the insertion of an intramedullary pin. If the fracture is recent, this can be performed with closed reduction, but if the injury is more than one week old, the site should be opened and the bone ends freshened with bone cutters. After insertion of the pin, the leg is held in extension by coaptation so that the pull of the gastrocnemius is relieved.

Kirk describes a method in which a metal plate is bound to the plantar surface of the tarsus and metatarsus with the upper end arched backward. The tuber calcis is then wired to this metal strip by means of a silver wire.

Perry, using somewhat the same method, places a stainless steel pin through the tuber calcis and attaches this to the metal splint running down the back of the leg. Adjustment can be made by means of a bolt on either side. (Cited by Kirk.)

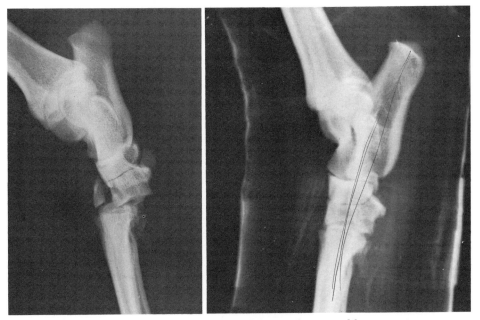

Figure 117. Fracture and separation of the tarsals repaired by coaptation.

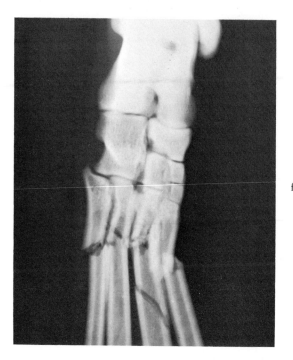

Figure 118. Fracture of all four metatarsals.

Bateman recommends wiring at the fracture site and supporting this by applying an Eggers-type stainless steel plate to the lateral surface of the tuber calcis and the tibia. This plate is inserted between the popliteal tendon and the tibia and is held in place by screws. It may be necessary to split the tendon in order to place the screws in the tibia.

FRACTURE OF THE CENTRAL TARSUS (SCAPHOID). Coaptation seems to offer the simplest treatment for this injury (Fig. 117). It can be applied with the use of the Mason metasplint, care being taken to pad well over the fractured bone so that pressure can be held against it. Reduction is not complete but it is usually adequate.

Bateman has described an acrylic prosthesis to replace the fractured scaphoid. This requires surgical removal of the fractured bone and its replacement with a specially formed prosthesis. He also has employed a metal wedge to replace the loose segment. This wedge is held in place by a small screw set in the tibial tarsal. This is later removed when the space has filled with fibrous tissue.

FRACTURE OF THE METATARSUS AND PHALANGES. Multiple fractures are the most difficult to manage, particularly when all metatarsal bones (Fig. 118) are involved. These may require some manipulation through angulation and "toggling." Reduction is less important when there is a single fracture. Coaptation with a Mason metasplint is usually ideal fixation for these fractures. In single fractures the other bones also lend some support.

REFERENCES

Anderson, W. D., Schlotthauer, C. F., and Jones, J. M.: Method for treatment of fractures of the femoral neck of the dog. I. An experimental study. J.A.V.M.A., *122*:158–160, 1953.

Archibald, J., and Ballantyne, J. H.: A practical prosthesis for the canine and feline femoral head. N. Am. Vet., *34*:496–501, 1953.

Armistead, W. W., and Lumb, W. V.: Management of distal epiphyseal fractures of the femur. N. Am. Vet., *33*:481–483, 1952.

Bateman, J. K.: Broken hock in the greyhound: Repair methods and the plastic scaphoid. Vet. *93*:146, 1937.

Bateman, J. K.: Broken neck in the greyhound: Repair methods and the plastic scaphoid. Vet. Rec., *70*:621–623, 1958.

Bateman, J. K.: A fresh approach to the repair of the os calcis in the greyhound. Vet. Rec., *60*:674, 1948.

Boyd, H. B., and Salvatore, J. E.: Acute fracture of the femoral neck: Internal fixation or prosthesis? Jour. Bone Joint Surg., *46A*:1066–1068, 1964.

Brinker, W. O.: Some troublesome lesions of the coxofemoral joint amendable by surgery. Vet. Med., *50*:77–78, 1955.

Brinker, W. O.: Factors influencing the result in fractures of the femoral neck. An. Hosp., *2*:160–166, 1966.

Brown, R. E.: A surgical approach to the coxofemoral joint of dogs. N. Am. Vet., *34*:420–422, 1953.

Carlin, J.: Fracture of the lower femoral epiphysis in the dog. N. Am. Vet., *17*:9, 42–45, 1936.

Cawley, A. J., Archibald, J., and Ditchfield, W. J. B.: Fractures of the neck of the femur in the dog. I. A technique for repair of fractures of the femoral neck. J.A.V.M.A., *129*:354–358, 1956.

DeAngleis, M., and Hohn, R. B.: The ventral approach to excision arthroplasty of the femoral head. J.A.V.M.A., *152*:135–138, 1968.

Ehmer, E. E.: The treatment of femoral fractures in dogs. N. Am. Vet., *15*:6, 40–42, 1934.

Fitzgerald, T. C.: Blood supply of the head of the canine femur. Vet. Med., *56*:389–394, 1961.

Frye, F. L.: Use of a needle cannula for repair of trochanteric fracture in two cats. J.A.V.M.A., *153*:182–183, 1968.

Gay, W. I.: Preliminary evaluation of femoral head prosthesis in the presence of coxitis. J.A.V.M.A., *126*:85–90, 1955.

Gay, W. I.: Evaluation of hip prostheses used in canine patients. Sm. An. Clin., *1*:294, 1961.

Gorman, H. A.: A hip prosthesis for the dog. Thesis for M.S. degree, Ohio State University, 1955.

Gorman, H. A.: Hip joint prostheses. Vet. Scope, 7:3–9, 1962.

Hickman, J., and Spickett, S. G.: Avascular necrosis of the femoral head in the dog. Proc. Roy. Soc. Med., *58*:366–369, 1965.

Hohn, R. B.: Surgical approaches to the canine hip. An. Hosp., *1*:48–55, 1965.

Hurov, L., and Seer, G.: External Kirschner clamp fixation with intramedullary pinning for distal epiphyseal fracture repair. Canad. Vet. Jour.,9:31–40, 1968.

Hutton, W. C., and England, J. P. S.: The femoral head prosthesis of the dog. J. Small Animal Pract., *10*:79–85, 1969.

Jenny, J.: A motion picture review of modern fracture treatment. Proc. Int. Vet. Congress, *2*:946–951, part 1, 1953.

Jenny, J.: Resection of the femoral head in developmental hip disorders in dogs. Sc. Proc. A.V.M.A., pp 170–171, 1963.

Jonas, S.: Compound comminuted fracture of the patella. N. Am. Vet., *34*:189–191, 1953.

Keene, R. B., and Yarborough, J. H.: Surgical correction of the central tarsal bone in the racing greyhound. Vet. Med. Small Animal Clin., *61*:980–984, 1966.

Kemp, H. B. S.: Avascular necrosis of the femoral head in dogs. J. Bone Joint Surg., *50B*:431, 1968.

Kirk, H.: Modern methods of fracture repair in large and small animals. Vet. Rec., *64*:319–328, 1952.

Knowles, J. O.: Fracture repair by bone pinning. Vet. Rec., *61*:648–652, 1949.

Knowles, A. T., Knowles, J. O., and Knowles, R. P.: Clinical application of pinning in fracture reduction. Vet. Med., *44*:259–265, 1949.

Lawson, D. D.: The use of Rush pins in the management of fractures in the dog and cat. Vet. Rec., *70*:760–763, 1958.

Leighton, R. L.: The use of vitallium screws in the fixation of fractures of the malleolus in dogs. Cornell Vet., *47*:396–399, 1957.

Miller, M. E.: Unpublished work.

Miller, M. E., Christensen, G. C., and Evans, H. E.: Anatomy of the dog. Philadelphia, W. B.
    Saunders, 1964.
Myers, S.: Repair of femoral head fractures in the dog. Southeastern Vet., *13*:105–108, 1962.
Nilsson, F.: Operativ behandling av fractura colli femoris och epiphyseolysis capitis femoris
    hos hunden. Svensk Vet., *46*:158–168, 1941.
Ormond, A. N.: Treatment of hip lameness in the dog by excision of the femoral head. Vet. Rec.,
    73:576, 1961.
Piermattei, D. L.: Femoral head ostectomy in the dog: Indications, technique and results in ten
    cases. An. Hosp., *1*:180–188, 1965.
Piermattei, D. L., and Greeley, R. G.: An Atlas of Surgical Approaches to the Bones of the Dog
    and Cat. Philadelphia, W. B. Saunders, 1966.
Schroeder, E. R.: The treatment of fractures in dogs. N. Am. Vet., *14*:5, 27–31, 1933.
Schroeder, E. R.: Recent progress in canine orthopedic surgery. N. Am. Vet., *20*:8, 54–61, 1939.
Seer, G., and Hurov, L.: Simultaneous bilateral coxofemoral excision arthroplasty in the dog.
    Can. Vet. Jour., *9*:70–73, 1968.
Singleton, W. B.: Limb fractures in the dog and cat. V. Fractures of the hind limb. J. Small
    Animal Pract., *7*:169–175, 1966.
Spruell, J. S. A.: Excision arthroplasty as a method of treatment of hip joint diseases in the dog.
    Vet. Rec., *73*:573–575, 1961.
Tovee, B. E., and Geudron, E.: The use of radioactive phosphorus in the determination of the
    viability of the femoral head in dogs after subcapital fractures. J. Bone Joint Surg., *36A*:1,
    185, 1954.
Vaughan, L. C.: Acrylic femoral head prosthesis in the cat. Vet. Rec., *67*:804–805, 1955.
Vincent, Z. D.: The repair of tibial fractures by intramedullary pinning. Vet. Rec., *64*:64, 1952.

Chapter 6

Fractures in the Pectoral Limb

FRACTURES OF THE SCAPULA

Although the occurrence of fractures of the scapula has commonly been considered relatively rare, statistics at our clinic for the past 20 years indicate that fractures in this bone constitute 1.3 per cent of the total fractures seen. They occur as the result of direct force and may sometimes be overlooked, particularly in the presence of other fractures in the same limb.

The three common sites where fractures occur are across the body (Fig. 119), through the neck, or longitudinally separating the acromion and some-

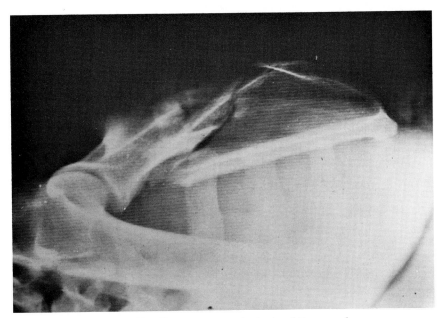

Figure 119.   Fracture across the body of the scapula.

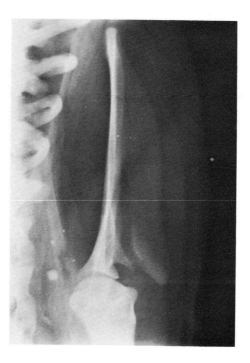

Figure 120. Fracture of the spine of the scapula.

times the entire spine from the body (Fig. 120). Most fractures of the scapula are simple with slight displacement and little evidence of swelling or hemorrhage.

The patient is quite likely to show both a swinging and a standing leg lameness. With fractures of the neck there may be a definite drop to the shoulder with inward rotation of the leg. In such a case, the elbow protrudes noticeably. With the exception of neck fractures, crepitus is not a prominent sign and pain varies depending on the proximity of the injury to the shoulder joint. Both an A-P and a lateral roentgenogram should be taken for diagnosis.

The prognosis is usually good because of the muscle support over the scapula. However, in cases of neck fracture showing paralysis of the leg, recovery is doubtful even with good fracture healing.

For most fractures of the scapula, including many neck fractures, a good body cast, which includes the flexed forelimb, is quite sufficient. Plaster of Paris may be used, or surgical padding if overlaid with adequate tape. The forelimb is brought into flexion and coaptation is applied so that the leg is encased to the elbow and bound to the body. The cast should be placed completely around the body, with bandaging on either side of the opposite foreleg for anchorage. When the cast is completed it is well to bandage the suspended appendage to avoid swelling of the foot. If Aire-Cast is used, one should allow for shrinkage.

FRACTURES OF THE HUMERUS

For purposes of convenience, fractures of the humerus may be divided into fractures of the proximal segment, fractures of the middle segment, and fractures of the distal segment. Taken as a whole, fractures of the humerus represent 6.9 per cent of the total fractures seen in the dog. Of this number, 5.7 per cent are fractures of the shaft and 1.2 per cent are fractures involving the condyles.

Fractures of the Proximal Segment

These fractures are rare and are usually in the form of a proximal epiphyseal separation. An injury of young dogs resulting from indirect force, this separation, according to Schroeder, is brought about by dogs jumping from moving cars. The fall is broken by an extended forelimb that is abducted. Another type of injury, sustained when the animal lands squarely on the foot, will be discussed under Intercondylar Fractures.

The long distal segment displaces cranially and medially to the proximal segment and there is some overriding. Damage to soft parts in the brachial region can cause temporary or permanent paralysis. Fortunately, the traumatizing segment is seldom sharp and therefore is more likely to bruise than to lacerate.

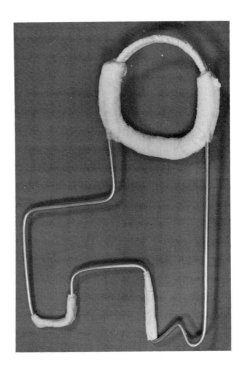

Figure 121. A Thomas splint fashioned to fit the forelimb.

The dog carries the limb with the lower parts flexed and the shoulder extended and abducted. There is intense pain on palpation and little resistance to abduction or adduction.

Reduction of the overriding segment is extremely important if permanent lameness is to be avoided, because a large callus may form, causing pressure around the brachial plexus which may be severe enough to cause paralysis. The distal segment is "toggled" against the small proximal segment, while at the same time the small segment is secured by grasping the scapula. Angulation is obtained by abducting the lower segment. After reduction is completed, fixation is accomplished by longitudinal skeletal traction in a Thomas splint. The splint is fashioned as outlined in the chapter on Methods and Materials and the bars are shaped as shown in Figure 121. Traction is obtained by placing a pin or wire through the olecranon and fastening this to the bottom bar. The splint should remain in place for three to six weeks.

Fractures of the Middle Segment

Fractures are common in the middle of the humerus, and are transverse, oblique, spiral, or comminuted. They are most frequently caused by a direct force. Hemorrhage and swelling are always present, frequently with severe injury to the nerves and blood vessels of the upper arm. The proximal

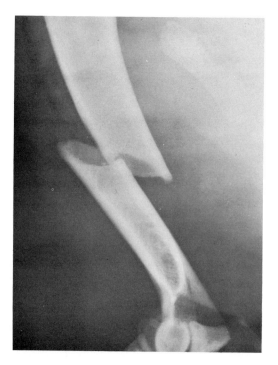

Figure 122. A typical midshaft fracture of the humerus. The displacement of the distal segment is cranial and medial.

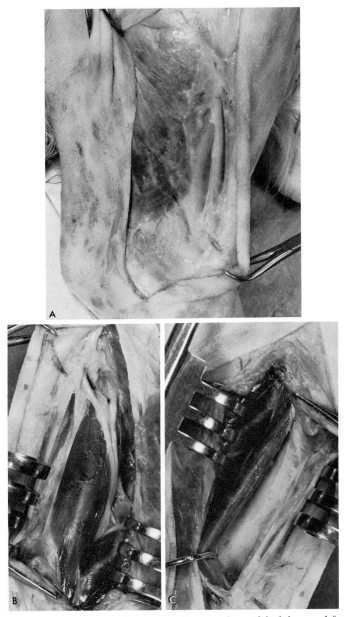

Figure 123. Lateral approach for open reduction of a midshaft humeral fracture. A, The skin is incised from the point of the shoulder to the elbow. B, The triceps is reflected caudally, exposing the radial nerve and the brachialis. C, Caudal reflection of the brachialis uncovers the humerus.

segment is abducted so that the overriding of the distal segment is cranial and medial. There is also outward rotation and adduction of the lower segment (Fig. 122).

The toes point outward and there is a definite shortening of the limb. The elbow is dropped and the carpus is partially flexed. On manipulation of the limb, both pain and crepitus can be elicited. There is firm swelling over the area when the fracture is several days old. This is softer in recent fractures and may even crepitate as result of emphysema in compound fractures.

Treatment varies according to the type of fracture. A transverse fracture may be reduced by either an open (Fig. 123) or a closed method and an intramedullary pin inserted. If the open reduction method is used and the pin is inserted retrograde, no external landmarks are needed; but if the reduction is closed, the greater tubercle is used as the location for inserting the pin. The pin should be of adequate size and length so that the point can be embedded in the cortex of the medial condyle. It is best to bury the pin beneath the skin even though it is to be extracted after healing. Burying is done by retracting the pin slightly, cutting it, and then driving it into place with a punch. Care should always be taken not to penetrate the distal cortex. It is sometimes necessary to apply some form of coaptation to prevent long axis rotation, and this can be accomplished by binding the brachium to the body or by a simple cast around the limb itself. Usually this can be removed after a week or 10 days. If the fracture is oblique, spiral, or comminuted, half

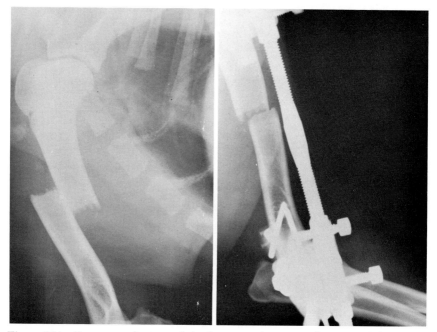

Figure 124. Transverse fracture of the humerus showing reduction and fixation with a Stader splint. Other forms of splintage would be applicable in this instance.

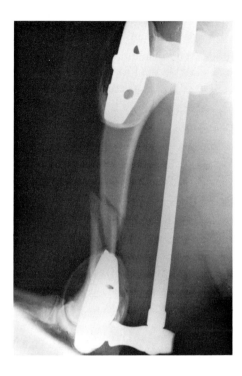

Figure 125. Fixation of a midshaft fracture of the humerus with a Schroeder splint.

pin splintage is indicated unless the fractured ends are rough enough to impact firmly (Figs. 124 and 125). The point for insertion of the number 1 pin can be located by flexing the leg to approximately right angles with the scapula. If a line is then projected from the spine of the scapula across the humerus, it will indicate the proper pin location. The number 4 pin is

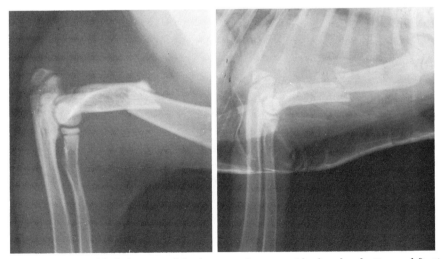

Figure 126. Midshaft fracture of the humerus in a cat with closed reduction and fixation by coaptation. In this case tape encircles the chest after padding.

inserted into the lateral epicondyle. Approximate reduction should be achieved before the extension bar is put into place.

In some instances of transverse fractures in young or small animals, it is possible to perform a closed reduction followed by coaptation fixation in which the upper limb is bound to the rib cage with right angle flexion at the shoulder and the elbow (Fig. 126). It is seldom possible, however, to obtain good fixation by coaptation alone.

Supracondylar and Intercondylar Fractures

Definition

Fractures occurring in the region just above the condyles of the humerus are usually referred to as supracondylar and those in which the fracture line occurs through the trochlea are called intercondylar fractures. Sometimes both kinds of fractures occur simultaneously, and these are often designated as T or Y fractures.

Incidence

Although these fractures constitute less than 1 per cent of all fractures, they have received much attention from orthopedists because of the difficulties encountered in reduction and fixation.

Etiology

The etiology of fractures occurring in the distal end of the humerus is most interesting because of the forces involved and the anatomic relationship of the ulna to the condyles of the humerus. A simple, uncomplicated supracondylar fracture is caused by a direct force against the lateral epicondyle, whereas a simple fracture through the medial supracondylar shaft is caused by an indirect force applied to the ulna in a horizontal direction and just distal to the lateral epicondyle. The semilunar notch, because it is deep-seated when extended, puts pressure against the medial condyle, causing it to split through the supracondylar shaft and the trochlea. This is a type of fracture most commonly seen when the injury is the result of impact with a moving object (e.g., an automobile).

When an indirect force is applied in a vertical direction, through the semilunar notch, the fracture line traverses the trochlea and the lateral supracondylar shaft, thereby separating the lateral condyle. Most of these fractures are the result of jumping from a high place or from a moving car and alighting on the extended forelimb. This produces a shearing action on the lateral condyle.

Pathology

Most of the fractures in the elbow region are simple with a wide separation of the condyles when either or both of the supracondylar shafts are broken. This separation is likely to complicate the fracture by permitting a luxation of the joint. Hemorrhage is mild except in supracondylar fractures, in which both swelling and hemorrhage may be extensive because of the rich blood supply to this area. Injury to the ulnar nerve may be caused by the fracture or by manipulation during reduction.

Signs

The forelimb is carried with the elbow in extension and the carpus flexed. If the medial condyle is fractured, the foot may partially supinate because of the contraction of the supinator on the lateral side and the separation of the pronator teres on the medial side. Sometimes, when only one condyle is fractured, the dog will show a swinging leg lameness but only slight standing leg lameness. This is particularly true when the lateral condyle is fractured. Usually there is only mild distortion of the limb with possibly some adduction of the foot and almost imperceptible abduction of the elbow. The joint feels wider when compared with its mate, and palpation produces both pain and crepitus.

Diagnosis

The diagnosis is confirmed by a roentgenogram taken in two planes, although the A-P view is usually diagnostic (Fig. 127).

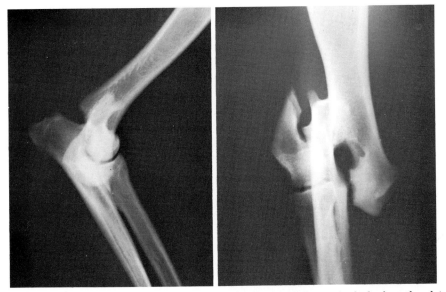

Figure 127. A fracture of the lateral supracondylar shaft taken in both the lateral and A-P planes. It is clear which position offers the best diagnostic features.

Prognosis

A guarded prognosis should always be given because of the involvement of a prominent joint and the difficulty of holding the fragments in proper fixation (Fig. 128). Unless the repair is good, there may always be some lameness even when the joint is functional. The prognosis is good, however, in a simple supracondylar fracture, since it does not involve the joint and is usually uncomplicated.

Treatment

SUPRACONDYLAR FRACTURES. Intramedullary pinning of this type of fracture may succeed occasionally, but because of the instability of such a fixation it is not especially recommended. Usually the distal fragment is short and cannot be completely transfixed because of the proximity of the joint. Jenny has suggested the use of two Kirschner wires. One is inserted through each epicondyle at an angle so that it follows the supracondylar shaft and crosses over to the opposite cortex at the true shaft (Fig. 129). These wires protrude from the elbow so that compression can be exerted by lacing the ends together with rubber bands or soft wire. The entire elbow is then supported in some form of coaptation with the limb held in partial flexion.

On rare occasions, the arm can be held in coaptation with the fracture reduced against the body, but this is usually not very satisfactory. A description of this type of fixation was given earlier in this chapter.

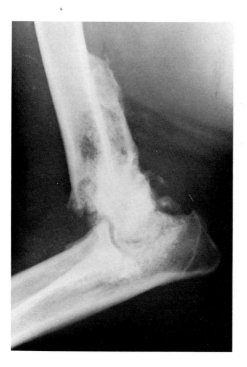

Figure 128. Ankylosis of the elbow resulting from excessive callus around the joint following poor reduction and fixation of a supracondylar fracture of the humerus.

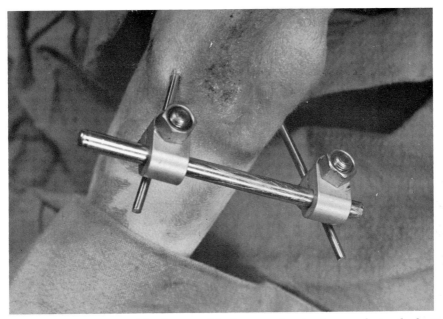

Figure 129. A supracondylar fracture of the humerus showing the use of wires for fixation. The Rush pin has also been recommended for this purpose.

The Thomas splint with skeletal traction from the olecranon makes a satisfactory splintage, particularly if Thomson beaded wires are used to control the bone segments (Figs. 130 and 131).

A firm fixation can be produced by using half pin splintage. The upper pin assembly is placed as usual but the lower assembly is placed on the olecranon process. The elbow is flexed so that the lower assembly is at right angles to the upper assembly before the extension bar is attached. This is sometimes referred to as a T splint. With this method there is no absolute control over the distal segment unless Thomson beaded wires are used. These wires can be anchored to the extension bar. It is possible to maintain impaction of the segments by this method, but the joint is fixed in flexion until the splint is removed.

Stader has described the use of a condyle pin in conjunction with the Stader splint. A Kirschner wire is drilled through the distal segment so that it penetrates both epicondyles. The ends of the wire are then connected to a clevis, which in turn is attached to the distal end of the Stader extension bar. The proximal pin bar is installed in the usual position on the upper humerus.

The Kirschner condyle pin, attached to the Kirschner half pin splint, makes a very satisfactory fixation. The condyle pin is inserted through the epicondyle and fastened in place with ferrules. The pin is then cut on the medial side but left long enough on the lateral side so that a clamp can be attached and anchored to the extension bar as shown in Figure 132.

INTERCONDYLAR FRACTURES. The intercondylar fractures are the most

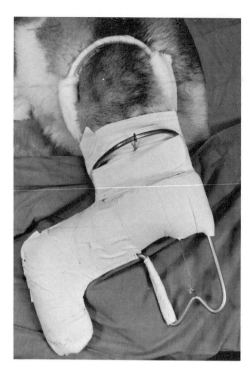

Figure 130. The Thomas splint applied to the forelimb in conjunction with the use of Thomson beaded wires for the control of the bone segments.

Figure 131. Diagram showing how traction is applied with Thomson beaded wires so that segments of the humerus are stabilized.

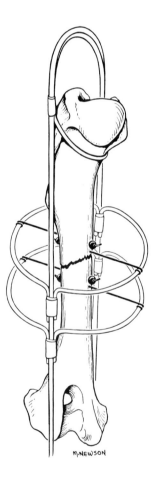

M. NEWSON

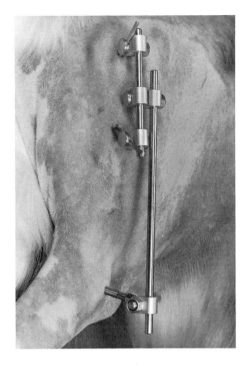

Figure 132. The use of a Kirschner condyle pin in conjunction with a Kirschner splint for fixation of a supracondylar fracture of the humerus.

difficult of all humeral fractures to maintain in proper alignment. There are two fracture areas to be reduced and immobilized; in the event of a T or Y fracture there are at least three such areas. Some form of internal fixation is necessary because the small fragments are important components of a primary joint and therefore must be held in firm fixation.

The method described by Jenny and referred to on page 154 has met with a measure of success in the handling of these fractures, whether single or double. If only the lateral condyle is involved and the displacement is not great, it is sometimes possible to apply a cast to the elbow and suspend the limb in flexion until the fracture is healed (Fig. 133).

Fixation with a condyle pin has been used with good results in both single and double condyle fractures. While the joint is held in slight flexion, the fracture is reduced manually and held in place with a condyle clamp (Fig. 134). A small pin is then drilled through both epicondyles. Starting just cranial to the center of the lateral condyle and drilling in a slightly caudal-distal direction so as to avoid the joint capsule and emerge in the center of the medial condyle, the pin is inserted far enough so that it protrudes well beyond the skin. After the skin adjacent to the pin has been incised, the ferrules are applied. The hexagonal ferrules with the Allen screws should be placed on the outside. The condyle clamp is then released and reapplied so that it fits over the pin. Pressure can be applied to the ferrules with the clamp, bringing the bone fragments into apposition, whereupon the Allen screws are tightened. The pin can then be cut next to the outside ferrule

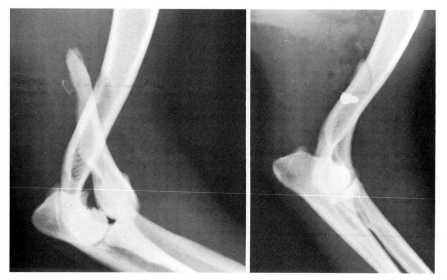

Figure 133. An intercondylar fracture with a splitting of the distal shaft of the humerus. This has been repaired by using a screw in the shaft area of the segment and immobilizing the elbow in coaptation.

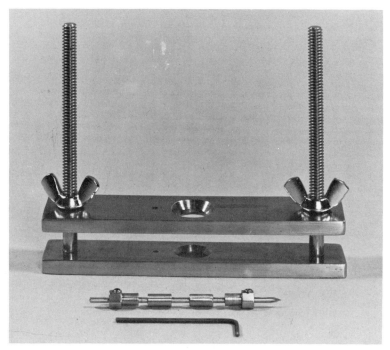

Figure 134. The Kirschner condyle clamp with its accessories. The large opening is used for applying the pin while the bone segments are being held in position by the clamp. After the ferrules are applied to the pin, but before tightening the Allen screws, the clamp is loosened and reapplied so that the small holes fit over the ends of the pin.

unless the fracture is T or Y, in which case the pin should be left long on the lateral side so that half pin splintage can be attached.

If a single condyle is fractured, it can be reduced openly and a screw placed through the epicondyle to immobilize it (Fig. 135). A crescent-shaped incision is made directly over the displaced epicondyle and the fracture site is exposed. The approach may be either medial or lateral. In the medial approach, it may be necessary to reflect the medial head of the triceps, and in the lateral approach some of the extensors will require separation. The condyle clamp is applied after reduction and the condyles are drilled to accommodate a vitallium or stainless steel screw long enough to engage both cortices.

If both condyles are fractured, it is frequently possible to apply a bone plate to one side of the bone, using the distal screw for fixing the two condyles to each other and the plate for fixing them to the shaft.

Mostosky and coworkers have described a surgical approach to the elbow joint for the repair of intercondylar fractures which they designate as "trans-olecranon." This is a caudal approach in which the olecranon process is transected. It has the advantage of a good joint exposure so that accurate reduction of the fracture can be made.

The skin incision is made on the caudo-lateral aspect of the elbow between the lateral epicondyle and the olecranon (Fig. 136). It extends a

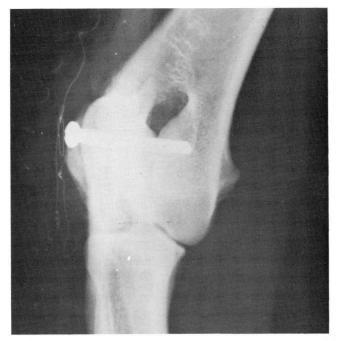

Figure 135. A stainless steel screw used in the fixation of a single condyle. This screw actually engages both cortices. Apparent shortness of the screw is due to the position of the limb.

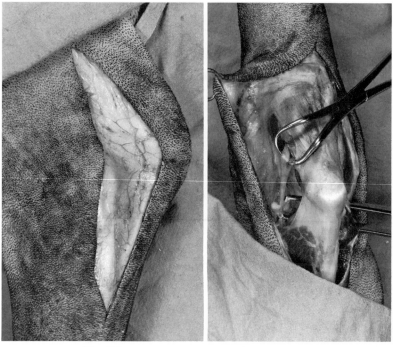

Fig. 136   Fig. 137

Figure 136. The location of the skin incision for the trans-olecranon approach to the elbow.
Figure 137. Exposure and reflection of the ulnar nerve.

reasonable distance above and below the elbow. The olecranon is exposed along with the condyles of the humerus and the insertions of the triceps and tensor fascial antebrachii.

At this point it is well to locate the ulnar nerve so that it will not be injured. It can usually be found just caudal to the medial epicondyle and should be gently freed from surrounding muscles and held to one side so that the medial head of the triceps can be separated from the humerus (Fig. 137).

By blunt dissection, starting at the medial aspect of the elbow, the muscle attachments to the olecranon are separated from the anconeus and brachialis muscles. The separation of the triceps and the antebrachii is then completed from the lateral side, making certain that they are freed from the caudal surface of the humerus.

It is well to drill the olecranon longitudinally for the fixation screw before transecting the olecranon process (Fig. 138). This will insure a perfect realignment on closure. Mostosky has recommended that the transection be performed with a Gigli saw. The bone is cut just distal to the muscle insertions, and the entire muscle mass along with the bone segment is reflected to expose the anconeus (Fig. 139). This muscle is often lacerated in such a way that the joint is exposed, but if it is not, it should be freed on the

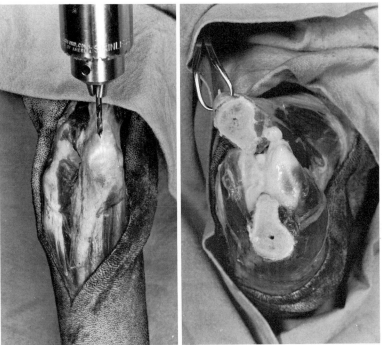

Fig. 138   Fig. 139

Figure 138.   Drilling the olecranon to accommodate the screw prior to sawing the bone.
Figure 139.   The reflected muscle mass and bone segment exposing the joint.

medial side and reflected laterally. The olecranon ligament is also frequently torn but this is of no great consequence. The joint capsule is usually torn but further separation may be necessary to expose the joint properly.

The fracture is cleared and reduced. An intercondyloid screw is used for fixation. During the drilling for the screw placement, the condyles may be held in place by a condyle clamp (Fig. 140). Mostosky has recommended the use of two Vulsellum forceps, which he feels are superior to the condyle clamp because they afford "better visualization and less physical obstruction" to the surgical field. The forceps also prevent rotation of the condyles during placement of the screw.

If the fracture is a T or Y, fixation of the supracondylar separation should be carried out before closing the incision. The capsule is closed, if possible, and the olecranon segment with its muscle attachments is replaced. A screw is inserted into the previously drilled hole (Fig. 141); if the patient is large a second screw may be placed parallel to the first. The closure is completed by replacing and suturing the muscle, fascia, and skin.

Regardless of the method used for reduction and fixation of fractures in the elbow joint, it is important that the fractured segments be rigidly fixed. At the same time, movement of the joint during healing is helpful in maintaining flexibility.

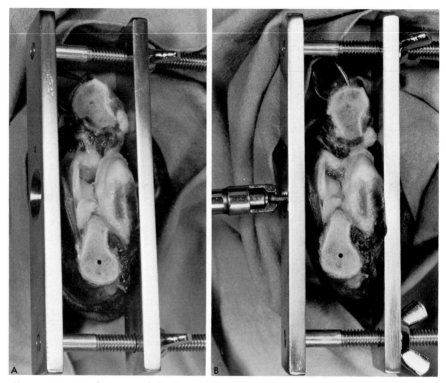

Figure 140. Reduction and fixation of the fracture. A, The condyle clamp applied to hold the reduced fragments in place. B, Applying the screw with an orthopedic screw driver through the large opening in the condyle clamp.

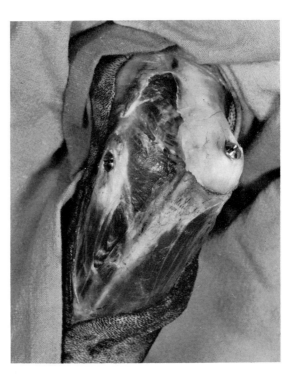

Figure 141. The replaced triceps showing the placement of both the screw in the condyles and the screw in the olecranon.

FRACTURES OF THE RADIUS AND ULNA

Definition

Most fractures of the radius involve the ulna, but the converse is not always true, as, for example, in fracture of the olecranon process. In such a case, the ulna alone is involved. However, since fractures of the forearm usually involve both bones they will be discussed concurrently.

Incidence

Fractures of the radius and ulna occurring together constitute 9.8 per cent of all fractures. Fracture of the radius alone is seen in 5.1 per cent of the cases, and fracture of the ulna alone occurs 3.7 per cent of the time. These figures are based on the statistics of our own clinic and may vary somewhat in other clinics. All types of fractures are seen, the large majority of them occurring in the distal half (Fig. 142), the one exception being the olecranon process. Green stick fractures of the radius are not unusual in young dogs, especially those that show some signs of rickets. Transverse and oblique fractures are common, these being mostly simple and only occasionally compound. Comminuted fractures seem to be more common in older dogs. Short distal segments and distal epiphyseal separations are sometimes seen, and these are often referred to as "Colles" fractures because they

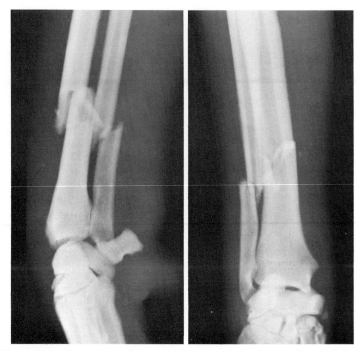

Figure 142. Two views of a typical fracture of the distal radius and ulna.

resemble the fracture of that name in humans. When fractures of the upper radius occur, they are usually either transverse or epiphyseal.

Etiology

Most of these fractures are the result of direct force, primarily by automobiles. Occasionally farm dogs are injured above the carpus by harvesting machinery, but most of these injuries are below the carpus.

Pathology

Hemorrhage and swelling are seldom severe. Frequently the swelling is greater distal to the fracture than at the fracture site itself, probably because damage to the soft tissues around the fracture has interfered with circulation beyond that point, particularly with the venous flow.

The distal portion of the radius heals slowly and is frequently the site of a non-union. There seems to be less vascularity in this region, and the soft tissue covering lacks the body necessary to amass a large hematoma. The tendency for transverse fractures to occur in the lower radius is another factor contributing to the poor healing reputation of this bone. Comminuted fractures frequently do well because of the large amount of bone surface exposed, thereby making available larger quantities of calcium (Fig. 143).

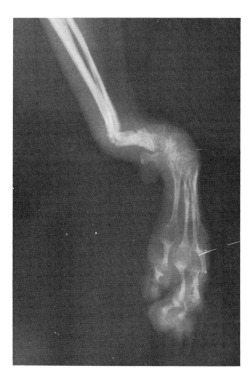

Figure 143. A non-union fracture of the radius.

Signs

The limb is carried at all times. There is slight flexion at the elbow and carpus. A curvature of the limb is usually apparent, with the concavity on the cranial side. The foot is rotated outward, with noticeable adduction distal to the fracture. When only the radius is fractured, the cranial surface of the limb is convex, with rotation and adduction minimized.

Pain and crepitus are constant signs, but swelling is more variable. In some cases the swelling may be moderate, but in others it may be slight. There is frequently some swelling of the foot.

When the olecranon process is broken there is a flat appearance to the caudal surface of the elbow. The dog shows difficulty in flexing the carpus and extending the elbow. Many times the elbow is held in a fixed position, slightly abducted and semi-flexed.

Diagnosis and Prognosis

The diagnosis is usually obvious but should be verified by roentgenograms. A guarded prognosis should be given, particularly in simple transverse fractures, because of the slow repair rate of the radius.

Treatment

Transverse fractures of the radius or radius and ulna can be manually reduced by angulation and "toggling." A good coaptation splint is usually sufficient fixation (Fig. 144). Since this portion of the limb is straight, it is difficult to maintain coaptation splintage in proper position without applying it too tightly. Pressure necrosis over the bony prominences of both the elbow and carpus must be avoided. The swollen foot must be covered with an even, well-padded pressure. In order to avoid excessive pressure on the limb, the coaptive material can be anchored to the body. Strips of adhesive applied to the lateral side of the splintage and carried over the shoulder, caudal to the opposite leg, across the chest, and then around the cast will prevent any slipping. Padding can be applied before taping if it seems desirable.

Such splintage as yucca or basswood should be applied to the lateral and medial sides of the fracture to prevent lateral distortion of the distal segments during healing. If plaster is used, it has been suggested by Jenny that the cast be molded so that the distal part curves medially. This will compensate for the lateral distortion so commonly seen in this type of fracture.

Frost recommends closed reduction and fixation with splints made of 24 gauge aluminum for small dogs and 16 gauge for larger dogs. These strips of aluminum are bowed across the short dimension to form a trough similar to the Mason metasplint extension. After they have been covered with tape, they are applied to the medial and lateral aspects of the padded limb.

Half pin splintage offers an excellent method of fixation for oblique or comminuted fractures as well as for compound fractures requiring frequent dressing (Fig. 145). The splintage should be applied to the cranial side of the radius, since this offers a flat surface and thereby facilitates pin insertion.

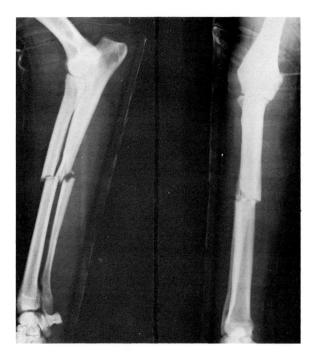

Figure 144. A satisfactory reduction and fixation with coaptation of a fracture of the radius and ulna.

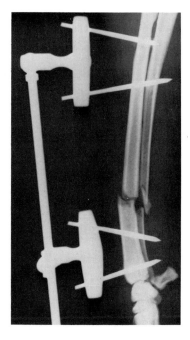

Figure 145. This application of the Schroeder splint illustrates half pin splintage of the radius and ulna. Pins 2, 3, and 4 are penetrating much too deep.

This placement of the pins has a further advantage of better counteracting the lateral pull of the distal segments by being at right angles to this force.

Insertion of the number 1 pin should be far enough distal so that it does not interfere with flexion of the elbow joint. This is the one exception to the rule calling for pin placement as near the bone extremities as possible. When difficulty is encountered at the distal end because of a very short segment (Colles fracture), the pin bar can be fastened to a block of wood which is bound to the carpus (Fig. 146). The fracture is reduced and the extension bar is applied in the usual manner. It is well to keep a light pressure bandage on the foot to prevent further swelling.

According to Vincent, the Rush pin provides a satisfactory method of repair for middle and distal shaft fractures. This method requires open reduction. The incision is made on the cranial side of the limb and the radius exposed for a good distance proximal to the fracture and for a short distance distal to it. A hole large enough to accommodate the pin is drilled through the cranial cortex well above the fracture site. The bit is started at a 90° angle. After the initial hole is made, it is elongated in the longitudinal direction so that the pin can be directed distally along the medullary canal. The pin is driven to the fracture site and the fracture reduced, whereupon the driving is continued until the pin reaches the distal cortex of the distal segment.

It is important to select a pin of proper length because the hook end should be preserved for extraction when the bone is healed. For best results, the pin should traverse nearly the entire length of the medullary canal.

The Leighton shuttle pin can be used to advantage if the distal end is

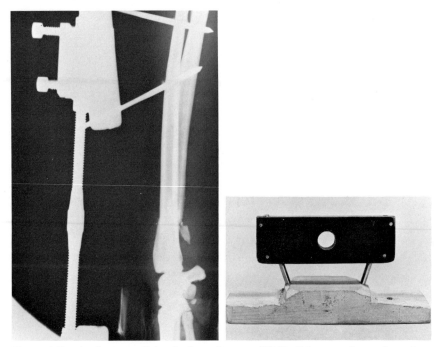

Figure 146. Application of the Stader splint to a "Colles" fracture. Inset shows how the distal pin bar is assembled.

short and it is found difficult to keep the bone ends in apposition. This should receive some external support to prevent angulation. Application of this splint is described on page 64 (Fig. 147).

Short distal segments can result in non-union unless properly immobilized, especially in the toy breeds. In these small dogs, it is often expedient to perform an open reduction and fix with an intramedullary pin. The incision in such a case should include the carpal area so that the distal end of the radius can be exposed. Great care should be taken to select a pin that is small enough. Very frequently the medullary canal of the distal radius in the toy breeds is extremely small and the bone is easily split when an oversize pin is introduced.

The carpal joint is held in extreme flexion and a single pointed pin is drilled through the distal end of the radius. As soon as it reaches the fracture site, the ends are apposed and the pin is continued proximally until it reaches the cortex. It is then "backed off" about 0.5 cm. The pin should be cut as close to the bone as possible and the end smoothed by filing. A punch is used to set the pin level with the bone surface so that there will be no interference with the joint.

If a pin can be prepared in advance so that it is the proper length and size, there is less likelihood of problems with making a smooth, blunt end.

Fractures of the ulna through the olecranon process can best be handled by intramedullary pinning (Fig. 148). The pin should be inserted through a

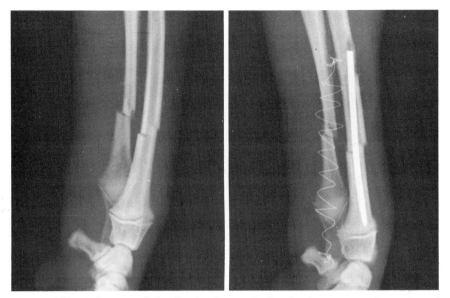

Figure 147. A fracture of the distal radius and ulna fixed in position by using a short intramedullary pin in a manner similar to the Leighton method.

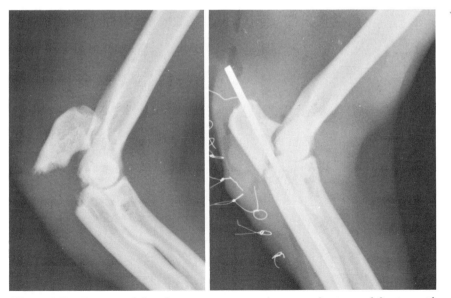

Figure 148. Fracture of the olecranon process with open reduction and fixation with an intramedullary pin.

stab incision over the point of the elbow. When the pin is securely embedded in the proximal segment, the angle is shifted until the two segments
are reduced. Drilling with the pin then proceeds until there is solid anchorage. Since the ulna narrows rapidly, it is possible to force the pin too far and
thus cause damage at the distal end, especially if a large diameter pin is
used. Small-caliber pins are preferable, with some external support to keep
the forelimb extended. This relieves tension on the proximal segment.

Open reduction can also be used (Fig. 149). The incision in such cases
should be made on the lateral side of the elbow and extended parallel to the
ulna an appropriate distance.

Fracture of the ulnar shaft with separation of the interosseous ligaments
frequently results in luxation of the radius. The radial displacement is cranial, so that it interferes with flexion at the elbow. The radius can be
replaced manually but it luxates as soon as the digital pressure is released.
This is frequently referred to as a Monteggia fracture-dislocation.

Open reduction and fixation with a screw to the ulna produces a sound
repair (Fig. 150). The skin is incised on the cranio-lateral side of the forearm
and the radius exposed by separating the common and lateral digital extensors. The bone is drilled in a caudo-lateral direction so that both the radius
and ulna will be tapped. The bit should be slightly smaller than the screw. It

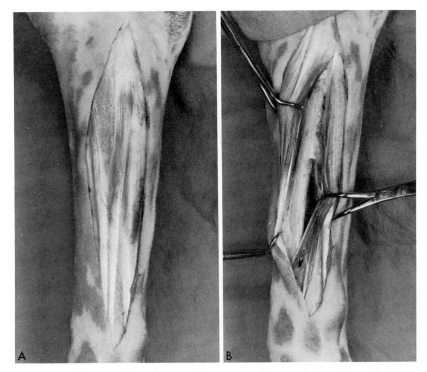

Figure 149. The cranio-lateral approach to open reduction of the radius and ulna. A, The
skin incision. B, Separation of the common and lateral digital extensors, exposing the radius.

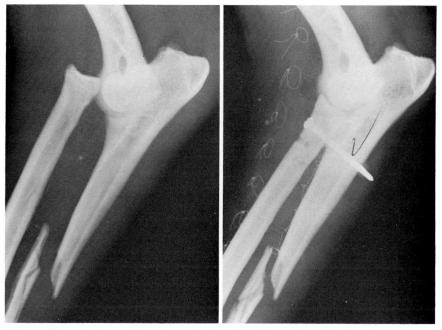

Figure 150. Fracture of the ulna with luxation of the radius. This has been repaired by means of a stainless steel screw. A slightly shorter screw could have been used and the insertion made about one inch distal to the present site. The two drill holes below the screw indicate unsuccessful attempts to align with the ulna.

is difficult to estimate the exact length of screw required, but it should be long enough to contact the caudal cortex of the ulna. A rough estimate can be made by measuring the roentgenogram. Both Ormrod and Hickman prefer the caudal approach, in which the screw is placed through the ulna first and then through the radius. The preferable way of repairing this fracture-luxation, according to Ormrod, is to repair the ulnar fracture with an intramedullary pin and then fix the radius in place by circumferential wiring around the radius and ulna.

FRACTURES OF THE CARPUS AND METACARPUS

Carpal fractures are extremely rare except those occurring in the accessory carpal (pisiformis). This fracture is seen occasionally in greyhounds as a result of racing; usually it affects the outside limb.

A small fragment is separated from the distal side of the carpal bone, thereby causing an intermittent lameness. The lameness appears to be most prominent after racing and will disappear after resting, only to reappear again when the limb is exerted.

Bateman recommends the resection of the extremely small muscle (abductor digiti quinti) which arises on the distal face of the carpal bone. This tiny muscle, by its contraction, distracts the fracture and thereby prevents healing. A small skin incision is made on the lateral side of the carpus, starting at the pisiformis and extending distally over the tendinous portion. The muscle is elevated through the incision and a small section is removed.

Inasmuch as fractures of the metatarsus and phalanges have been discussed under Fractures in the Pelvic Limb, the reader is referred to Chapter 5, since information concerning fractures in the metacarpus and phalanges is identical to that mentioned in the previous chapter.

Fractures of the volar sesamoids at the distal end of the metacarpus should be mentioned, since they have been reported in greyhounds. It is not uncommon for these sesamoids to fracture transversely and to displace into the interosseous space, thereby causing lameness. Bateman advocates removal of these fractured sesamoids by making a vertical incision directly over them and dissecting them free.

REFERENCES

Bardens, J. W.: Bone stapling to correct anterior deviation of the radius. Illinois Vet., 8:9, 1965.

Bateman, J. K.: Fracture of the accessory carpal (pisiform) bone in the racing greyhound and its repair. Vet. Rec., 62:155, 1950.

Bateman, J. K.: Fractured sesamoids in the greyhound. Vet. Rec., 71:101, 1959.

Few, A., and Hoerlein, B.: Traumatic luxation and fracture of the carpus. Auburn Vet., 17:68, 1961.

Frost, R. C.: The closed reduction and repair of radio-ulna fractures in the dog. J. Small Animal Pract., 6:197, 1965.

Knight, G. C.: Internal fixation of the fractured lateral humeral condyle. Vet. Rec., 71:667, 1959.

Knight, R. W. J., and Pittaway, E. M.: Fracture of the olecranon process of the ulna in a dog. Vet. Rec., 67:754, 1955.

Leighton, R.: Permanent intramedullary fixation of the distal fractures of the radius and ulna in dogs. Southwestern Vet., 16:97–100, 1963.

Mostosky, U. V., Cholvin, N. R., and Brinker, W. O.: Transolecranon approach to the elbow joint. Vet. Med., 54:560–568, 1959.

Nielson, H. M.: Recent experiences in the treatment of fractures by surgical methods. Vet. Rec., 61:791–795, 1949.

Ormrod, A. N.: Limb fractures in the dog and cat. IV. Fractures of the forelimb. J. Small Animal Pract., 7:155–162, 1966.

Roach, L. M.: A new method for repairing fractures of the olecranon. J.A.V.M.A., 127:120–121, 1955.

Robinson, G. W.: Supracondylar fracture of the canine humerus. J.A.V.M.A., 152:1673–77, 1968.

Schmidtke, D., and Schmidtke, H.-O.: Treatment of supra- and intercondylar fractures. J. Small Animal Pract., 10:593–597, 1969.

Schroeder, E. F.: Fractures of the humerus in dogs. N. Am. Vet., 15:31–40, May, 1934.

Stader, O.: Intracondylar and supracondylar fractures of the distal end of the humerus. N. Am. Vet., 38:156–159, 1957.

Sumner-Smith, G.: Fixing intercondylar fractures of the humerus of the dog. Vet. Rec., 74:293, 1962.

Vincent, Z.: Observations on the use of stainless steel Rush pins and Steinmann pins in the treatment of fractured radius and ulna in the dog. J. S. African Vet. Med. Assoc., 34:451–456, 1963.

Walker, R. G., and Hickman, J.: Injuries of the elbow joint in the dog. Vet. Rec., 70:1191–1194, 1958.

Chapter 7

Fractures of the Skull, Spine and Pelvis

FRACTURES OF THE SKULL

Incidence

Fractures of the flat bones of the skull occur often and are more frequent in cats than in dogs. Most of these fractures are seen in the mandible; it alone accounts for 6.3 per cent of all fractures. The maxillae are fractured only 0.7 per cent of the time, and the bones of the calvarium account for 1.4 per cent of all fractures. Other bones of the skull are fractured occasionally.

For the sake of convenience in describing fractures in this region, the bones of the skull have been divided into three groups. The mandible, because it is the most frequently fractured, has received the most attention. Bones of the face are treated as a second group and bones of the calvarium as a third group.

Etiology

The usual cause of skull fractures is collision with moving automobiles. They also result from kicks, usually in farm dogs. Some occur following a jump or fall from a high place. Mandibular fractures are sometimes the result of fights. With the exception of some fractures in the rami of the mandible, skull fractures are the result of direct force.

Pathology

The flat bones of the calvarium are composed of an outer and an inner layer of cortical bone, between which lies a layer of varying thickness composed of cancellous bone containing many veins. When fractures occur, the outer layer separates along a few fissure lines (Fig. 151) and often

173

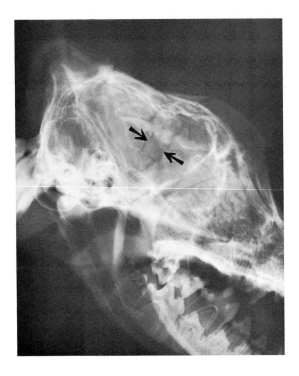

Figure 151. Fracture of the parietal bone. Note the fissures which are typical of fractures in this region.

depresses, but the inner layer tends to shatter. Hemorrhage can be abundant from the cancellous layer as well as from the bone and brain coverings. Damage to the brain, either direct or indirect, can occur in this region and may assume more importance than the fracture itself. Sometimes the brain injury is the result of direct force from the fracture, or it may be due to pressure from the ensuing hemorrhage (Fig. 152). There may also be disturbance of the circulation to the brain or to the flow of cerebral spinal fluid. Mortality is high because of the increase in intracranial pressure and the infection which frequently complicates these cases.

Fractures of the mandible occur most frequently at the symphysis and are compound. Those occurring in the body are frequently compound on the buccal and lingual surfaces but seldom through the skin. Fractures of the ramus are less likely to be compound and displacement is less pronounced. Severe laceration of the masseter and temporal muscles can occur when the fracture line is through the ramus.

Fractures of the facial bones tend to produce more hemorrhage because they surround an extremely vascular area. Displacement of these bones is seldom great but is usually sufficient to cause damge to adjacent tissues.

Signs

When a fracture of the calvarium is suspected, one should watch closely for any change in consciousness if the patient is not already unconscious. Depending on the type of injury, there should be some change in respiratory

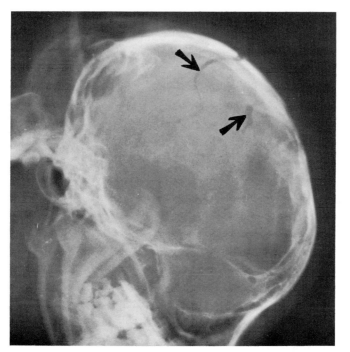

Figure 152.   Fracture of the skull. This injury resulted in fatal hemorrhage in the brain.

and pulse rate. Some part of the skull may be depressed or there may be swelling due to subcutaneous bleeding. Crepitus can seldom be elicited; furthermore, it is dangerous to attempt this type of palpation. It is not uncommon to have a fracture without external damage to the skin. Bleeding from the ears and nose and ecchymosis beneath the conjunctiva are common signs.

Fracture of the facial bones usually is evidenced by distortion and hemorrhage from the mouth and nose. Malocclusion is frequently seen. The patient often has great difficulty in breathing.

The signs are usually obvious in fractures of the mandible. Movement of the jaws is distorted, there is malocclusion, and when both the ramus and symphysis are fractured there is rotation with lateral displacement on that side. Symphysial fractures alone may allow some rotation on both sides. Fractures through the body affect the occlusion of the teeth rostral to the injury, and if the fracture is bilateral the rostral jaw may drop. Dropping of the entire jaw usually indicates fracture of the ramus or luxation.

Diagnosis

Examination of the mouth yields sufficient evidence for a diagnosis of mandibular fractures, except those located in the ramus. Other fractures of the skull require roentgenograms taken in several planes. Sometimes fractures of the calvarium are difficult to depict unless the head is rotated so that other bones of the skull do not interfere. Fractures in the upper rami also require careful exposure.

Prognosis

Perhaps the most important factor to bear in mind in evaluating a head injury is the damage and possible sequelae to the contents rather than the bony structure itself. Injury to the brain and infections which may reach brain coverings should be carefully considered, along with the primary fracture.

A guarded prognosis should be given when bones of the calvarium are fractured. These bones heal slowly, sometimes requiring from two to three months. In the adult dog, replacement of large bone losses does not take place. If there is pus at the fracture site, elevated temperature, or coma, the prognosis is poor. Fractures of one or more of the facial bones may result in some deformity but otherwise the outcome is good.

Mandibular fractures of the body and symphysis, except in cases of osteodystrophia fibrosa (rubber jaw), can usually be given a good prognosis, but fractures of the ramus should be prognosticated with caution.

Treatment

Needless to say, bones of the calvarium that have sustained fractures without displacement should not be disturbed but should be protected from further damage. Depression fractures require relief as soon as possible to alleviate pressure on the underlying brain tissue and to prevent laceration from sharp fragments.

Asepsis is extremely important when working so close to the brain.

Swelling and edema of the brain can be controlled somewhat by administering 50 per cent sucrose solution intravenously prior to surgery. However, 50 per cent sucrose may be toxic to the kidneys and therefore should only be given for 24 hours. The sucrose is administered in 100 ml. doses every six hours.

Hoerlein has found Mannitol to be very effective in reducing brain edema in dogs without appreciable elevation of cerebrospinal fluid pressure and without toxicity to the kidneys. He recommends 1.0 gm./kg. of body weight given intravenously in a 20 to 25 per cent solution over a period of 10 to 15 minutes.

Corticoids are indicated for about two weeks.

Extreme caution should be exercised in administering anesthetics to these patients, since their tolerance is usually low. Morphine is contraindicated because of its depressive action.

The skin incision is made directly over the area and the bone fragment is exposed. A splinter forceps works well for grasping the fragment, which should be lifted without prying. Care must be taken not to tip the opposite edge inward so that it inadvertently places pressure on the underlying soft tissues. Blood clots should be carefully removed from the brain covering and the area gently cleansed with saline solution. Care should be taken not to produce hyperemia by rough handling or the use of excessively warm washing solution. If the fracture occurs over a sinus, gentleness is not quite so important, but should nevertheless be practiced. Large fragments should be sutured in place unless the periosteum is completely disrupted. This is done by drilling small holes and lacing across the fracture line with chromic catgut, silk, or fine wire.

Bones of the face can usually be manipulated into position with the fingers. Sometimes healing takes place without fixation but it may be necessary to use wire. When the fracture is unilateral, anchorage can be obtained by drilling a Kirschner wire or a bicycle spoke through the maxilla caudal to the canine teeth. The heavy wire can then be wrapped around the canine teeth after the fracture is reduced. This method can also be used when the hard palate is split. If slightly modified, it can be used in other facial fractures.

Fractures of the mandible (Fig. 153) require less ingenuity to reduce than those of the face, but present a far greater problem of immobilization. Several methods of fixation have been proposed for the mandibular symphysis, but probably the simplest and most rigid is the insertion of a pin across the symphysis just caudal to the rostral mental foramen. This places the pin rostral to the canine teeth but in solid cortical bone without damage to nerves and blood vessels. It firmly binds the two segments together so that

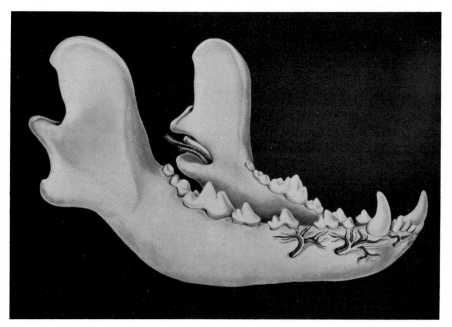

Figure 153. The mandible, showing the location of the principal blood vessels in the rostral end.

there is no movement between them. The fracture can be held in firm
apposition by placing a wire around the ends of the pin and tightening it
across the labial surface below the lower incisors (Fig. 154). The pin ends
are then cut so that about ¼ inch protrudes on either side. The pin and wire
are removed when healing is complete.

Amman's method for fixation of symphysial fractures is to pass a double
strand of stainless steel wire around the mandible (Fig. 155). The wire is
inserted in the gum at the labial surface of one canine by means of a curved
needle and emerges at the midline beneath the chin. It is then reinserted in
the same opening and pushed through the soft tissues until it emerges at the
labial surface of the opposite canine. The double ends can then be twisted
around the canine on either side. To further stabilize the fixation, a wire can
be placed across the mouth by anchoring to the wires attached to the canine.

Schunick and Richman have recommended the use of small vitallium
plates with small wood-type screws for both symphysial and body fractures.
These plates are made in two shapes (Fig. 156). They are applied directly to
the gum except in compound fractures. In the latter case the gum is reflected
and the plate applied directly to the bone. The gum flap is then resutured to
cover the bone.

Wiring of the canine teeth is commonly practiced, but it is inferior to
pinning because it does not ordinarily produce complete immobilization.
This method is better adapted to cats and small dogs because in them

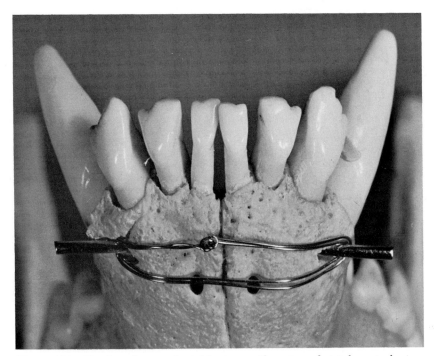

Figure 154. Fixation of a symphysial fracture with a pin and stainless steel wire.

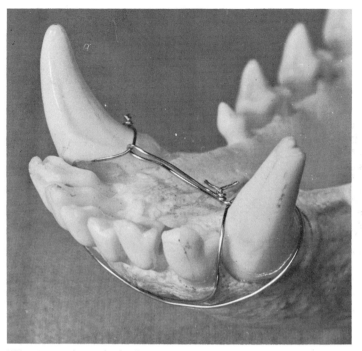

Figure 155. Amman's method of using wire for fixation of symphysial fractures of the mandible.

displacement pressure is slight. The wire may be passed directly around the teeth after notching the base or it may encircle the mandible just caudal to the canine teeth in a "figure eight" fashion (circumferential wiring) (Fig. 157).

Fractures through the body of the mandible, whether unilateral or bilateral, can usually be held in good apposition by half pinning. The Kirschner splint is easily adapted to the mandible. The pins should be set as low as possible so that they will penetrate more cortical bone and also avoid the alveolar nerves and blood vessels. Because the cortical bone is thin in the mandible, it is important that the pins be well seated to avoid loosening.

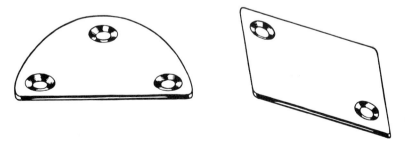

Figure 156. The type of plates used by Schunick and Richman for mandibular fractures.

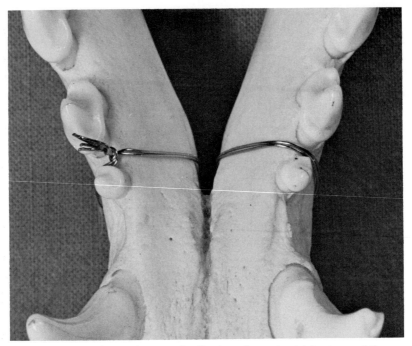

Figure 157. Circumferential wiring for fixation of symphysial fractures of the mandible. This wire is placed in form of a figure eight.

When properly applied, half pinning will give the most secure fixation. The same rules for half pins apply here as in the long bones. For detailed information, see Chapter 4, Methods and Materials.

Intramedullary pins can be used in body fractures with good results. The pins should be small and flexible enough to follow the medullary cavity. They should be started in the short segment and inserted the full length of the body. If the pin is to be started in the rostral segment, the lower lip is pushed downward and a site selected which is in line with the mandibular body both longitudinally and horizontally. Sometimes this point may be well toward the midline and deep on the labial surface. When the caudal segment is pinned first the point of insertion is on the ventral border just beneath the angular process of the ramus. This does not present a very wide target. To avoid slipping and soft tissue damage, the pin should be started slowly, with very mild pressure, until it is well engaged.

The protruding pin should be cut as short as possible when the cranial approach is used, but the end may be left longer on the caudal approach. Migration can be prevented by attaching a coupling and covering it with tape. Intramedullary pins in the mandible should be removed after healing whenever possible. When intramedullary pinning does not completely immobilize the fracture, further support may be had by applying a leather muzzle.

Various methods of wiring body fractures have been proposed and some have merit because of their versatility. Others should be used only as last resort measures because of the damage they inflict on surrounding tissues. Thomson beaded wires can be applied in comminuted fractures in conjunction with half pinning. They will provide anchorage or traction in a medio-lateral direction. Two wires applied to the same segment in opposite directions will immobilize that segment because of the counter-traction of the beads (Fig. 158).

Heavy (20 gauge) stainless steel wire is sometimes used to wire between teeth on opposite sides of a fracture and between the lower and upper arcades. This is referred to as intermaxillary wiring. Because of the shape of the dog's teeth, it is frequently difficult to prevent the wires from slippping even when the loop method is used (Fig. 159). With the loop method, a small loop is twisted into a strand of wire and is then placed between two adjoining teeth so that the loop is at the interdental space. Both ends of the strand are passed through the loop after encircling the teeth. The direction of the ends is then reversed so that they again encircle the teeth and are fastened by twisting together. When a similar loop has been anchored on the opposite side of the fracture or in the opposite arcade, a wire can be passed through the two loops for anchorage. If necessary, several anchorages can be made on either side of the fracture, as well as across the fracture, and the wiring can be strengthened by placing two loops at each spot.

Fractures in the ramus are the most difficult mandibular fractures to reduce and immobilize. The heavy musculature interferes with accurate

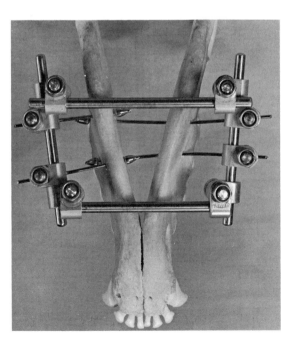

Figure 158. The application of Thomson beaded wires to the body of the mandible.

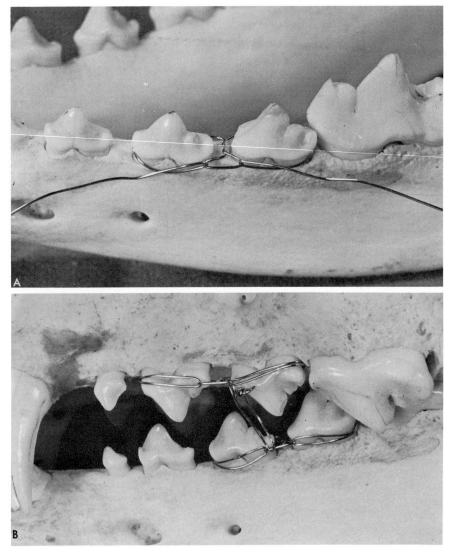

Figure 159. Intermaxillary wiring for fixation of mandibular body fractures. A, A loop in the wire is placed between two teeth and the ends carried around the teeth, passed through the loop, and then reversed so that they encircle the teeth and fasten on the medial side. B, Upper and lower arcades wired together after each arcade has been wired as shown in A.

reduction and unless the fracture is near the angle of the jaw, the upper segment is almost impossible to hold in place. Half pin splintage will provide a reasonably good fixation if it is carefully applied and the fracture is not too high. Immobilization of the jaw will aid considerably, and this can be accomplished by intermaxillary wiring. A leather muzzle provides reasonably good assistance, and since this can be removed at feeding time it eliminates the necessity of feeding with a tube.

The author has found that the upper segment of a fracture through the ramus can be controlled by using Thomson beaded wires. Actually it is an adaptation of the half-pin method of splinting (Fig. 160).

Palpation of the fracture site and the upper segment of the mandible can easily be accomplished with the index finger inside the mouth. The rostral edge of the ramus is located just beneath the oral mucous membrane. A small stab wound is made to expose the bone about 0.5 cm. caudal to the rostral edge and dorsal to the fracture line. This site should be over the thickest part of the ramus.

A Thomson beaded wire is drilled through the bone and punctured through the skin. Before seating the bead against the bone, the trailing end of the wire should be cut close to the bead and the cut edge smoothed with a file. The wire is then pulled tight against the bone. A second wire is placed in similar fashion about 2 or 3 cm. dorsal to the first. This distance will vary with size of the dorsal segment. The mucous membrane should cover the beads after they are in place. It may even be necessary to place a stitch or two to insure proper coverage.

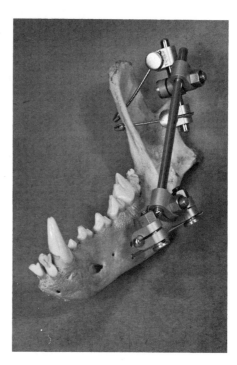

Figure 160. Placement of Thomson beaded wires in conjunction with the Tower splint for controlling fractures through the ramus of the mandible.

A pin bar is attached by couplings to the wires about 1 cm. external to the skin of the cheek. Before tightening, the couplings are pushed toward the ends of the pin bar so that the wires are diverging in the dorso-ventral direction. This prevents movement of the bone segment in the medio-lateral direction.

The second pin assembly, consisting of pins number 3 and 4, is placed on the lateral side of the mandibular body. It should be placed as far ventral as possible and the pins should penetrate both cortices. This assembly will be at an angle to the first, but the two can easily be fastened together with one or two extension bars.

Aftercare is the same as for any half-pin splintage. Ample time should be allowed for healing because this type of fracture does not ossify rapidly.

In general, aftercare in mandibular fractures depends largely on the type of fixation. In uncomplicated fractures where intramedullary and half pin splintage is employed, the food should be soft but does not have to be liquid. Whenever wiring alone is used, the food should be liquid, even though the jaws can be opened, since wiring usually is not strong enough to withstand the pressure of chewing. Concentrated meat broth, milk, and gruel can be used as liquid foods.

Daily cleansing of the mouth should be practiced so that infection can be avoided. This also provides an opportunity for inspection to see that alignment is maintained.

FRACTURES OF THE SPINE

Definition

In the dog and cat, fractures of the spine fall into two natural categories, those in which cord damage is present or imminent and those in which cord damage is not probable. There is always a possibility of cord involvement if the vertebral body, spinous process, or mammillary body is fractured. Fracture of the transverse process is less likely to involve the cord. Cord damage may be the direct result of the fracture or it may occur from dislocation or displacement of the vertebral bond. Fractures may occur anywhere along the spine but seem to be most common in the caudal thoracic and in the lumbar vertebrae. Other areas, in descending order of frequency, are sacral, coccygeal, and cervical. Fractures of the cervical vertebrae probably occur less frequently because there is more or less free movement in this area. Spinal fractures constitute 5.7 per cent of all fractures seen in our clinic.

Etiology

In cases of body fracture and compression, the cause is usually an indirect force which brings about a violent flexion of the spine. When the transverse process is fractured, the cause is usually a direct force. If there is

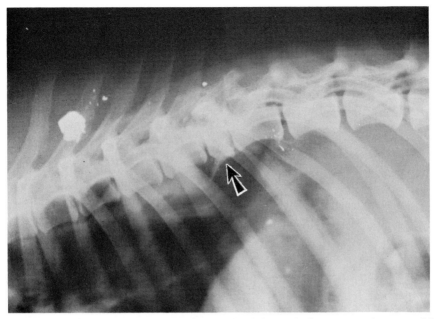

Figure 161. Compression fracture of the body of the tenth thoracic vertebra, caused by a bullet which can be seen to the left. The cord was undamaged.

displacement or luxation, the cord may be severed or subjected to extradural pressure. In many such cases there is irreparable damage. If, on the other hand, the result is a compression fracture of the body, the cord may not be too severely injured (Figs. 161 and 162). Hemorrhage is common at the site of fracture and often causes undesirable pressure. If one of the articular processes, such as the mammillary process, is fractured, the vertebra may luxate, thereby causing severe damage to the cord (Fig. 163). Except for damage to nerve roots, fractures of the transverse process seldom seriously endanger the nervous system.

Signs

With cervical fractures, the patient is frequently unable to stand. There is spasticity of the head muscles and wrinkling of the skin over the forehead. Cyanosis is common and the breathing may be rapid. Movement of the head in any direction will usually cause pain and crying. Nystagmus and subconjunctival hemorrhage are usually present.

When the fracture is in the thoracic or lumbar region, the forelegs are extended and rigid and the hindlimbs are flaccid. The back is arched at an acute angle over the fracture area, with some lateral deviation if the fracture displacement is great. The patient has an anxious expression but seldom indicates pain unless palpated. Pain can be elicited at the fracture site and in the abdomen in lumbar fractures. Cyanosis may also be present in these cases. If only the transverse process is fractured, the signs, aside from pain,

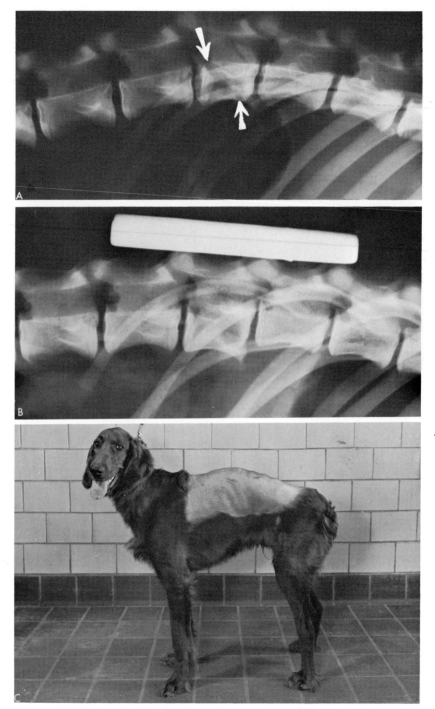

Figure 162. Compression fracture of the body of the first lumbar vertebra with slight displacement. A, Preoperative roentgenogram. B, Postoperative roentgenogram with bone plate fixation. C, The patient three weeks after surgery.

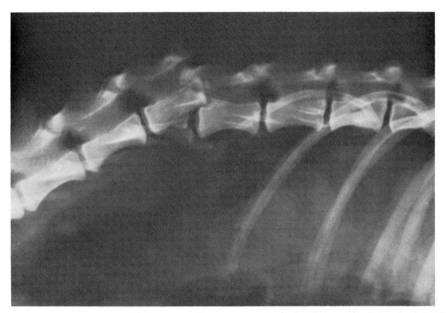

Figure 163. Fracture of the mammillary process with displacement of the third lumbar vertebra and severance of the spinal cord.

may be obscure. There may be asymmetrical paralysis if the ventral root is damaged or under pressure. Coccygeal fractures usually produce paralysis of the tail (Fig. 164).

Diagnosis and Prognosis

The diagnosis can be definite only after roentgenograms in at least the lateral and ventro-dorsal positions have been studied. According to Gage, if the radiographic displacement is less than one-third the diameter of the canal and there is adequate neurological function, surgical correction may be attempted.

The prognosis should be guarded in all fractures of the body and articular processes even though the signs at the moment do not seem serious. Such cases have to be judged on their potential rather than actual damage. It is quite possible for the displacement to shift or for a luxation to develop which would result in severance of the cord. Reflex actions of the feet following a stimulus have no bearing on the integrity of the cord. Wagging of the tail and positive, purposeful movements of the legs is good evidence that the cord is not severed. Compression fractures of the body usually respond if the initial damage to the cord is not great. A good prognosis can usually be given when there is an uncomplicated fracture of the transverse process. If the cord is severed, the patient is a hopeless paraplegic.

Treatment

Little has been done to advance the treatment of fractured vertebrae. Body casts of plaster of Paris or Aire-Cast have been used, but these alone

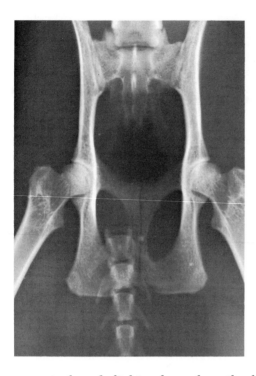

Figure 164. Fracture of a coccygeal vertebra in a cat with gross separation and paralysis of the tail.

seem to be of slight value when the body and articular processes are involved. Early surgical treatment usually is indicated. In most cases this would be within 24 to 48 hours. Cervical fractures require early decompression and immobilization. Hoerlein, who has investigated the treatment possibilities more extensively than anyone else, recommends the use of internal fixation supported by external splintage. According to him, bone grafts require long periods of time before they offer much support. In the meantime, some type of external support must be maintained. Bone plates with screws do not hold well in the spinous processes but bone plates with bolts applied to the dorsal spines provide excellent fixation (Fig. 165). Some external splintage in addition to the vitallium plates is helpful, especially in larger dogs.

A long incision must be made over the spinous processes and the muscles separated from them so that one or more spines on either side of the fracture are completely exposed. A No. 1 or 2 spinal fusion plate, Wilson type,* is then placed alongside the spines to serve as a template for drilling on one side of the fracture. A plate is then placed on either side of the spines and a bolt put in place. When the fracture has been reduced, it is held in position by an assistant while a spine on the opposite side of the fracture is drilled and bolted. After these bolts have been tightened it may be possible to further strengthen the fixation by bolting another spine.

---

*The Wilson type spinal fusion plate is vitallium and manufactured by Austenal of New York City. The bolts furnished for this plate are also vitallium and have lock nuts. Stainless steel plates, Auburn type, are manufactured by Richards of Memphis, Tennessee. Bolts for these plates are stainless steel.

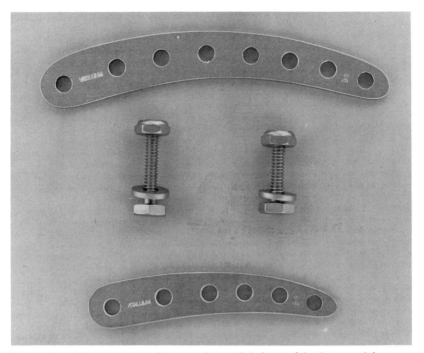

Figure 165. Wilson type spinal fusion plate with bolts used for fixation of the spine.

The reduction is best accomplished by grasping the spinous processes with heavy forceps. In some cases it is possible to drill through the process close to the body with a bicycle spoke. This can then be fitted with a cross-bar which serves well for lifting but does not give the exact control that forceps will provide. Traction and counter-traction are applied so as to distract the fracture. When this has been achieved, the upper segment of the spine should be forced downward while the other segment is forced upward until the fracture is reduced.

After the incision has been closed and covered with a sterile dressing, a body cast should be applied to further strengthen the internal fixation. Aftercare consists of constant nursing to be sure that the skin and appendages are kept in good shape so that decubital sores do not develop and that the bladder and bowels are kept empty. Exercise should be provided in the form of an exercise cart to prevent excessive muscular atrophy. Keeping the animal on its feet for several hours a day will also help in preventing decubital sores.

FRACTURES OF THE RIBS AND STERNUM

Fractures of the thoracic cage occur less frequently than one might suppose. They constitute about 1.4 per cent of all fractures. Some may escape detection, however, because of the support given by unbroken ribs and the fact that very little distortion results from the fracture of a single rib. Sternal fractures (Fig. 166) are far less common than rib fractures (Fig. 167). The cause is always some form of external violence.

Displacement is usually not great unless a number of ribs are broken. Quite often the pleura is ruptured, but the real danger lies in puncture of the lung. When this occurs, there may be subcutaneous emphysema or the case may terminate fatally with collapse of both lungs. Considerable hemorrhage can accompany the fracture if the intercostal vessels are damaged, and this may lead to hemothorax.

When there is severe damage, the signs are usually acute. The patient is cyanotic, the respiratory rate is greatly increased, and there is a hacking cough. If several ribs are fractured, the chest is often distorted. In fractures of the sternum, the chest may be flat. Swelling over the area is extremely variable. Pain can generally be elicited on palpation, but crepitus is frequently more difficult to produce.

The diagnosis is often difficult without the aid of a roentgenogram. This should be taken in lateral recumbency with the suspected side toward the cassette and with short exposure time to eliminate movement of the ribs.

The prognosis is usually good unless there is lung damage. In such a case it may vary from guarded to grave.

A body cast is used when several ribs are involved, and the patient is rested as much as possible. Chest movements are painful and retard healing. Anything that minimizes these movements is beneficial. Healing requires two to three weeks in young animals and three to eight weeks in older animals.

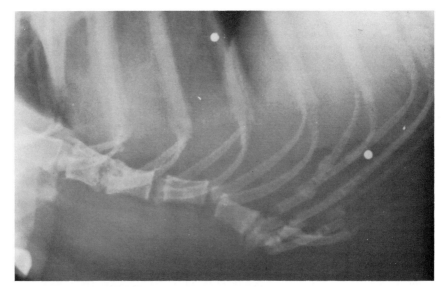

Figure 166. Fracture of the sternum. The result of crushing with an automobile. The shotgun pellets are incidental.

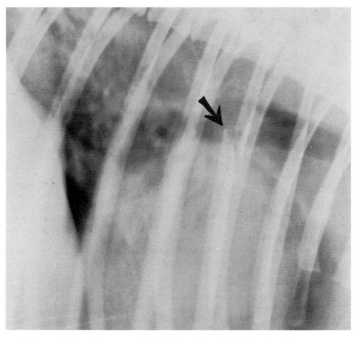

Figure 167.   Fracture of the fifth rib with slight displacement.

FRACTURES OF THE PELVIS

The term "pelvic fracture" usually encompasses fractures of any of the three pelvic bones as well as those involving the acetabulum. Although the true pelvis includes the sacrum and four coccygeal vertebrae, fractures of these bones have been included under Fractures of the Spine. Separation of the sacro-iliac ligament is frequently included in the syndrome of pelvic fractures although not specifically referred to as a fracture. Pelvic fractures are common, especially those involving the ilium; other bones of the pelvis are less commonly fractured. Frequently, more than one bone is involved. Symphysial fractures are seen most frequently in young dogs but sacro-iliac separation is seen in dogs of all ages. Of the fractures seen at our clinic, pelvic fractures comprise 22.6 per cent, and of these 80 per cent involve the ilium. Ilial fractures usually occur from a direct force applied laterally, and ischial fractures often result from a direct force from a caudal direction.

Fractures of the pelvis are often multiple but seldom are compound. Displacement is variable and seems to depend somewhat on the violence of the original force. Muscular tension has some effect on the amount of displacement but apparently plays a secondary role. Soft tissue damage can be severe, particularly if the fracture is in the region of some of the larger nerves or adjacent to organs in or near the pelvic canal, such as the rectum, bladder, or vagina. Hemorrhage is frequently noticeable beneath the skin on the ventral side, forming large ecchymotic blotches. If nerve damage is extensive, there may be paresis or paralysis which may be unilateral or bilateral.

When pressure is applied to the tuber coxae or the tuber ischii, it should be met with resistance in the normal pelvis. Mobility when the ischii are palpated indicates fracture of the pubic symphysis and possibly of the body of the ischium. In the same manner, the integrity of the ilium and the sacro-iliac articulation can be tested.

With fractures of the shaft or wing of the ilium the patient is usually able to sustain weight but walks with great difficulty (Fig. 168). Sometimes the leg is held in flexion. There is often a flattening of the rump with an inward rotation of the leg. When the body of the ischium or the tuber ischii is fractured there is usually intermittent lameness for five to seven days (Fig. 169). In those cases involving separation of the symphysis, and especially when bilateral sacro-iliac separation is also present, the patient is often unable to rise or bear weight on the hind legs (Fig. 170). This is not ordinarily caused by paralysis, but rather by a lack of stable anchorage from which the muscles can apply leverage. The animal lies in a sprawled position, making leg movements when encouraged but unable to support its hind parts. Fractures through the acetabulum are characterized by a unilateral lameness of varying degree. The limb is abducted and joint movement is limited. The trochanter major is depressed and the leg appears shorter than its mate. The femur head is displaced inward, producing an intrapelvic luxation (Fig. 171), and the hip may appear flattened. Pain is a constant sign

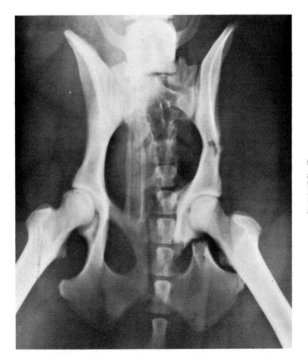

Figure 168. Fracture of both the ilium and the ischium as well as the acetabular branch of the pubis. This usually creates a severe lameness because of lack of anchorage for the hip.

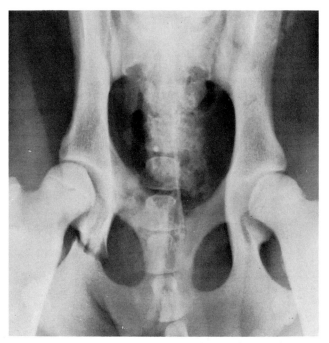

Figure 169. Fracture through the body of the ischium. There is also a fracture of the acetabular branch of the pubis on the same side.

Figure 170. Multiple fractures of the pelvis, including a sacro-iliac separation, a fracture of the ischium, and a fracture of the acetabular branch of the pubis. When such an injury is bilateral, the patient is unable to rise.

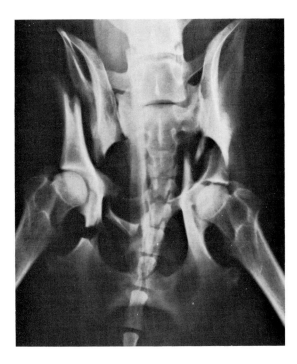

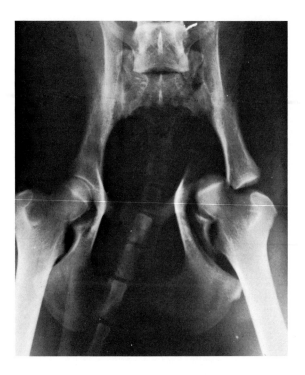

Figure 171. Fracture of the acetabulum with intrapelvic luxation of the femur.

in most pelvic fractures, but crepitus may be difficult to elicit except in impacted fractures of the acetabulum.

A tentative diagnosis can frequently be made by rectal palpation, but all findings should be confirmed by roentgenogram. Whenever possible, the patient should be positioned so that a symmetrical view of the entire pelvis is obtained. This is best done by making a ventral-dorsal exposure with the hindlegs extended caudally without rotation.

If the fracture does not involve the hip joint, the prognosis is fair to good. If a deformity of the pelvic canal is likely to result, a guarded prognosis should be given, particularly if the patient is a brood bitch or one likely to be used for breeding. Severe damage to the hip joint or adjoining structures calls for a guarded or a poor prognosis.

Treatment

Until recent years, very little attention had been given to the treatment of pelvic fractures. Rest and nursing care were sufficient for those fractures in which displacement was slight and the injury uncomplicated. Some animals with more extensive fractures recovered after a long convalescence, but with gross deformities. Nature alone was responsible for many "miraculous" recoveries.

Rest and good nursing care are still the treatment of choice in those cases in which displacement is slight, the patient is young, and slight pelvic deformities will be of little consequence. More heroic measures are usually reserved for those fractures in which there is gross displacement that will result in unsightly deformity or interference with the natural function of the animal.

With the advent of bone pinning, methods for the control and fixation of these fractures were found. It has long been known that casts are usually contraindicated in pelvic fractures because they tend to compress the pelvis and cause excoriation of the skin through the retention of moisture and movement of the limbs.

Stader, Knowles, Olsen, and others have reported good results with the use of half pin splints. The main principle involved in half pin fixation of the pelvis is the selection of a sound, well-aligned bone area for anchorage to which fractured segments can be tied. Insertion of pins must be made in those parts of the pelvic bones having the heaviest cortex so that the pins are less likely to split the bone or become loosened because of inadequate cortical bone. For the best holding power the pins should be inserted at converging or diverging angles. Further stabilization may be had by inserting Kirschner wires, Thomson beaded wires, or bicycle spokes through parts of the pelvis near the surface so that a clevis can be formed with a pin bar of the half pin splint, thereby preventing the pins from retracting.

With certain modifications in angle and placement, the following points on the pelvis can be used for half pin insertion, either single or double as the fracture may require or the case allow.

THE ILIUM.   The tuber sacrale, particularly in the region of the caudal dorsal iliac spine. Pins should be inserted ventro-medially so that the body of the sacrum is engaged. This will give a very firm anchorage.

The body of the ilium on the dorsal aspect of the greater ischiatic notch. The bone is deep and slopes ventro-caudally. Care should be taken to place the pins cranial to the acetabulum (Figs. 172 and 173).

THE ISCHIUM.   The tuber ischii is comparatively thin and therefore pins placed parallel to the long axis do best.

The body of the ischium on the dorsal aspect of the lesser ischiatic notch. This insertion should not be attempted without incising the skin and exposing the bone by blunt dissection. The presence of the sciatic nerve makes this pin placement hazardous unless the point selected is immediately cranial to the tuber ischii.

The areas for pin placement form the corners of a rectangle which can be connected together, cross-braced, or diagonally braced with extension bars according to the number and location of the fractures (Figs. 174 and 175). It should be pointed out that many times these pin assemblies loosen when placed in pelvic bones, and therefore anything that will improve the anchorage is helpful. As indicated in Chapter 4, threaded pins serve no useful purpose. Along the dorsal iliac spine and the tuber ischii, where the bone is near the skin surface, wires may be of assistance. They are easy to insert in these areas, and by fastening the ends over the pin assemblies the half pins can be held securely in place.

Kirschner wires and Thomson beaded wires may be used in place of half pinning when the fracture site is near the surface. The skin over the fracture

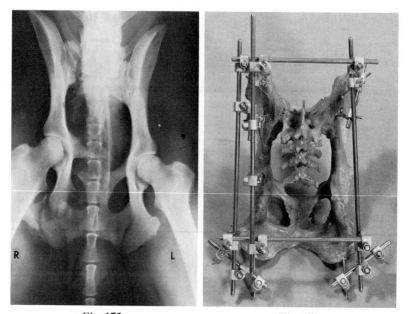

Fig. 172   Fig. 173

Figure 172.   Multiple fractures of the pelvis with a free ilium on the right side.
Figure 173.   A method of controlling the fracture shown in Figure 172.

area is incised and the bone exposed on either side of the fracture site. One
or two wires are placed transversely through the bone on either side of the
fracture. The number will depend upon the amount of traction required. The
wires are bent so that they will protrude through the incision or through stab
wounds in the skin. After closing the incision and covering it with sterile
gauze pads, a Richards Plasti-Coat splint is laid over the area so that the
wires will protrude through the holes. The Plasti-Coat splint is aluminum,
with a foam padding and numerous holes for ventilation. It should be
applied with the padding toward the skin.

A padded aluminum strip is placed between the wire loop ends with the
padded side down. All wire ends should now be paired and each pair
tightened by twisting until the desired tension is obtained. Care should be
taken to avoid pressure necrosis of the skin.

It is sometimes possible with impacted fractures of the acetabulum to
apply a Thomas splint with good results. The fracture is reduced with
straight traction on the leg. When the impaction has been reduced, the leg is
placed in a Thomas splint with either skin traction or skeletal traction. This
traction keeps the femur in place while at the same time the ring of the
splint places counter-traction on the bodies of the ischium and ilium.
Usually 10 days to two weeks with this type of splintage is sufficient to
stabilize the hip, and healing will continue unaided if the patient receives
careful attention.

Cawley and Archibald have suggested the use of intramedullary pins.
This method is best applied to single fractures, particularly those occurring

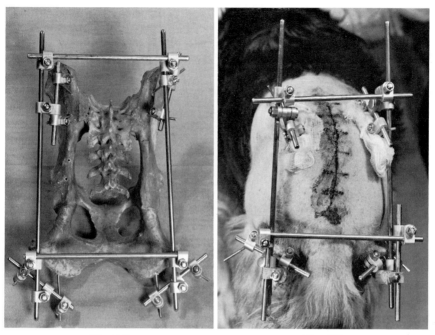

Fig. 174   Fig. 175

Figure 174.   Extension bars placed in a rectangle. Note the pins in the ilium are at right angles to those in the ischium. Strength is gained by such placement of the pins, and the holding power of the pins themselves is increased by inserting them into the heaviest cortical bone.

Figure 175.   Position of the splint on a patient.

in the wing or body of the ilium and in the body of the ischium. The pinning is done in conjunction with open reduction.

For fractures occurring in the wing of the ilium, an incision is made from the middle of the tuber sacrale to the trochanter major. After the bone over the dorsal iliac spine has been exposed by blunt dissection, the periosteum is incised and separated from the bone to expose the fracture site.

The intramedullary pin is inserted on the medial aspect of the cranial dorsal iliac spine so that it will traverse the bone parallel to its long axis. When the pin reaches the fracture, it is reduced and the drilling continued until the pin is firmly set in cortical bone cranial to the acetabulum. The pin is cut close to the bone and the periosteum and fascia are closed over the bone.

Retrograde pinning may be used if the fracture is in the body of the ilium. The skin incision begins at the dorsal midline and, passing just cranial to the trochanter major, continues two-thirds of the way along the lateral surface of the thigh. This is the same incision site as is used for exposure of the hip joint, and the underlying tissues are separated in the same way. After exposure of the bone at the fracture line, an intramedullary pin is inserted into the cranial segment near its dorsal border and is drilled until it appears beneath the skin at the tuber sacrale. The pin is then exposed and withdrawn far enough to allow the fracture to be reduced. It is then driven into the caudal segment until firmly embedded. The pin is cut as short as possible and covered with skin. The incision is closed in the usual manner.

It is frequently possible to align fractures of the body of the ischium by closed reduction. An intramedullary pin can then be introduced into the tuber ischii and directed dorso-medially so that it follows the body of the bone until it embeds in cortical bone, usually just dorso-medial to the acetabulum. Great care should be taken that the pin is kept in the bone and not allowed to damage the sciatic nerve.

The method used in repairing the pelvis should be chosen carefully, the most conservative but still adequate method taking precedence.

REFERENCES

Alexander, J. E., Archibald, J., and Cawley, A. J.: Pelvic fractures and their reduction in small animals. Mod. Vet. Pract., *43*:9, 41–45, 1962.

Alexander, J. E., Archibald, J., and Cawley, A. J.: Fractures of the acetabulum. Mod. Vet. Pract., *43*:10, 39–43, 1962.

Alexander, J. E., Archibald, J., and Cawley, A. J.: Multiple fractures of the pelvis in small animals. Mod. Vet. Pract., *43*:11, 33–36, 1962.

American Medical Association: Primer on Fractures. 6th ed., Special Exhibit Committee on Fractures. New York, Paul B. Hoeber, Inc., 1951.

Amman, K. and Müller, A.: Zur fixationstechnik der unterkiefersymphysenfraktur des hundes. Berl. U. Münich tierärztl Wchnschr., *69*:447–448, 1956.

Bancroft, F. W., and Marble, H. C.: Surgical Treatment of the Motor-Skeletal System. 2nd ed. Philadelphia, J. B. Lippincott Co., 1951, Part II.

Brinker, W. O.: Fractures of the mandible. Vet. Med., *44*:53–55, 1949.

Cawley, A. J., and Archibald, J.: Intramedullary pinning of pelvic fractures. I. The ilium. N. Am. Vet., *36*:747–751, 1955.

Clark, H. B., and Hayes, P. A.: A study of the comparative effects of "rigid" and "semirigid" fixation on the healing of fractures of the mandible in dogs. J. Bone Joint Surg., *45A*:731–741, 1963.

Dammrich, K.: Pathology of growth and reconstructive processes in the cranium bones in animals (dogs and cats). Dt. tierärztl Wschr., *73*:590–596, 1966.

Gage, E. D.: Surgical repair of a fractured cervical spine. J.A.V.M.A., *153*:1407–1411, 1968.

Hoerlein, B. F.: Clinical spinal conditions of the dog. Vet. Med., *51*:575–580, 1956.

Hoerlein, B. F.: Methods of spinal fusion and vertebral immobilization in the dog. Am. J. Vet. Res., *17*:695–709, 1956.

Hoerlein, B. F., Few, A. B., and Petty, M. F.: Brain surgery in the dog—preliminary studies. J.A.V.M.A., *143*:21–29, 1963.

Hofer, W., and Danwalder, M.: Treatment of mandibular fractures in cats. Schweitz. Arch. Tierheilk., *104*:559, 1962.

Hohn, R. B., and Jones, J. M.: Lateral approach to the canine ilium. An. Hosp., *2*:111–113, 1966.

Hurov, L.: Spinal fracture plating. Can. Vet. Jour., *4*:128–132, 1963.

Johnson, H. W., and Farquharson, J.: Fracture of the mandible and its treatment in the dog. J.A.V.M.A., *94*:647–649, 1939.

Knowles, A. T., Knowles, J. O., and Knowles, R. P.: Clinical application of splints in fractures of the pelvis. Vet. Med., *44*:308–310, 1949.

Olsen, M. L.: Canine Surgery. 4th ed. Evanston, Ill., American Veterinary Publications, Inc., 1959.

Pozzi, L.: Treatment of fractures of the mandible in the dog. Atti. Soc. Ital. Sci. Vet., *14*:214, 1960.

Schmidtke, H-O.: Über die behandlung von unterkieferfrakturen bei hunden mittels intraoraler draht und kunststoffschiewing. Deutsch. tierärztl Wchnschr., *63*:215–220, 1956.

Schunick, W., and Richman, S.: A new technique for treatment of fractures of the mandible in dogs. Vet. Med., *35*:356–358, 1940.

Zedler, W.: Fracture of the pelvis in dogs and cats. Berl. Münch. tierärztl. Wschr., *74*:265, 1961.

PART THREE

Luxations

Luxation and dislocation are synonymous terms referring to the separation or change in relationship of the articular surfaces of bones. The word "luxate" is taken from the Latin "luxare," which means to dislocate. The author prefers this term because of its compactness, especially when used with compound words designating joints, e.g., coxo-femoral luxation *versus* coxo-femoral dislocation.

Articular separations are classified as *luxations* (dislocations), *subluxations* (incomplete dislocations), and *total luxations* (complete dislocations) according to the degree of separation and displacement. A luxation can be defined as a complete separation of the articular surfaces at a joint. A subluxation is a partial separation or a change in relationship with some of the articular surfaces still in contact (Fig. 176). A total luxation is the complete separation of a bone at all articular surfaces, for example, luxation of the scaphoid bone or central tarsal. Luxations are also classified as *acute* and *chronic* or *recurrent* depending upon whether the displacement is a single, recent occurrence, a luxation of long standing, or a recurrence following reduction. Both *simple* and *compound* luxations can also occur, but most of the luxations in dogs and cats are simple.

In general, the joints involved in luxations are synovial joints, vertebral joints being the one exception. Luxations of the fibrous joints have been treated as fractures in this book since functionally such joints promote

199

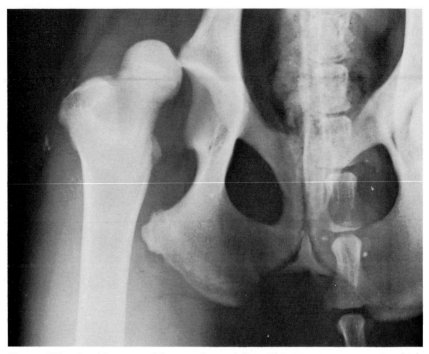

Figure 176. A subluxation of the coxo-femoral joint. This is an extreme case in which only the smallest areas of the articular surfaces are in contact.

rigidity rather than provide movement. Discussion of fibrous joint separations will therefore be found under Part Two, Fractures.

In general, the distal bone comprising a joint is spoken of as being luxated when there is separation at the joint. Exceptions to this are the patella, the scaphoid, and a vertebra.

It has been the experience of our clinic that luxations occur far less frequently than fractures, the proportion being one to five. Many times fractures and luxations occur in the same injury. This is particularly true of the spine, in which a luxation seldom occurs without fracture of one or more articular processes.

Acute luxations occur as the result of direct or indirect force; chronic or recurrent luxations are generally the result of degeneration of the restraining structures of the joint, such as the joint capsule or ligaments. Force may have played a part in the original injury which brought about degeneration, but it is only a minor contributing factor in the ultimate luxation. A good example is furnished by the femorotibial joint, where the cranial cruciate ligament degenerates and ruptures, thus allowing the tibia to subluxate. Congenital deformities may also be responsible for luxations at times, as demonstrated in certain patellar luxations.

The articular surfaces are made to withstand force, and the structures surrounding the joint are primarily designed to hold these surfaces in apposition. When excessive force is applied to a joint from an unnatural direction the capsule tears and the ligaments rupture. Ligaments readily give way under stress applied with leverage at an unaccustomed angle. Small fragments of bone may separate at the points of insertion of the ligaments, and in some cases the articular surface may be damaged. Blood vessels and nerves are commonly injured in the process, so that hemorrhage, swelling, and paralysis frequently follow a luxation. Damage to soft tissue components of the joint usually complicates the healing process far more in luxations than in fractures because these structures form the main support of the joint and they are slow to heal. In very short ligaments where reapposition is virtually impossible (cruciate), healing does not take place. Arthritic changes are common in joints in which chronic or recurrent luxation has occurred. Periarticular bone formation may impede the action of the joint and in some cases produces ankylosis, especially in hinge-type joints.

DIAGNOSIS

Great care should be given to the diagnosis, since in certain joints a fracture may be confused with a luxation and in others a luxation may be mistaken for a sprain. On the whole, fractures and luxations are easily distinguishable, but irreparable damage can be done by attempting to reduce a luxation which is actually a fracture. By the same token, ignoring a sprain which is actually a luxation may result in a crippled patient.

The signs are severe pain, limited movement, deformity, loss of function, swelling, and deviation in length of the extremity. These vary in degree and extent according to the location of the luxation and its severity. For instance, luxation of the patella produces very few of these signs and then only in a mild way. On the other hand, luxations of vertebrae produce all the signs except deviation in length.

Changes in position of the bone ends may be noted on palpation or may be indicated by position of the limb. Variations in the length of extremities are common in coxo-femoral luxations and, to a lesser degree, in elbow luxations. Crepitus is not a prominent sign but may be present in a muffled form which is usually slightly different from that encountered in fractures. Muscle spasm increases the rigidity and may increase the deformity. It is a contributing factor in the limitation of movement as well. Roentgenography provides confirming evidence and will uncover complications such as fractures.

TREATMENT

Reduction should not be undertaken until the full extent of the injury is known and the exact relationship of the articulating bones is established. In addition to the physical examination, one or more roentgenograms should be taken in order that the luxation can be properly visualized. Excessive force should not be necessary even in old unreduced dislocations. Manipulation should be confined to those movements necessary for diagnosis and those of a purposeful nature that will lead to reduction. Too often the joint is subjected to much aimless jostling in the name of treatment. In unreduced luxations, there are often adhesions which require some force to separate. This should be done if possible by movements and manipulations which will not involve the joint. If muscle spasm is extensive it must be overcome by gradual traction so that the muscles become fatigued. Seldom are the muscles in unreduced luxations as inextensible as they are in long-standing fractures. If joint cavities are impaired by the interposition of soft tissues, an open reduction may be indicated. It may also be necessary to open the joint when a luxated bone has become lodged by penetrating muscle or fascia.

Luxations should be reduced at the earliest opportunity appropriate to the general condition of the patient. Occasionally, a simple reduction can be accomplished immediately without danger to the patient, but most reductions must be delayed until danger from shock or internal hemorrhage has passed. Luxations which are reduced early are less likely to recur, all other things being equal; however, reduction should not be undertaken without due consideration for the patient. Except for those rare instances when immediate reduction can be effected, a general anesthetic is indicated. The anesthesia should reach a surgical plane so that the patient is entirely relaxed and all pain is abolished. This will facilitate the mechanics of reduction by overcoming much of the muscle spasm. Local anesthetics are less effective, particularly when used alone, because the patient is still apprehensive. A short-acting barbiturate is frequently sufficient, but longer-acting anesthetics should be used if the procedure is likely to be prolonged or the aftercare is likely to require rest and quiet for a few hours.

Some luxations will require fixation following reduction, and these will be considered under the specific treatments. In other cases, if the ligament and capsule damage is not great the reduction may be self-retaining. In all instances, whether splinted or not, it is important that the patient be allowed to recover from the anesthetic while lying on the uninjured side so that no unnecessary strain is put on the injury when he attempts to rise. It may even be necessary to use some sedation or tranquilization for a few days in order to prevent undue strain. Ambulation and mild acts of exercise should be encouraged fairly early in the healing process to prevent muscle atrophy and to improve circulation to the injured parts.

Chapter 8

Luxations in the Pelvic Limb

COXO-FEMORAL LUXATION (LUXATION OF THE HIP)

Coxo-femoral luxations are usually classified according to the relationship the femur head bears to the acetabulum following dislocation. They are cranial, dorsal, caudal and intrapelvic. Since intrapelvic luxation occurs only when there is a fracture of the acetabulum, it has also been discussed under pelvic fractures. It is recognized that, with the exception of intrapelvic luxations, the position of the femur head must be lateral to the acetabulum, and therefore this descriptive term has been purposely omitted. According to our statistics, 39 per cent of all luxations seen in the dog and cat involve the hip joint. The most common hip luxation is the cranial, with the dorsal next in frequency and the caudal a poor third.

Etiology

An indirect force transmitted through the femur on an adducted joint is the usual cause of luxation of the hip. This force may be caused by many things, the automobile being the most frequent agent. When force is transmitted on an abducted joint the result could be an intrapelvic luxation with fracture of the acetabulum. A more likely result is a capital or neck fracture of the femur. The intrapelvic luxation occurs more frequently as the result of a direct force against the joint from a lateral direction.

Luxation occurs when the leg is extended, as in jumping or falling, with the weight suddenly shifted so that the center of gravity lies lateral to the hip. The ligamentum teres is long and does not confine the femur head to the acetabulum, so that such a force has a shearing action on this ligament. Furthermore, the joint capsule is relatively weak and tears under strain. The ultimate position of the femur head largely depends on the amount of flexion at the hip at the time of impact.

203

Pathology

With few exceptions, the capsule is torn. In the cranial luxation, the ligamentum teres is ruptured and the femur head rests on the lateral surface of the body of the ilium. It is craniolateral and possibly slightly superior to the acetabulum (Fig. 177). In dorsal luxations, the femur head rests above the acetabular rim in a dorso-lateral position (Fig. 178), and in caudal luxations it is found caudal and lateral to the acetabulum along the body of the ischium (Fig. 179). Muscles in the immediate vicinity are damaged and are the source of hemorrhage. With a cranial luxation, most of the damage is in the ilio-psoas and the rectus femoris. The gluteal muscles suffer most when the luxation is dorsal, and when it is caudal the quadratus femoris is damaged. In some cases of caudal luxation the sciatic nerve may be paralyzed through pressure or trauma. Hemorrhage fills the acetabular fossa, along with fragments of capsule and remnants of the ligament. This gradually organizes into a fibrinous mass which may interfere with reduction if allowed to remain more than a few days. At other times, the torn capusle will heal as a diaphragm across the acetabulum if the luxation remains unreduced. Damage to the articular surface of either the femur head or the acetabulum can occur, but this is quite unlikely to produce ankylosis unless the periarticular tissues are severely damaged and the resulting exostosis is excessive.

Circulation to the head is maintained through the continuity of bone

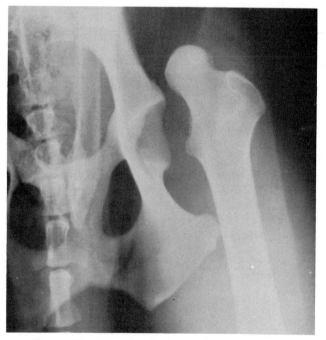

Figure 177.   Cranial coxo-femoral luxation in a dog.

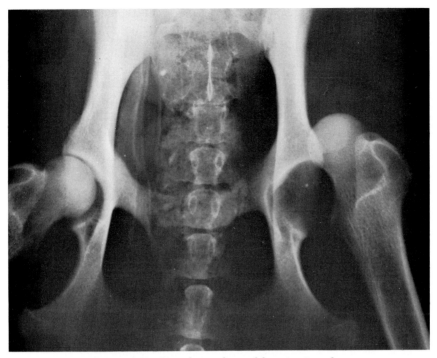

Figure 178. Dorsal coxo-femoral luxation in a dog.

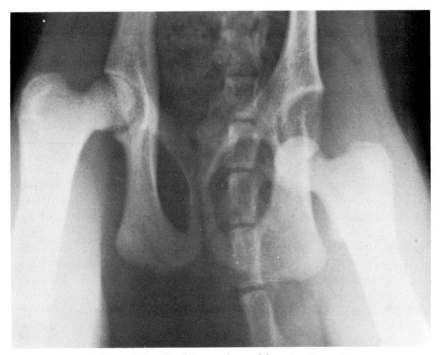

Figure 179. Caudal coxo-femoral luxation in a cat.

even though the capsule and ligament are separated. Necrosis of the head is seldom seen even in young dogs. When it does occur, it can usually be traced to a fracture of the neck that went undiagnosed.

Signs

If possible, the patient should be examined first in a standing position. Observations should be made from a few feet distant concerning the hip conformation and a comparison made between the injured side and the sound side. Look for elevation of the trochanter and any abnormal carriage of the limb. The limb is abducted in all cases except in caudal luxation. The thigh is rotated outward in cranial luxation and inward in caudal luxation; in fact, the inward rotation is so pronounced that the stifle and toes usually point toward the opposite forelimb. In dorsal luxation and in intrapelvic luxation rotation is slight.

In those patients that can move without harm to the injured parts, a similar examination is made while they walk. Determine the weight-bearing capacity of the limb, whether it is abducted or adducted, and whether it is rotated inward or outward.

When the findings indicate that a further examination is necessary, the patient is anesthetized for closer inspection and palpation of the injury. Usually, a short-acting barbiturate is sufficient to relieve pain and muscle spasm as well as to overcome apprehension and struggling on the part of the patient. A methodical examination of the hips should then be made as follows:

1. Palpate the trochanter major. This is often the key to a correct diagnosis. Determine whether it is elevated or depressed. The trochanter is elevated if, on palpation, it appears to be dorsal to a line drawn from the tuber coxa to the tuber ischii. Elevation of the trochanter is seen in all luxations except the intrapelvic. It is also seen in fractures of the femoral head and neck. It may also be present in multiple pelvic fractures in which the acetabulum is separated both cranially and caudally.

Next, determine whether the trochanter is rotated. Normally, the trochanter can be felt facing outward at right angles to the long axis of the body. A comparison with the trochanter on the sound side is often helpful. Both should be equidistant from the tuber ischii. If the trochanter is nearer to the tuber ischii than its mate it is said to be rotated outward. If it is farther away, it is rotated inward. Outward rotation is seen in cranial luxations and inward rotation in caudal luxations.

Finally, the trochanter is used to test the soundness of the hip joint. Palpate deeply with the thumb fixed between the trochanter major and the tuber ischii while the femur is rotated around its long axis. In a sound joint the trochanter major will pinch the thumb when rotated toward it, but the luxated femur will slide away when the trochanter begins to press against the thumb. Other movements, such as abduction, adduction, flexion, and extension will be of assistance in detecting luxations, although some of the signs are also present in fractures of the femoral neck. All of these signs are based on the fact that in the normal hip the femur head is seated in the acetabulum and is a fixed pivot. When the thigh is moved, the trochanter describes a definite arc which does not vary. Fractures in or near the joint and luxations destroy this fixed point so that the feeling of precise movement is lost. Of these movements, perhaps the one with most differential value is abduction. It meets with resistance in luxations but seldom in femoral neck fractures.

2. Compare the legs for length (Fig. 180). The patient is placed in dorsal recumbency and the hind legs extended by grasping the hocks. On extension of the legs vertically, both will be approximately the same length when the luxation is cranial or caudal, but if the luxation is dorsal the injured leg will be shorter. In a like manner, if the legs are extended horizontally caudad, they will be essentially the same length in dorsal luxation but the injured leg will be shorter in cranial luxation and longer in caudal luxation. The leg in intrapelvic luxation is the same length or slightly shorter in both positions.

Diagnosis

A roentgenogram is necessary to confirm the physical findings and to eliminate the possibility of other complications. Usually a ventrodorsal view is sufficient. The hind legs should be extended parallel with the body and elevated to the level of the hips. A lateral view is seldom of any value. For each individual diagnosis, the findings may be summarized as follows:

CRANIAL LUXATIONS. (1) Thigh abducted, rotated outward. (2) Slight weight bearing (standing). (3) Trochanter elevated, rotated outward. (4) Leg length shortened horizontally.

DORSAL LUXATIONS. (1) Thigh abducted, very slight outward rotation. (2) Slight weight bearing (standing). (3) Trochanter elevated. (4) Leg length shortened vertically.

CAUDAL LUXATIONS. (1) Thigh adducted, rotated inward. (2) No weight bearing. (3) Trochanter elevated, rotated inward. (4) Leg length lengthened horizontally.

INTRAPELVIC LUXATIONS. (1) Thigh abducted, rotation variable. (2) No weight bearing. (3) Trochanter depressed. (4) Leg length shortened slightly both horizontally and vertically.

Prognosis

With the exception of the intrapelvic luxation, the prognosis is good provided reduction is accomplished within a reasonable time (two days). Unreduced or chronic recurrent luxations require a guarded prognosis insofar as normal function of the joint is concerned, but they may form pseudo-arthroses which will provide functional recovery, if not perfect conformation and gait.

Great care should be exercised in making a prognosis when the sciatic nerve is injured either from pressure of a caudal luxation or through attempts at open reduction. Unless the nerve has been severely damaged, a slow

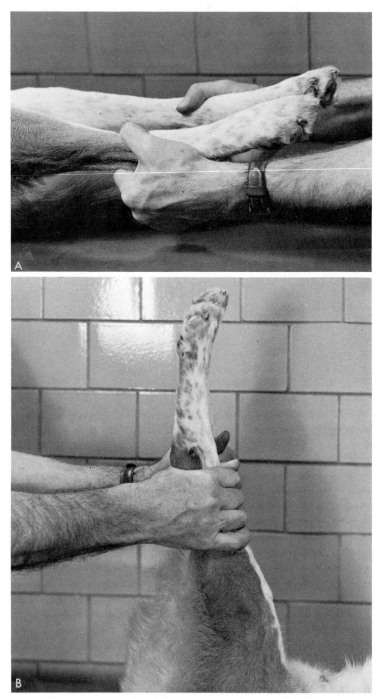

Figure 180. Comparing length of legs. A, The horizontal position. B, The vertical position.

recovery can usually be expected. The owner should warned, however, that the paralysis can be permanent, in which case the leg remains useless with the stifle depressed and the phalanges flexed.

Fractures around the rim of the acetabulum are often cause for a poor prognosis because of the difficulty of retaining the femur head. As a matter of fact, a prognosis should be withheld in any case in which reduction is difficult to maintain until such time as the outcome can be fairly certain.

Treatment

Reduction of coxo-femoral luxations should be carried out as early as possible. At times delay is expedient when there is danger from shock or the use of an anesthetic. General anesthesia is recommended whenever possible so that the muscles are relaxed and the patient is under control. If the reduction appears to be a simple one, it can sometimes be accomplished while the animal is still under anesthesia from the roentgenogram.

The patient is placed in lateral recumbency with the luxation uppermost. Some sort of anchorage is then applied to the pelvis. This may be in the form of a well-padded rope passed on the medial side of the thigh, over the body, and fastened to the undercarriage of the table. An oversized Thomas splint or the Gordon extender works well (Fig. 181). These are held in place by pressing against the abdomen of the operator. If an assistant is available he may either manually restrain the pelvis or use the aforemen-

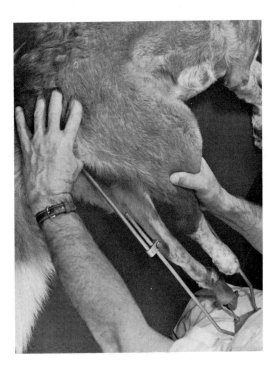

Figure 181. Reduction of a coxo-femoral luxation using the Gordon extender for anchorage. Note position of the operator's hand and rotation of the thigh.

tioned rope. Whatever restraint is put on the pelvis, the injured leg should remain free so that it can be manipulated.

If the luxation is cranial or dorsal, the leg is grasped just below the stifle and flexed. At the same time, the operator places his other hand so that the fingers are over the trochanter and the thumb is beneath the thigh in the region of the acetabulum. The leg is abducted and rotated inward so that the cranial aspect of the femur will lie medially. In most instances, the femur head will now be located dorsal to the acetabulum with the shaft and neck cranial. By applying traction at the stifle and guiding the head with the opposite hand, the luxation should reduce. This maneuver may have to be repeated several times because either the muscles are not sufficiently relaxed or the acetabulum is missed on the first attempt. Usually reduction can be accomplished by this method, particularly if the luxation is recent.

When the luxation is caudal, the procedure is the same except that the leg is rotated outward so that the femur head is moved cranial. If this fails to bring the head into close proximity to the acetabulum, the rotation can be reversed and the head forced cranial with the thumb of the opposite hand.

The reason for this procedure is to place the femur head in such a position that it can be easily guided into the acetabulum without sliding cranial or caudal along the rim. It also prevents unnecessary leverage being put against the head and neck as it is pulled over the rim during the final stage of reduction.

Sometimes the head returns to normal position with enough force to produce a decided thud. This usually means that the retaining structures of the joint are not too badly damaged and the femur head will remain in position without further treatment. At other times, the head repositions without sound or vibration of any sort. Such reductions should be regarded with suspicion, since they are likely to reluxate.

Reductions should be confirmed and tested for soundness. The thigh and trochanter should regain their normal position. The leg length should correspond to that of its mate in all positions. Abduction of the leg should be unhampered but there should be definite resistance to moderate pressure of the femur against the acetabulum. According to Schroeder, about 20 per cent of all hip luxations will be recurrent. In fact, some do not reduce by manual manipulation. In recent luxations, this is usually due to extensive damage to muscles, joint capsule, ligamentum teres, and in some instances to the glenoidal cartilage.

If reduction is accomplished and the luxation recurs during the testing for soundness, closed reduction and fixation will usually give satisfactory results. One of several methods can be used.

Ehmer has described a method of bandaging and casting the leg in flexion, which can be used either unilaterally or bilaterally. The bilateral cast is variously referred to as the "butterfly cast," the "spread cast," or the "airplane cast." In this method the bandage is applied in a figure eight and impregnated with sodium silicate. The leg is flexed and bandaged in this position; we have found orthopedic padding and tape to be excellent materials for this purpose. It should be further supported by bandaging to the body. Some abduction will be required, and the leg should be rotated inward in cranial luxations and outward in caudal luxations. It is helpful in this regard to bandage around the thigh toward the body for inward rotation and around the thigh away from the body for outward rotation. When severe abduction is required, both legs are bandaged, abducted, and taped to a board or metal frame placed across the rump. This board should be well padded. Bindings should be placed on the ventral side of the pelvis to support the body weight, and these too should be padded, particularly for males where the bindings pass over the penis and scrotum (Fig. 182). We have devised runners for this splint, made from aluminum rod, which keep the body slightly elevated and avoid soiling (Fig. 183). Ordinarily, such a cast is kept on only long enough for the femur head to become established (five to 10 days), since long periods of confinement may be detrimental.

Schroeder used the Thomas splint with a high degree of success. Skeletal traction could be applied with bone tongs or a bicycle spoke attached to the cranial bar of the splint by means of heavy rubber bands (Fig. 184). He also devised an aluminum abduction rod which was attached to the splint and to the body so that the leg could be held in abduction with proper rotation and a fixed degree of flexion.

In line with this method of fixation, Obel devised a method of hip flexion to force the femur head in a medial direction. He found that the force required to luxate the femur increased from 2 kg. to 12 kg. when the angle between the femur and the body was reduced from 80° to 0°. The metatarsus

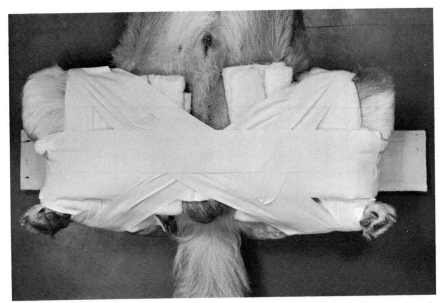

Figure 182. An Ehmer type cast for holding the legs in horizontal flexion. This shows how the bindings should be applied to the male.

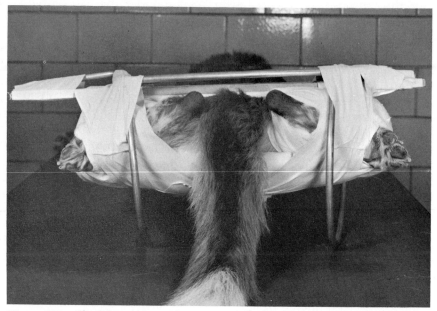

Figure 183.   The Ehmer cast with runners applied so that the patient can move about more easily.

is bandaged to prevent injury and then is covered with plaster. A leather belt is taped to this cast. When the luxation is reduced, the belt is drawn tight around the body so that the hip is in acute flexion and the plantar surface of the foot is pressed close to the body.

Stader recommended a closed reduction with half pin fixation. A similar method has been used by Brinker, employing the Kirschner splint. Half pinning can be used in several ways to maintain fixation of the coxo-femoral joint. The anchorage is made in the pelvis with a pin or pins in both the ilium and the ischium. If the Stader pin bar is used, it can be inverted so that the pins are divergent. Anchorage can also be obtained by pinning on either side of the acetabulum and connecting these pin bars. A pin is then inserted into the femur on the lateral aspect just below the trochanter major. When this pin is connected by means of a swivel to the anchoring bars, lateral pressure can be applied to the femur head (Fig. 185). This type of fixation inhibits only abduction and adduction, allowing flexion and extension at the hip while fixing the femur head in the acetabulum.

DeVita uses a method of retaining the femur head by creating a barrier dorsal to the femoral neck. A long intramedullary pin is inserted through the fascia immediately ventral and adjacent to the tuber ischii. It is then passed over the femur neck just lateral to the head and dorsal to the joint capsule and pushed forward until it contacts the wing of the ilium. Slight digital pressure is put on the pin to prevent slipping as it is embedded in the bone for anchorage of the cranial end. Great care must be taken in passing the pin that (1) the luxation is reduced, (2) the leg is adducted, and (3) the sciatic

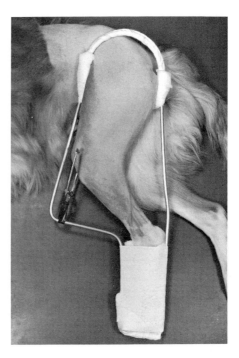

Figure 184. The Thomas splint with bone tongs applied to the distal femur, thereby supplying fixation for a hip reduction.

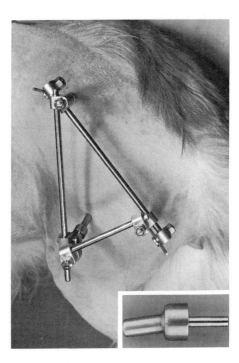

Figure 185. The use of a triangle half pin assembly and a swivel joint to hold a chronically luxating hip in place. Inset shows the swivel enlarged.

nerve is not injured. The progress of the pin can usually be checked by digital palpation. Migration of the pin can be controlled by inserting a half pin into the tuber ischii at right angles to the DeVita pin and coupling the two pins together (Fig. 186). This method of femur head retention is quite effective, except in cats, in which the wing of the ilium does not flare enough for the pin point to engage the bone.

Yarborough has modified this technique by inserting two pins at right angles to each other over the neck of the femur (Fig. 187). One pin is applied to the body of the ilium cranio-dorsal to the joint but from a caudo-lateral direction. The other pin is applied to the body of the ischium caudo-dorsal to the joint from a cranio-lateral direction. These pins are so placed that they cross each other dorsal to the femoral neck, thereby creating a barrier to luxation. The ends of these pins remain exposed and must be removed when the joint is healed.

Whenever difficulty is encountered in the closed reduction of recent luxations, and in most unreduced luxations, there should be no hesitation to perform an open reduction. It serves as an exploratory operation as well as a therapeutic measure. Very often the interfering factor is fibrous granulation tissue in the acetabulum or a torn capsule blocking the reposition of the femur head.

Occasionally the femur head is entangled in muscle, joint capsule, or fascia. Frequently both the acetabulum and the femur head require the surgical removal of granulation tissue. Usually this can be separated from the

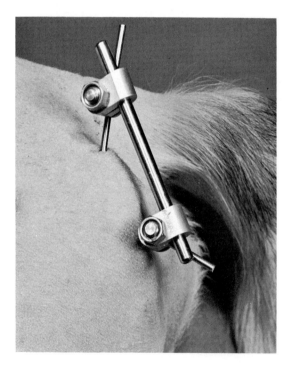

Figure 186. The DeVita pin in place with half pin anchorage.

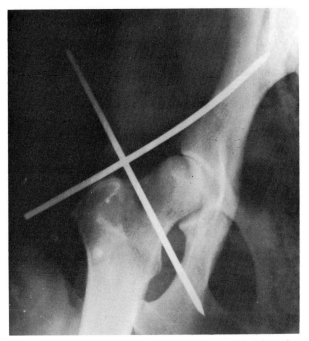

Figure 187. Yarborough's method of retaining the femur head in the acetabulum.

underlying cartilage with comparative ease. It should be done as carefully and gently as possible. We use gauze sponges to rub away the final fragments.

In performing an open reduction, care should be taken to preserve all structures, especially those having a direct bearing on reconstruction of a sound hip. The skin incision and approach to the joint should be dorsal, extending from the dorsal midline to the middle of the thigh. This prevents disturbance of the sciatic nerve, which lies on the caudal side of the femur. Bottarelli has described this approach, but his exposure is far too small for an unhampered repair. The fascia lata is separated by sharp dissection from the biceps femoris, and the tensor fascia lata is split. The gluteal muscles are transected close to the trochanter major, allowing a ¼-inch tendinous stump to remain attached to the bone. The femoral nerve and the cranial femoral artery should be located and retracted to avoid injury. In many instances landmarks may be somewhat obscured by the luxation. The acetabulum will be more difficult to locate in cranial luxations because it lies ventral and caudal to the femur head and is therefore covered by the shaft. The joint capsule is torn, as well as some of the muscles. In unreduced luxations some of these structures are not easily identified in the presence of fibrous tissue.

The same approach can be used in dorsal and caudal luxations and, because of the location of the femur head, the acetabulum is more accessible. By rotating the femur outward, the head can be exposed for complete inspection before reduction.

Archibald et al. have described the open approach in three cases. Two were successful and one was not. The capsule was not sutured in any of these, but the two successful cases were splinted.

It has been our experience that open repair is highly successful provided that the acetabulum is intact and the hip was normal before luxation. In most instances splintage is unnecessary provided that: (1) The capsule is securely sutured (Fig. 188). This is frequently impossible because it is so badly lacerated. Fascia in the immediate area should then be used as a substitute. (2) Muscles and fascia supporting the joint are carefully repaired and securely fastened. The suture material should be of a non-absorbable type so that the suture line will remain strong. Simple interrupted sutures disrupt more easily than mattress or retaining type sutures. (3) The patient is careful with the leg. If the animal is hospitalized and kept away from other animals and excitement which might tend to make him forget the injured leg, he will usually not use it vigorously until it is strong enough. Tranquilizers may also be of some benefit. Using the leg with moderation should improve the healing.

Knowles has proposed a method of reconstrucing the ligamentum teres by the use of fascia or plastic. Stainless steel wire can also be used (Fig. 189). This method need not be a permanent repair of the ligament, since the important structures requiring repair are the capsule and surrounding muscles. Repairing the ligament therefore retains the femur head long enough for these structures to heal. The procedure in this case is to perform

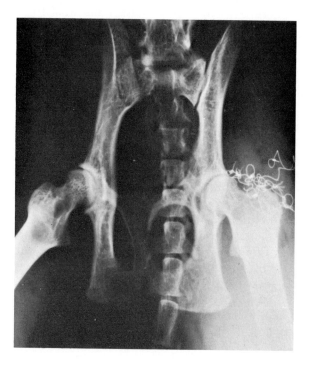

Figure 188. A reduced chronic luxation in a cat showing the sutures placed in the capsule and in the gluteal attachments (multifilament stainless steel wire).

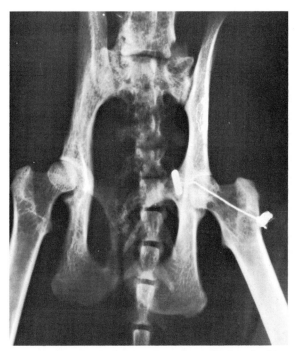

Figure 189. A stainless steel toggle applied to the hip.

an open reduction. While the leg is held in a normal position, following reduction, a drill jig is used to align the bit. From a starting point at the base of the trochanter major, the bone is drilled through the center of the neck, head, and acetabulum with a 5/32-inch bit. A toggle is threaded with fascia or heavy plastic suture and installed on the end of a cannula. With the leg held in a fixed position, the bit is removed and the cannula introduced. When the toggle has reached the pelvic canal, a stylet is pushed through the cannula to disengage the toggle and permit it to lock in the pelvis. As soon as the toggle is secure the cannula is removed. The trochanter major is drilled sagittally and one end of the fascial strip is threaded through the hole. The femur head is pushed firmly into the socket and the fascial ends are tied. The tying should be firm but not tight enough to hinder movements of the joint. If a stronger ligament is required, heavy plastic suture or stainless steel wire may be used. The stainless steel will break in time but usually not until the joint has healed. Another toggle or button can be used for anchorage on the lateral side of the femur instead of tying through the trochanter, if it is so desired.

We have modified this method somewhat by the following procedure: The toggle is made from 1/4-inch sections of intramedullary pin drilled transversely and threaded with stainless steel wire. After the bone drilling is completed, the femur head is lifted from the socket and the toggle is thrust through the opening in the acetabulum with alligator forceps. As soon as the toggle is secure, the alligator forceps are thrust through the femur opening from the lateral side and the wire is retracted. Another toggle is then threaded on the wire. The head is replaced and held firmly by taking up the slack in the wire and tying to the outside toggle.

If one prefers the use of fascia, it can be obtained directly from the patient by dissecting a strip about ½ inch wide from the fascia lata during the exposure of the operative site.

Bild has suggested the use of a fascia bank, which will preserve this material for several months. A donor dog is prepared and the skin over the thigh reflected aseptically. The fascia lata is cut in half-inch strips and each is placed in a tube containing 10 ml. of sterile physiologic saline, 200,000 units of penicillin and 0.25 gram of streptomycin. The liquid is decanted after 30 minutes. The tube is sealed and placed in a freezer at −10° Fahrenheit. Frozen fascia is dropped into sterile physiologic saline at room temperature whenever it is required.

Dobbelaar recommends bone grafting along the dorsal rim of the acetabulum to prevent luxation following reduction. Preserved homoplastic bone grafts are inserted in the dorsal margin of the acetabulum by drilling holes and driving bone pegs into them. A heavy callus will form along the ridge which prevents luxation.

PATELLAR LUXATIONS

Patellar luxations are usually of the recurrent type and almost invariably medial in direction. They constitute 20.5 per cent of all luxations seen at our clinic. Although observed in all breeds, they occur most frequently in the smaller breeds. The congenital abnormalities of the trochlea, distal femoral shaft, and tibial head are responsible for most of the chronic luxations seen in the toy breeds.

Etiology

An indirect force is usually the immediate cause. This force is transmitted to the weakened fascial attachment on the lateral side of the patella by sudden extension of the stifle while the tibia is rotated inward. Such an accident could occur while the animal is turning at high speed. The principal attachment is the patellar ligament with its insertion on the tibial tuberosity. Medially and laterally, the patella is held in the trochlear groove by fascial attachments which are not true ligaments. Any undue medial curvature of the distal femur will cause the tendon of the quadriceps femoris to subtend the arc thus formed. This in turn puts excessive strain on the lateral aponeurosis, thereby weakening it enough so that when sudden force is applied it separates. Direct force is not a customary cause, although luxation of the patella sometimes occurs in conjunction with fractures near the stifle which are caused by direct force. We have seen one case in which poor reduction of a distal epiphyseal femoral fracture caused lateral luxation of the patella.

Shuttleworth indicates that most patellar luxations are the result of bony malformations due to rachitic tendencies, particularly in the smaller breeds. Even in recent luxations in which the condition is not chronic, femoral curvature may have been a predisposing cause. Congenital luxation is frequently seen in the toy breeds and is usually caused by a shallow trochlea or some other congenital malformation, such as a medial deviation of the tibial crest or a medial rotation of the tibial shaft. In fact, the greatest number of patellar luxations are seen in the small breeds and are hereditary in origin. Singleton believes that some of the most severe malformations are congenital (the pup is born with practically no trochlea and the patella luxated medially, thereby causing the tibial head to rotate before epiphyseal fusion takes place).

The collateral ligaments should be checked during examination, since some laxity in this regard may be responsible for rotation of the tibia and subsequent patellar luxation. Some rotation of the tibia on the femur is possible in a relaxed flexed position, but none should be present when the limb is extended.

Pathology

In congenital luxations and in those caused by deformity of the stifle, the patella remains luxated without evident discomfort to the patient. Recent and recurrent luxations may cause some pain, at least momentarily. The patella may vary in position from the medial trochlear ridge to a point well back on the condyle. Arthritic changes are frequently present in the femoropatellar joint, and the joint capsule may be displaced medially. Of all luxations this probably shows the least gross change.

Signs

Lameness is common in all but the congenital cases in which the gait is distorted by deformity. This is not a true claudication. In recurrent cases the lameness is intermittent, and frequently the dog moves on three legs with both a standing and a swinging leg lameness. The leg is held in flexion with the stifle pointing inward and the hock outward. Recent luxations are painful and some may be swollen, although this is not a common sign.

On palpation, the patella will be found over the medial ridge of the trochlea and can usually be replaced by passive extension of the femorotibial joint. In recurrent cases the patella may remain in place for some time after repositioning, but in congenital cases, particularly if the medial trochlear ridge is absent, it reluxates immediately, or at least as soon as the leg is flexed.

Diagnosis

Digital palpation affords the best means of diagnosis. Roentgenograms will help in locating arthritic changes but are of little help otherwise, unless the injury has resulted from direct force. In such a case the joint should be checked for fractures. When the joint is palpated, the patella can easily be felt and the amount of luxation determined by extending the leg and forcing the patella from side to side in the trochlea. Acute luxations show a more medial movement than chronic or congenital luxations. They are also easily replaced on extension of the leg. In many instances the luxated condition of the patella is quite evident.

Singleton has conveniently classified the congenital luxations according to degree of tibial rotation and severity of deformity.

Grade 1. Intermittent luxation.   Limb carried occasionally. Patella can be luxated manually with no crepitation. Very slight rotation of the tibia. No abduction of the hock.

Grade 2. Limb is carried.   Almost constant luxation. Patella reluxates when manual pressure is released. Tibia rotated 30°. Slight deviation of tibial crest. Hock slightly abducted.

Grade 3. Patella permanently luxated.   Rotation of 30°–60°. Flexion and extension of the joint produces abduction and adduction of the hock. Trochlea very shallow.

Grade 4. Tibial rotation of 60°–90°.   Patella lies above the medial condyle of the femur. Trochlea is absent or convex.

Prognosis

Luxations that are secondary to other injuries of the stifle may not respond well to treatment. Congenital malformations should be approached with caution. Some are amenable to surgery and some are not. When the luxation is recent and the conformation of the leg is fairly normal, a good result can usually be expected if the surgical repair is correctly done.

Treatment

Lacroix has recommended medial desmotomy. This has been satisfactory in small dogs when the luxation is slight and of a recurrent type. The operative site is located on the medial side of the stifle. A stab wound is made in the skin at about the middle of the medial border of the patella with a No. 12 Bard Parker blade or a knife with a similar curved blade. The blade is carried beneath the skin until the proximal border of the patella is reached. It is then directed caudad through the medial fascial attachment and drawn distally until the medial attachments of the patella are severed. The completed desmotomy is verified by luxating the patella laterally. If all medial attachments are not severed, the patella cannot be forced over the lateral lip of the trochlea. With both medial and lateral attachments separated, the patella remains in the trochlea unless manually displaced. A bandage is placed over the small incision for 12 hours to control bleeding. No other aftercare is necessary.

In those cases in which the patella is misshapen or luxated because of congenital absence of a trochlea, or ankylosed for some reason, Craver has reported successful treatment through surgical removal of the patella. This method has a definite place in patellar surgery, but it has been much abused through indiscriminate use.

The skin incision for this operation should extend along the medial border of the patella and about ½ inch beyond in either direction. The incision is then carried through the fascia and periosteum on the midline over the patella. A periosteal elevator is used to peel the patella carefully from the enveloping tendon. This is often a very tedious and difficult task. When the patella has been removed, the tendon is sutured with interrupted chromic catgut sutures. Fascia and skin are closed in the usual fashion and the leg is placed in extension in a Thomas splint for one week. Only mild exercise should be given during this period. The leg will gradually return to normal following removal of the splint.

Shuttleworth is of the opinion that chronic luxations do not result from "traumatic" luxation. He feels that some anatomic abnormality exists which prevents the correct alignment of the patella. In order to correct the position of the patella, he suggests a cuneiform osteotomy on the lateral side of the distal femur. This corrects any curvature and allows the patella to move in the trochlea without angular traction.

A skin incision is made over the femur on the lateral side of the thigh and extending from the trochanter major to the stifle. The fascia lata is divided and the biceps separated from the quadriceps to expose the femur. A wedge-shaped piece is sawed from the femur so that the existing curvature will be obliterated. This osteotomy does not completely transect the bone, a small cortical attachment being left on the medial side. Small holes are then bored on either side of the osteotomy and the breech is closed by wiring the two sides together. Before the incision is closed, the patella is checked to see that it is moving correctly. The customary incision closure is followed by rest for several days without splintage of any kind.

With certain modifications, the method proposed by Stader produces the best results in most instances in which the luxation is not due to congenital malformation, because it creates a strong repair and is sound mechanically. This procedure, designed to bring about a strengthening of the lateral attachments, must be done on an exact pivotal point of the patella as it moves in an arc on the trochlea in order to maintain a constant restraining force against the pull of the medial attachments.

A skin incision is made from the trochanter major to the head of the tibia following the natural curve on the lateral side of the leg (Fig. 190A). Beginning at the lateral border of the patella, a strip of fascia lata is dissected to its upper limits and freed from the tensor fascia lata. The fascial incisions are best made with scissors and should take a caudal direction before gradually curving dorsal. The strip varies in width depending on the size of the dog, but is usually about one half to one inch. At the patellar border great care should be taken to see that the strip produces an exact lateral pull. This can be adjusted by careful dissection (Fig. 190B).

An aneurysm hook is passed around the lateral fabella, starting caudal and emerging cranial (Fig. 190C). The hook is pendulated to enlarge the

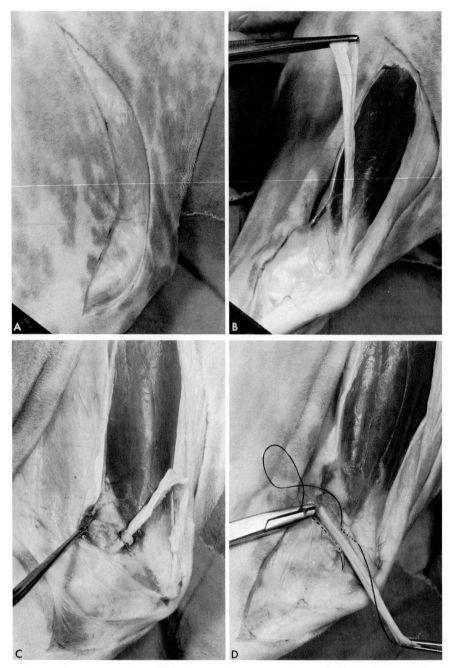

Figure 190.   The Stader method of correcting luxation of the patella. A, The skin incision.
B, The strip of fascia freed at its upper end but attached to the lateral side of the patella. The
underlying vastus lateralis muscle appears in the opening left by the separation of the fascia
after the strip is removed. C, The aneurysm hook has been placed around the fabella and the
fascia is attached to it ready to be drawn around the fabella. D, Application of the first stapling
stitch for anchorage of the new ligament.

opening enough to accommodate the strip. After the strip has been attached to the hook with suture wire it is drawn around the fabella by withdrawing the hook. Sufficient tension should be placed on the fascial strip to hold the patella in place before suturing. This tension should never be excessive but just enough to balance the pull from the medial side. Anchorage is obtained by doubling the strip on itself and applying a stapling suture of multifilament steel wire over the doubled fascia (Fig. 190D). It is locked in place by folding the free end over the suture and applying another stapling stitch.

The opening in the fascia is closed to prevent muscle hernia and the skin is covered by a light dressing after closure. A good method of dressing is to circumscribe the incision with liquid adhesive and then to apply a gauze sponge which can be trimmed to the shape of the incision. No splintage is used and mild exercise is encouraged. Hard exercise should not be undertaken before two weeks have elapsed.

Singleton describes a method that was first used by Hauser and later by Knight to correct congenital luxations. This is a transplantation or translocation of the tibial crest laterally so that the patella will traverse the trochlea in a straight line. We have used this method with some modifications since 1959 with a high degree of success. *It should be borne in mind that this type of defect or deformity is hereditary and that the necessary precautions should be taken to insure that such a patient is not used for breeding or showing.*

An incision is made on the cranial aspect of the limb, starting 3 cm. proximal to the patella and continuing distally until the tibial crest is entirely exposed (Fig. 192A). Careful dissection of the subcutaneous tissues will delineate the patellar ligament and the tibialis cranialis muscle lying on the lateral side of the tibial crest. This muscle is reflected laterally to expose a flat surface of bone into which the tibial crest can be transplanted (Fig. 192B).

Using the Hall air drill (Fig. 191), the crest is undercut to the depth of the cortex. This piece of bone should include the attachment of the patellar ligament and a long triangular piece of the tibial crest (Fig. 192C). In younger dogs whose bone is still soft, it is frequently possible to make this cut with a sharp, curved blade bone chisel. After the bony attachment has been freed, the joint capsule is opened along the edge of the ligament and the patella so that the trochlea can be inspected (Fig. 192D) and the ligament adjusted to its new position. If the trochlea is shallow or absent, the drill is used to shape a fresh groove deep enough to carry the patella. This groove should be planed with a burr until it is very smooth (Fig. 192E).

With the leg in extension, the segment of tibial crest is placed on the lateral side of the tibia at a point where the patella will slide in a straight line along the trochlea. The positioning should be done without tension, thereby compensating for the tension that will be present when the limb is flexed. The position is marked and a triangular piece of cortex, the size of the transplant, is removed from the tibia. The drill is the best instrument for shaping this opening, but various types of chisels may be used. It is impor-

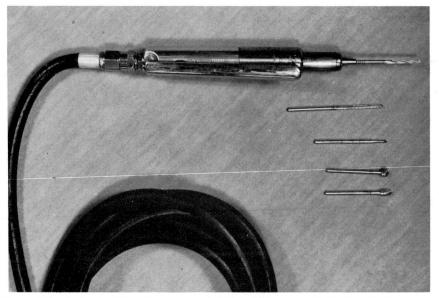

Figure 191. Hall air drill with some of the bits and burrs available for this instrument.

tant that the upper edge or base of the triangle be undercut so that the transplant will not slip under pressure.

The transplanted bone segment should fit snugly into the bed and the surface should be level with the surrounding bone. Since the transplanted bone is small and frequently relatively soft, we have refrained from drilling it in order to apply anchorage. Instead we drill through the tibia from side to side and apply two wires over the transplant and through the tibia. These wires are equally spaced and the proximal one is applied first (Fig. 192F).

Some ingenuity may be required to close the joint after the repositioning, particularly if the rotation is severe. The joint capsule can be tailored by making a flap on the medial side and moving it under the patellar ligament to the lateral side. The original dissecting incisions should be made slightly distal to the patella and patellar ligament so that enough capsular tissue remains for adequate suturing at closure. Occasionally it may be necessary to groove the tibial head so that the patellar ligament can move freely.

Pearson recommends the use of vitallium implants as a means of overcoming trochlear deficiencies, particularly on the medial side. He suggests this method of controlling the patella after the transplantation of the tibial crest where the medial trochlear ridge is lacking or the trochlear groove is too shallow.

This type of surgery requires a skin incision that begins at least 8 cm.

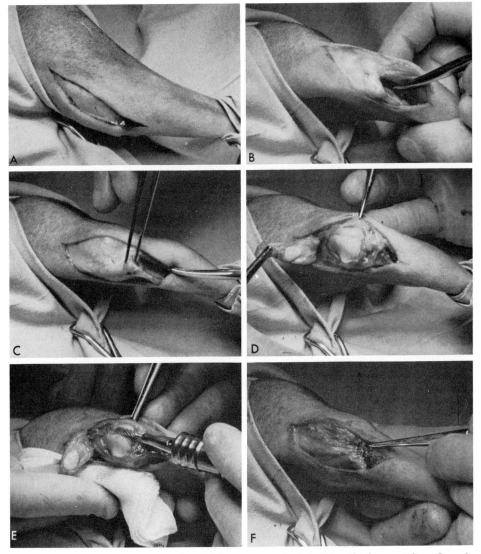

Figure 192. A, Skin incision for tibial crest transplant. B, The tibialis cranialis reflected. C, The tibial crest has been cut. D, The joint capsule is opened. E, Reshaping the trochlear groove. F, Wires holding the transplanted tibial crest in place.

above the patella in order to expose the medial condyle and lower shaft of the femur. The usual exposures are made and the patellar ligament with the sectioned tibial crest to be translocated is reflected. The trochlea is exposed and a proper size implant is fitted to the craniomedial side of the femur just proximal to the medial trochlear ridge. In order to function properly, the implant should fit the contour of the femur and extend cranially far enough to be level with the external surface of the tendon of the extended quadriceps. The implant is held in place by a screw which is anchored in both cortices.

The usual closure is made, except that the separation between the vastus medialis and the tendon of the quadriceps is allowed to remain open so that they can move without interference from the implant.

FEMORO-TIBIAL LUXATIONS

The stifle is composed essentially of two joints: the femoro-patellar, already discussed, and the femoro-tibial. The latter is a hinge-type joint with two menisci, each of which receives a condyle of the femur. The general relationship which the tibia bears to the femur is controlled by the two cruciate ligaments and the two collateral ligaments. To be sure, the meniscal ligaments play some part in strengthening the articulation but are not primarily concerned with the clinical entity under consideration. Meniscal injuries, however, are frequently seen in femoro-tibial luxations and will be discussed.

Complete luxation of this joint is uncommon and occurs only when all the ligaments are disrupted (Fig. 193). Subluxation, on the other hand, probably occurs more frequently than is suspected. A rupture of the medial collateral ligament allows the tibia to move laterally and abduct, whereas separation of the lateral collateral ligament permits the tibia to move medially and adduct. Rupture of the cranial cruciate permits forward movement of the tibia (not extension), and separation of the caudal cruciate permits backward movement (not flexion). Rupture of the caudal cruciate alone is rather rare.

Only 4.75 per cent of all luxations are in the femoro-tibial joint, and most of these are chronic or long standing subluxations. Sprains are fairly common in this joint, particularly those affecting the menisci and the meniscal ligaments.

Etiology

Direct force will sometimes cause a complete disruption of all the ligaments as well as the joint capsule, resulting in a complete luxation. Subluxation of this joint is much more common and is caused by direct force. In the case of the cruciates and the menisci, there is frequently a preliminary degeneration which weakens the part. It is believed that this degeneration is

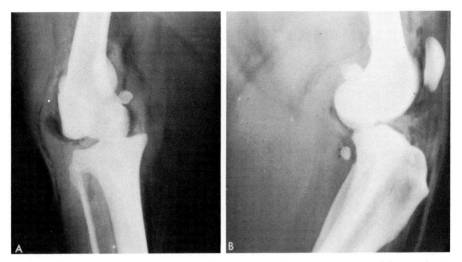

Figure 193. A complete luxation of the femoro-tibial joint. A, Cranio-caudal view showing sufficient displacement to indicate total disruption of the collateral ligaments. B, Lateral view showing enough cranial displacement of the tibia to indicate at least rupture of the cranial cruciate.

probably initiated by mild violence to the joint. It has also been suggested that aging brings about this degeneration. On the other hand, it is quite likely that an accumulation of mild injuries will accrue in the older dog to bring about the changes. Tears and bruises are inflicted on the avascular areas near the center of the menisci and in the cranial cruciate where it crosses the caudal cruciate.

An indirect force applied while the leg is in flexion will rupture the cranial cruciate. If there is some twisting motion with this action, a collateral ligament may separate and sometimes the meniscus is torn.

Overextension, such as might occur when a dog catches his foot in going over a barrier, also causes rupture of the cranial cruciate and perhaps the collateral ligament, depending on the amount of rotational twist placed upon the tibia.

Outward rotation of the lower limb while it is in flexion and under stress will disrupt the cranial cruciate and the medial meniscal ligaments, frequently with tearing of the medial meniscus. Inward rotation under the same circumstances will tear the ligaments of the lateral meniscus.

Pathology

When a complete luxation is present, all of the ligaments of the joint are torn or detached, including some of the meniscal ligaments. The joint capsule is disrupted and the menisci are torn. Most of the meniscal tears are longitudinal, fully isolating the avascular parts and instigating necrosis. Hemorrhage fills the joint and surrounding tissues. Edema of the joint region and pendant portions of the limb occurs with regularity.

If subluxation is present, the cranial cruciate is either partially ruptured and stretched or completely separated. This is usually the primary lesion. Following partial or total rupture of this ligament, the unnatural movement in the joint causes meniscal tears, stretching or separation of the collateral ligaments, partial rupture of the caudal cruciate, thickening of the joint capsule, and osteoarthritis around the periphery of the joint.

The meniscal lesions are usually longitudinal tears which interrupt the meager blood supply. The central portion is avascular, but some circulation reaches the intermediate parts from the outer circumference unless they are isolated by longitudinal tearing. Occasionally transverse tears occur, but these do not interfere with circulation. Necrosis of the central portion of the meniscus is common, particularly in older dogs when the joint has been subjected to strain for a number of years.

The caudal cruciate is seldom ruptured except in complete luxations with tearing of the joint capsule. There may be partial separation and stretching of this ligament in long-standing cases of rupture of the cranial cruciate. In this same type of case the joint capsule is frequently thickened. The synovial membrane may be hyperplastic and the joint distended with excessive synovia. Arthritic changes are often present and are frequently coupled with stretching or laxity in the lateral collateral ligament.

Signs

Lameness is a constant sign and is usually the reason for presentation by the owner. It may be so severe that the dog carries the limb at all times. In chronic cases the patient may show only a slight limp, but there may be atrophy of the thigh muscles. Needless to say, claudication is more severe in luxations than in subluxations. The lameness may appear suddenly and without any other evidence of injury.

The leg is carried in very mild flexion with the toe pointing forward. Active flexion of the stifle seems difficult and painful. On palpation, the joint may feel swollen, or it may be difficult to palpate because of a greatly thickened capsule. Pain may be elicited on palpation or on passive flexion.

Because of pain and apprehension it is frequently impossible to inspect the stifle properly until the patient is anesthetized. A short-acting barbiturate will produce sufficient relaxation for a thorough examination and roentgenogram. If angulation of the tibia in either a medial or a lateral direction is present or can be produced, the collateral ligament is disrupted on the side opposite to the angulation (Fig. 194). The so-called "drawer sign" is the best indication of cruciate disruption. This is produced by grasping the thigh lightly above the joint in one hand and the tibia in the other and attempting to move the tibia backward and forward while the joint is in a slightly flexed position (Fig. 195). The "anterior drawer sign" is manifested by a forward gliding of the tibia. This indicates rupture of the cranial cruciate. The "posterior drawer sign" is a gliding of the tibia in the opposite direction and is indicative of caudal cruciate separation.

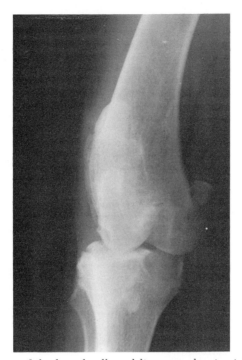

Figure 194. Rupture of the lateral collateral ligament, showing inflammatory reaction in the area.

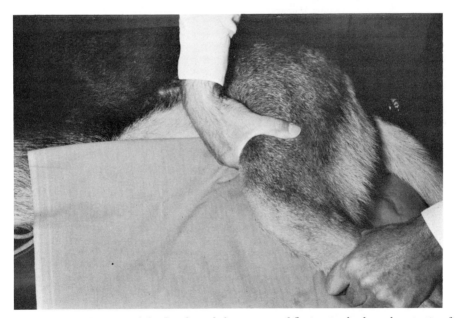

Figure 195. Position of the hands and the amount of flexion in the leg when testing for the "drawer sign."

Fig. 196　　　　　　Fig. 197

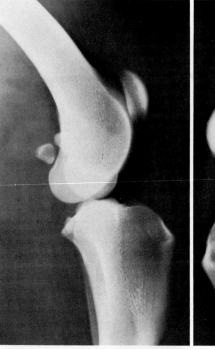

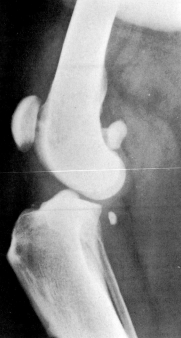

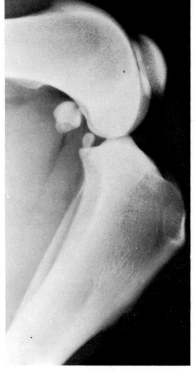

Figure 196. Roentgenogram of a stifle in slight flexion with a partial tear and stretching of the cranial cruciate ligament.

Figure 197. Roentgenogram of a stifle in slight flexion with a complete separation of the cranial cruciate ligament.

Figure 198. Roentgenogram of a stifle in flexion with a torn cruciate ligament. In this position the displacement is not as great because of the tension on the collateral ligaments.

Fig. 198

Manipulation of the joint often produces crepitus. It is also often possible to hear crepitation when the patient walks.

A lateral roentgenogram (Figs. 196, 197, 198) is helpful in detecting bony changes along the articular edges in long-standing cases. Meniscal injuries are difficult to detect in this way except as the space between femur and tibia is altered by disintegration of the cartilage.

Diagnosis

The "anterior drawer sign" provides the best diagnosis for rupture of the cranial cruciate, and medial or lateral angulation is indicative of stretched or torn collateral ligaments. Meniscal injuries are difficult to diagnose and are frequently uncovered by a process of elimination. If the signs strongly indicate the meniscus to be the seat of the trouble, an exploratory arthrotomy is in order. Many times the meniscal pathology is discovered when the repair of the cruciate is undertaken.

Prognosis

A fairly good prognosis can be given if surgical repair is undertaken before osteoarthritic changes have occurred. Healing of the ligaments and menisci is dependent upon surgical intervention; rest and conservative treatment will seldom produce permanent relief. Even when some osteoarthritis exists, the condition can be improved by surgical correction of the primary cause.

Treatment

Since the primary cause of subluxation and meniscal injuries in the femoro-tibial joint is rupture of the cranial cruciate ligament, it should receive primary consideration in any corrective procedure. It has been well established that, once ruptured, this ligament will not reestablish itself, and therefore surgical correction is required. Paatsama has described a method of fascial replacement which we have used with good results (Figs. 199 and 200).

A skin incision is made on the lateral side of the thigh from the trochanter major to the head of the tibia, exposing the fascia lata (Fig. 200A). Beginning at the lateral tibial condyle where the fascia is fairly well attached, a strip of fascia about one half to one inch wide is dissected dorsally to the tensor fascia lata muscle. The strip is transected at this point and tucked beneath the biceps femoris to prevent drying while the site is prepared for transplanting (Fig. 200B).

The entire length of the joint capsule is incised on the lateral side through the opening already made by removing the fascial strip. The incision should be made between the patella and the lateral trochlea and extended distally cranial to the tendon of the long digital extensor. The patella is reflected medially and the joint flexed. This exposes the interior for inspection (Fig. 200C).

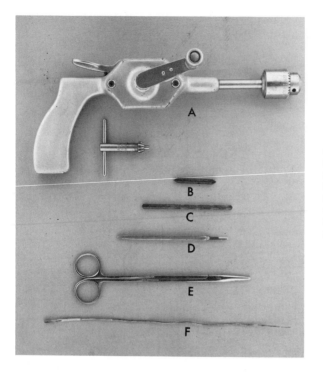

Figure 199. The instruments required for the Paatsama fascial transplant. A, Bone drill; B, "Starter bit" sharpened to avoid slipping; C, Regular bit about 3/16" diameter; D, Beaver knife for cutting the meniscus; E, Metzenbaum operating scissors; F, Seton needle.

Fat and excessive synovial membrane, together with the ruptured ends of the cruciate, are trimmed away. This is done by careful dissection with scissors. The menisci are then scrutinized for tears. If any are discovered, that portion of the meniscus is removed by cutting across it transversely with a No. 62 or a No. 64 blade in a Beaver Miniature Blade Knife (see Fig. 208). It is important that all damaged meniscus be removed. Paatsama also recommends the removal of the cranial horn of the medial meniscus so that a wall of regenerative tissue will be established to stabilize the joint. Meniscal healing takes place from the synovial membrane and grows inwardly but never completely unites with the cartilage along the transverse lines made by excision of the damaged meniscus. Partial meniscectomy should always be performed with this healing process in mind. Finally, any soft growths along the trochlear borders or around the patella should be excised.

An opening is drilled in the lateral femoral condyle to accommodate the new ligament, starting at a point above the insertion of the lateral collateral ligament and emerging at the femoral insertion of the cranial cruciate (Fig. 200D). To avoid slipping of the bit, a sharp-pointed starter bit or an intramedullary pin can be used initially. Drilling should be done with a bit of suitable diameter so that the fascial transplant can be easily threaded through the tunnel. The tibial opening is begun at the tibial insertion of the cranial cruciate and is directed toward the flat surface of the tibia just medial to the tibial crest and slightly distal to the medial condyle (Fig. 200E). The fascia is fastened to a seton needle or some other suitable instrument and twisted enough to convert the ribbon-like tissue into a cord. It is then threaded first through the femur and then the tibia (Fig. 200F). These openings will not be in an exactly straight line but the new ligament will be in approximately the same position as the original and its diagonal position will fortify it against excessive strain.

After the stifle is extended and the patella is replaced, the transplant is drawn tight across the tibial crest and anchored with two stapling sutures of multifilament steel wire (Fig. 200G). It is locked in position by doubling the free end over the sutures and applying another stapling suture. The joint now has reinforcement by way of a new cruciate and also a new lateral collateral ligament. Altogether, a very stabilizing effect is produced.

The joint capsule and the fascial opening are closed with stainless steel wire (Fig. 200H). The skin is closed in the usual fashion and the incision covered by gauze pads held in place with liquid adhesive. The leg is not splinted. Undue strain will not be placed upon the leg unless the patient is subjected to unnecessary excitement. Active use of the leg should begin in two weeks. In some chronic cases when the leg is not used because of muscular atrophy, it may be necessary to weight the foot with enough sheet lead to counterbalance the flexion and thereby set up active exercise in the leg.

In long-standing cases of subluxation, one or both collateral ligaments may be partially ruptured or stretched. Many times repair of the cranial cruciate will bring sufficient stabilization to the joint, but if it does not, a fascial transplant can be made. On the medial side the aponeurosis at the insertion of the sartorius muscle can be used and on the lateral side, the fascia lata. A slip approximately one half inch wide is dissected as near the caudal border of the joint as possible, leaving the ends attached. A stainless steel screw is then placed in the center of the condyle of the femur and the fascial strip is stretched over it. The opening in the fascia is closed with stainless steel sutures and the screw is set deep enough that it will not press against the skin.

When total luxation occurs it may be necessary to resort to several transplants in addition to meniscectomy. If such extensive surgery is required it is important that the joint be immobilized for two weeks until healing is well advanced. A Thomas splint or half pin splint could be used for support in such a case.

The Paatsama method of replacement of the cranial cruciate ligament has been our method of choice since it was described by Paatsama in 1952. The fascia, if applied as described, will form a strong, ropelike ligament which does not loosen with use and maintains its strength and usefulness for years. However, in certain individuals, especially older obese spaniels, the fascia is thin and friable and totally unsuitable for use as a ligament. In these cases it is necessary to use other material or other tissues in place of fascia lata. Fortunately the suitability of the fascia can be determined when the initial incision is made and an alternate method chosen to complete the repair if necessary.

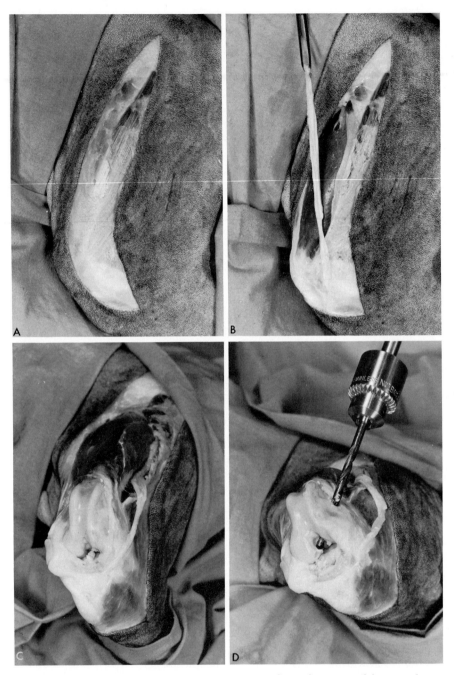

Figure 200. Illustrations of the Paatsama operation for replacement of the cranial cruciate ligament. A, The skin incision. B, The fascial strip which attaches to the head of the tibia. C, Exposure of the joint. The torn ligament is visible just beneath the trochlea. The inverted patella can be seen on the left and the new ligament on the right. D, Drilling the hole through the lateral condyle.

(*Illustration continued on opposite page.*)

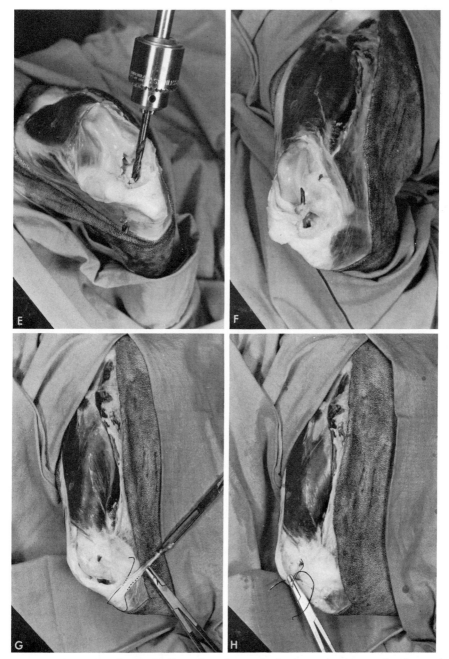

Figure 200 continued. E, Drilling the tibia with the bit emerging on the flat medial surface. The opening through the femur can be seen just to the left of the bit. F, Threading the twisted fascial strip. It has already been placed through the femur and shows to the right of the seton needle. It is now about to be pulled through the tibia. G, The fascial strip has been drawn across the tibial crest and a stapling stitch is being applied as the first step in anchoring. H, Closing the joint capsule. Closure of the fascial defect left by removal of the fascial strip will be the next step.

In 1957, Gibbens chose to use skin treated with quaternary ammonia solution as a substitute for fascia. Later, Leighton recommended the use of skin without special treatment. Others have tested skin as a routine ligament replacement with varying results. Our experience has indicated that skin has a tendency to stretch and thereby cause a loose joint. Furthermore, it is not uncommon to find cysts developing in the transplanted tissue. Hohn also reports the loss of strength in transplanted skin and degeneration.

Dueland has reported satisfactory results by using the patellar ligament to replace the cranial cruciate (Fig. 201). This method was first used in man by K. G. Jones. The skin incision is made craniolateral over the stifle region and the joint is opened by a parapatellar incision from the tibia to the proximal end of the femoro-patellar joint capsule.

After the usual inspection of the joint, the trimming of the ruptured ligament and whatever necessary meniscial surgery is finished, a central longitudinal section of the patellar ligament and the tendon of the quadriceps equal to one-third of the width of the patella is made. A wedge-shaped piece is then cut from the cranial aspect of the patella. This delicate operation should be done with a very fine saw or, better still, with a small high-speed drill. The cut should not be deep enough to penetrate the articular surface and should connect with the incision in the ligament and tendon. The tendon is freed at the proximal end, thus leaving a strip of tendon, bone, and ligament attached to the tibial tuberosity.

An oblique tunnel, approximately the diameter of the patellar wedge, is

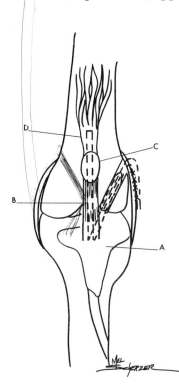

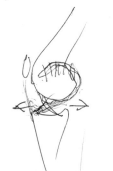

Figure 201. Replacement of the cranial cruciate ligament. Method of Dueland. A, Tibial crest. B, Patellar ligament. C, Patella. D, Tendon of the quadriceps muscle.

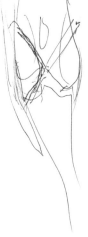

drilled through the lateral condyle of the femur. This tunnel corresponds to that made in the Paatsama operation.

Great care must be taken in threading the new ligament through the tunnel because it is easily frayed and the bone wedge will probably fit rather closely. The proximal end is sutured to the fascia while the leg is held in extension. Strande prefers to suture to the lateral collateral ligament.

This operation should not be undertaken unless one is prepared with the proper instruments and mental attitude for a very tedious piece of surgery, especially if the patient is one of the smaller breeds.

A number of methods have been devised for the replacement of the cranial cruciate ligament with synthetic material. The procedure in other respects is essentially the same as that used by Paatsama.

Ormrod uses a double strand of nylon threaded through ⅛ inch tunnels in the femur and tibia. The strand approximates the position of the cranial cruciate and is anchored on either end with stainless steel buttons (Fig. 202).

Singleton uses the same material but modifies the anchorage by drilling two converging tunnels in the lateral condyle of the femur and two separate tunnels in the tibia. The anchorage on the proximal end is obtained by inserting opposite ends of the loop of nylon into separate holes. They converge through the joint and are separated and threaded through opposite tunnels in the tibia before tying (Fig. 203).

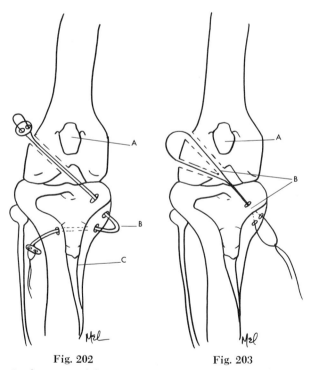

Fig. 202   Fig. 203

Figure 202. Replacement of the cranial cruciate ligament. Method of Ormrod. A, Patella. B, Two nylon strands. C, Tibial crest.

Figure 203. Replacement of the cranial cruciate ligament. Method of Singleton. A, Patella. B, Converging tunnels.

Johnson uses braided nylon and anchors the ends to stainless steel screws placed above the femoral tunnel and below the tibial tunnel. He does not feel that this method is suitable for small or toy breeds (Fig. 204).

Cameron and coworkers recommend the use of Teflon strips. The proximal end is anchored by means of a plastic button. The distal end is secured by passing through a tunnel in the tibial crest, folding over the crest, and suturing on itself (Fig. 205).

Zahm used a synthetic material called Supramid. Anchorage in this case is obtained by separating the ends of the loop and tying through a short cross-tunnel.

Butler uses Teflon to replace the ligament and reports that the synthetic strands are infiltrated with connective tissue. Anchorage on the proximal end is by suturing to the origin of the long digital extensor and on the distal end by passing through the tibial crest, doubling back, and suturing to itself.

Childers and others have claimed success by the use of Lembert-type stitches to imbricate the fascia over the lateral side of the stifle joint and thereby stabilize it.

Hohn and Miller have devised a method for stabilizing the joint by using the tendon of the long digital extensor. This tendon is attached to the cranio-lateral aspect of the lateral epicondyle of the femur.

An incision is made on the cranio-lateral side of the stifle. This incision should be approximately the same as that made in the Paatsama procedure. The joint is exposed and the usual surgical attention given to the cruciate remnants, arthritic lesions, and menisical injuries. The joint capsule is closed

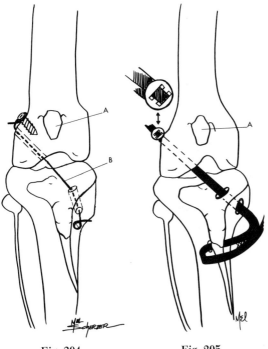

Figure 204. Replacement of the cranial cruciate ligament. Method of Johnson. A, Patella. B, Braided nylon.

Figure 205. Replacement of the cranial cruciate ligament. Method of Cameron, Sevy, Carren, Cooper, and McKeown. A, Patella.

Fig. 204   Fig. 205

and the tendon of the long digital extensor is uncovered for its entire length by reflecting the tibialis cranialis (Fig. 206).

After separating the lateral attachment of the patellar ligament from the tibial tuberosity and crest, a channel is made in the lateral third of the tuberosity to accommodate the tendon of the long digital extensor. Ross prefers to drill a tunnel from the proximal face of the tibia to the muscular groove. A very narrow slot is then cut along the long axis of the tunnel.

The freed tendon is gently lifted without pinching to a medial position over the slot. It may require some gentle manipulation to work the tendon through the slot into the tunnel, but once in place it should not slip.

While the route of the relocated tendon does not follow the restraining lines of the cranial cruciate, it does have a very stabilizing effect on the joint. This is the method of choice in our clinic when the fascia is not available or is of inferior quality.

Postoperative splinting of the limb for 12 to 18 days has been recommended.

Rathor has suggested that the use of the tendon of the peroneus longus as a replacement for the cranial cruciate ligament. This muscle lies just caudal to the long digital extensor. It originates from the lateral ligament of the stifle and the lateral aspect of the heads of the tibia and fibula. The tendon is fairly heavy and inserts on the fourth tarsal.

In this procedure the stifle is prepared in a manner similar to the Paatsama technique. The tendon of the peroneus is dissected free and divided near the hock. The cut end is drawn through the tibial tunnel and then through the femoral tunnel by means of a wire loop. The tendon is pulled taut, with the leg held in extension, and sutured to the crural fascia.

Strande, who has done considerable investigative work on the femoro-tibial joint of the dog, suggests the use of the flexor digitorum longus tendon. This tendon is paired with the tendon of the flexor hallucis longus to form the deep digital flexor tendon. According to Strande, the tendon of the flexor digitorum longus can therefore be cut without noticeably affecting the normal movement of the leg. The origin of this short narrow muscle is from the head of the fibula and the popliteal line of the tibia.

A long incision is made beginning on the lateral side of the limb above the stifle, crossing diagonally over the stifle to the medial side, and following the caudomedial border of the tibia to the medial malleolus. The tendon is cut at the medial malleolus and dissected free. The bone tunnels are placed as in the Paatsama procedure. The tendon is pulled through from the medial side of the tibia to the lateral side of the femoral condyle. The free end of the tendon is sutured to the lateral collateral ligaments while the leg is held in extension (Fig. 207).

Many methods of treatment have been proposed for the stabilization of the stifle joint following rupture of the cranial cruciate ligament. Each method has its own proponents and therefore a choice has to be made by the individual surgeon. There are certain general parameters which may be used in selecting the best procedure under each special set of circumstances. First, it seems reasonable to assume that autogenous tissues should be

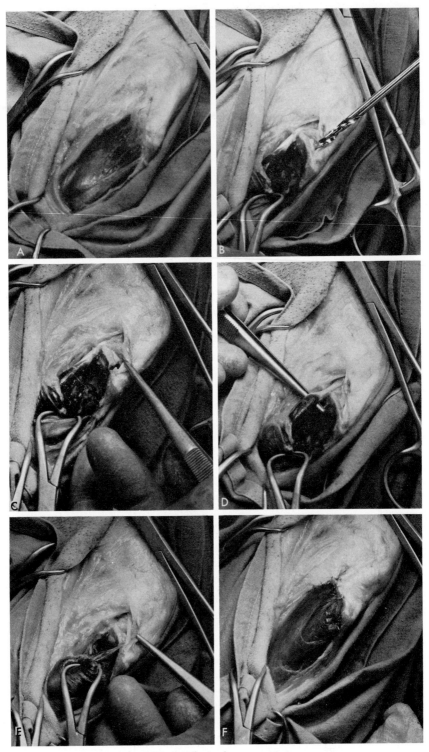

Fig. 206. See legend on opposite page.

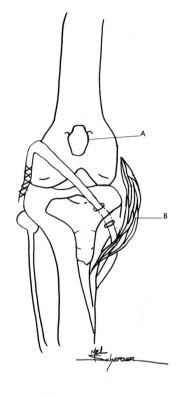

Figure 207. Stifle repair for ruptured cranial cruciate ligament. Method of Strande. A, Patella. B, Tendon of the flexor digitorum longus is passed under the semitendinosus near its attachment to the tibia.

tolerated better than foreign materials. It is also true that transplanted tissues will adapt better if some blood circulation is maintained. Second, no repair of the femoro-tibial joint should be undertaken without opening the joint and making the necessary repairs to structures within the joint (Fig. 208). Third, the joint capsule should be thoroughly cleaned of any debris before closing. Fourth, the method of anchorage of the ligament replacement is extremely important. The ligament should be tightened with the leg in full extension and the free end fastened to some structure which does not weaken or change in tensile strength when the joint is flexed. Fifth, splintage tends to interfere with circulation and is usually not necessary. The patient will carry the leg until it is sound enough to use. Sixth, there are no shortcuts to good surgery.

Figure 206. Method of Hohn and Miller for stabilizing the femoro-tibial joint. A, Exposure of the tibialis cranialis. B, Tibialis cranialis reflected and tunnel being bored through the tibial tuberosity to the bed vacated by the tibialis. C, Slot cut for access to the tunnel shows at the tip of the thumb forceps. The edge of the patellar ligament is drawn back to expose the slot. Tendon of the long digital extensor is to the left of the slot. D, Tendon being lifted to new position. Slot is covered by the patellar ligament and fascia. E, Tendon in place. It can be seen immediately to the left of the thumb forceps. The reflected tibialis cranialis muscle is being held by a towel clamp in the foreground. F, Tibialis cranialis replaced and sutured to the fascia.

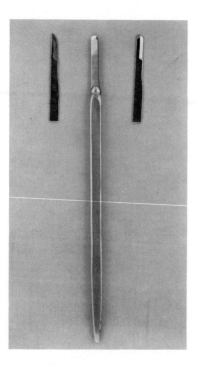

Figure 208. Beaver miniature blade knife. Excellent for trimming the menisci and other close work in joints.

LUXATIONS OF THE HOCK JOINT (TIBIO-TARSAL LUXATIONS, TARSAL LUXATIONS, TARSO-METATARSAL LUXATIONS)

The hock joint is a composite joint embracing the tibio-tarsal articulation, the intertarsal articulation, and the tarso-metatarsal articulations. Since the distal ends of the fibula and the tibia are fused, we have taken the liberty of designating the articulation of these two bones with the tarsus as tibio-tarsal. Luxations in the vicinity of the hock are frequently complicated by fractures which chip away a process involved in retaining the bone in position. Simple luxations are therefore exceptional in this region (Fig. 209). The tibio-tarsal joint luxates most frequently and accounts for 4.25 per cent of all luxations. Tarsal luxations are less common and are seen predominantly in racing dogs. The bones commonly affected are the tibial-tarsal (astragalus) and the central tarsal (scaphoid).

Etiology

Luxations at the tibio-tarsal articulation can be caused by either a direct or an indirect force. Indirect force is applied to the joint by twisting when it is in extension. Usually the leg is under a considerable strain at the time and it is not uncommon for a malleolar fracture to occur.

Indirect force is almost invariably the cause of tarsal luxations. Rupture of the interosseous ligaments during overextension, particularly when some rotational pressure is put on the foot, accounts for most of these injuries.

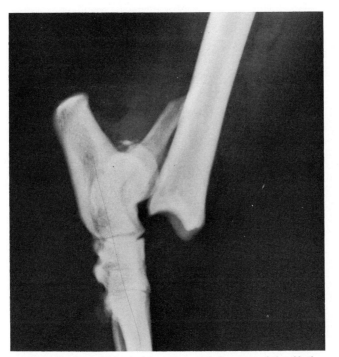

Figure 209. A tibio-tarsal luxation with fracture of the fibula.

Pathology

Ligaments immediately adjoining the joint are torn, with the usual swelling and some hemorrhage. Fractures are common, particularly in the tarsals; a scaphoid luxation seldom occurs without fracture. Displacement is usually not great in the tarsals but is slightly more severe in the tibio-tarsal joint.

Signs

The leg is held in flexion. It shows distortion if the luxation is in the tibio-tarsal joint. Tarsal luxations are usually not so prominent. Pain may be severe, especially on palpation. The foot is pointed downward with some inward rotation. The hock is bowed because of the displaced scaphoid. The tuber calcis is frequently rotated outwards. The Achilles tendon is flaccid. Palpation usually reveals the location of the luxation.

Diagnosis

A differential diagnosis must be made in order to eliminate fractures. Many times both conditions are present, and this can easily be determined by a roentgenogram taken in two planes.

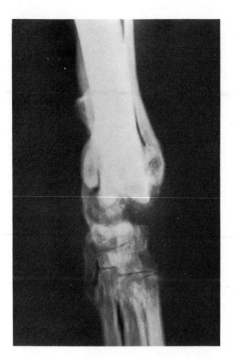

Figure 210. A tibio-tarsal luxation of long standing. Fibrosis and exostosis are plainly visible. It is quite unlikely that this can be satisfactorily reduced.

Prognosis

The prognosis is reasonably good, since the joints involved are not intensely active and some stiffness does not greatly hamper locomotion. Greater care is required in predicting the outcome of a tibio-tarsal luxation because of a possible distortion to the limb if it is not properly reduced (Fig. 210). Tarsal luxations require considerable time for healing, sometimes as long as three months.

Treatment

TIBIO-TARSAL LUXATIONS. Reduction is best achieved by moderate distal traction with the hock extended and the stifle partially flexed. Digital pressure is then applied to complete the reduction. Occasionally these injuries can be reduced and fixed with coaptation. The surgeon may use any of the many materials available. The cast should be left in place for at least three weeks.

The Kirschner intramedullary pin serves very well for fixation once the luxation is reduced (Fig. 211). The insertion is made on the plantar surface of the hock through a stab wound directly opposite the tibia. With the hock in mild flexion, the pin is drilled through the tibial and fibular tarsals into the medullary canal of the tibia. It should be inserted well up the canal so that there is adequate purchase on the tibial shaft. The plantar branch of the saphenous artery and the lateral plantar nerve lie close to the point of

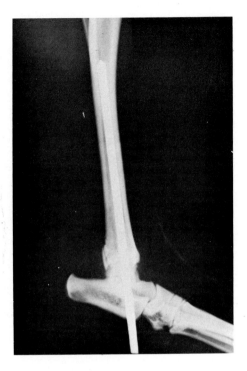

Figure 211. Reduction and fixation of the tibio-tarsal luxation seen in Figure 209 by the use of an intramedullary pin.

insertion, so that the pin must be started with caution. Coaptation should be applied for added support and particularly as a precaution against rotation.

TARSAL LUXATIONS. Complete reduction is sometimes difficult to achieve in the case of the scaphoid, and since a fracture is usually present the same methods of repair described under fractures in the pelvic limb can be used. The tibial-tarsal can usually be reduced by digital pressure when the hock is in extension. Coaptation will hold the luxation in place reasonably well (Fig. 212). If difficulty is encountered, the luxation can be fixed in position by wiring to the fibular tarsal.

In cases of subluxation at the tarso-metatarsal joint, Arwedsson has proposed a method of arthrodesis. A skin incision is made on the plantar surface lateral to the tendon of the superficial digital flexor. The incision should be long enough that there is a generous exposure. Fascia and intertarsal ligaments not already ruptured are incised. The joint cavity is opened by pressing the foot in the dorsal direction. All articular cartilage is removed with a high-speed drill or a curette. A sharp tooth scaler works well where the space is narrow. It is extremely important that all cartilage be removed.

Four full pins are used for fixation. One pin is drilled transversely through the tuber calcis and one through the body of the fibular tarsal. The third and fourth pins are placed mediolaterally through the proximal and distal ends of the metatarsals.

The tarsals and metatarsals are brought together and held by anchoring the pins with metal plates or with couplings and bars from a half pin

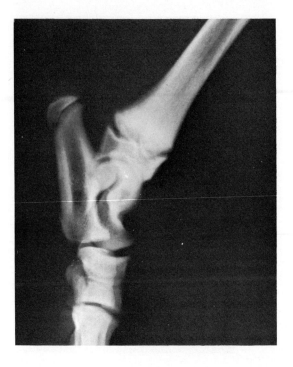

Figure 212. A case of subluxation of the tibial and fibular tarsals. This was held in coaptation for two weeks.

Figure 213. Diagram of screw placement for arthrodesis of tarsal bones. Method of Lawson.

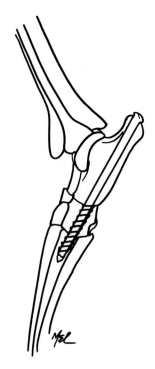

assembly. Plaster may be added for additional support or the splintage can be padded and taped.

Lawson has described six cases of intertarsal subluxation which were repaired by arthrodesis. Again the incision is on the plantar surface but is begun at the tuber calcis. After exposing the joint and removing the articular cartilage, the bones are brought into apposition with the use of a partially threaded screw. A channel with the same diameter as the screw is first drilled the length of the os calcis. Then, using a small bit, the fourth tarsal is penetrated. When the screw is passed through the fibular tarsal, the threads should not engage until there is contact with the fourth tarsal. This should draw the joint together tightly so that it will fuse (Fig. 213).

Luxations of the metatarsals and phalanges are usually self-evident and require only digital manipulation for reduction. A roentgenogram should be taken to avoid complications. Coaptation usually offers the best means of support until they are healed. This should remain in place for at least two weeks.

REFERENCES

Andres, R. L.: Recurrent patellar luxation in dogs. N. Am. Vet., 16:42, 1935.

Archibald, J., Brown, N. M., Naste, E., and Medway, W.: Open reduction for correction of coxofemoral dislocations. Vet. Med., 48:273–275, 1953.

Arwedsson, G.: Arthrodesis in traumatic plantar subluxation of the metatarsal bones of the dog. J.A.V.M.A., 124:21–24, 1954.

Bäckgren, A. W., and Olsson, S.-E.: Intraarticular fractures following traumatic coxofemoral luxation in dogs. Nord. Vet. Med., 13:197–204, 1961.

Blakely, C. L.: Multiple luxation of tarsal bones. N. Am. Vet., 32:347, 1951.

Blaney, A. J.: Surgical repair of a bilateral lateral luxation of the patellae in a dog. N. Am. Vet., 32:101, 1951.

Bottarelli, A.: Coxofemoral luxations in dogs. Clin. Vet., 61:407, 1938. Abstracted in N. Am. Vet., 21:428, 1940.

Brown, R. E.: The experimental use of stainless steel femoral head prostheses in normal dogs and cats. N. Am. Vet., 34:423, 1953.

Butler, H. C.: Teflon as a prosthetic ligament in repair of ruptured anterior cruciate ligaments. Am. J. Vet. Res., 25:55–59, 1964.

Cameron, T. P., Sevy, C., Carren, D., Cooper, L., and McKeown, D.: An aid in the repair of the anterior cruciate ligament. Vet. Med. Small Animal Clin., 63:337–340, 1968.

Campbell, J. R., Lawson, D. D., and Wyburn, R. S.: Coxofemoral luxation in the dog. Vet. Rec., 77:1173–1177, 1965.

Childers, H. E.: New methods for cruciate ligament repair. II. Repair by suture technic. Mod. Vet. Pract., 47:#13, 59–60, 1966.

Craver, N. S.: Removal of patella and its possibilities. N. Am. Vet., 19:55, 1938.

Dalton, P. J.: Recurrent coxofemoral luxations in the dog. Vet. Rec., 65:625–626, 1953.

DeAngelis, M., and Hohn, R. B.: Evaluation of surgical corrections of canine patellar luxations in 142 cases. J.A.V.M.A., 156:387–394, 1970.

Dibbell, E. B.: Dislocation of the hip in dogs and cats. N. Am. Vet., 15:37, 1934.

Dobbelaar, M. J.: Dislocation of the hip in dogs. J. Small Animal Pract., 4:101–110, 1963.

Dueland, R.: A recent technique for reconstruction of the anterior cruciate ligament. An. Hosp., 2:1–5, 1966.

Dyce, K. M., Merlen, R. H. A., and Wadsworth, F. J.: The clinical anatomy of the stifle of the dog. Brit. Vet. Jour., 108:346–353, 1952.

Ehmer, E. E.: Special casts for the treatment of pelvic and femoral fractures and coxofemoral luxations. N. Am. Vet., 15:31, 1934.

Flo, G. F., and Brinker, W. O.: Fascia lata overlap procedure for surgical correction of recurrent medial luxation of the patella in the dog. J.A.V.M.A., *156*:595–599, 1970.

Foster, W. J., Imhoff, R. K., and Cordell, J. T.: "Closed-joint" repair of anterior cruciate ligament rupture in the dog. J.A.V.M.A., *143*:281–283, 1963.

Geary, J. C.: Luxation of the patella: Radiographic aspects. Auburn Vet., *22*:27–29, 1965.

Geyer, H.: Treatment of cruciate ligament rupture in dogs: a comparative study. Schweiger Arch. Tierheilk, *109*.240–251, 1967.

Gibbens, R.: Patellectomy and a variation of Paatsama's operation on the anterior cruciate ligament of a dog. J.A.V.M.A., *131*:557–558, 1957.

Greene, J. E., Hoerlein, B. F., and Leonard, E. P.: Orthopedic surgery. N. Am. Vet., *34*:50, 1953.

Hohn, R. B., and Miller, J. M.: Surgical correction of rupture of the anterior cruciate ligament in the dog. J.A.V.M.A., *150*:1133–1141, 1967.

Jennings, W. E.: Dislocation of the hip joint in the dog. Cornell Vet., *24*:260, 1934.

Johnson, F. L.: Use of braided nylon as a prosthetic anterior cruciate ligament of the dog. J.A.V.M.A., *137*:646–647, 1960.

Jones, K. G.: Reconstruction of the anterior cruciate ligament. A technique using the central third of the patella ligament. J. Bone Joint Surg., *45A*:925–932, 1963.

Jones, V. B.: Dislocation of the patella in the dog. Vet. J., *91*:281, 1935.

Knowles, A. T., Knowles, J. O., and Knowles, R. P.: An operation to preserve the continuity of the hip joint. J.A.V.M.A., *123*:508, 1953.

Kodituwakku, G. E.: Luxation of the patella in the dog. Vet. Rec., *74*:1499–1506, 1962.

Kodituwakku, G. E.: Observations on injuries to some stifle joint ligaments in dogs. Ceylon Vet. Jour., *10*:128–131, 1962.

Lacroix, J. V.: Recurrent luxation of the patella in dogs. N. Am. Vet., *11*:47, 1930.

Lacroix, J. V.: A coxofemoral luxation. N. Am. Vet., *16*:47, 1935.

Lawson, D. D.: Inter-tarsal subluxation in the dog. J. Small Animal Pract., *1*:179–181, 1961.

Lawson, D. D.: Toggle fixation for recurrent dislocation of the hip in the dog. J. Small Animal Pract., *6*:57–59, 1965.

Leighton, R. L.: Repair of ruptured anterior cruciate ligament with whole thickness skin. Small Animal Clin., *1*:246–259, 1961.

Loeffler, K.: Joint anomalies as a problem in dog breeding. Dtsch. tierargtl Wschr., *71*:291–297, 1964.

Loeffler, K.: Damage to the Cruciate Ligaments of the Knee Joint of Dogs: Anatomy, Clinical Fractures and Experimental Investigations. Hanover, M. and H. Schafer, 1964.

Loeffler, K., and Meyer, H.: Hereditary luxation of the patella in toy spaniels. Dtsch. tierargtl Wschr., *68*:619–622, 1961.

Loeffler, K., and Reuleaux, I. R.: Zur chirurgie der ruptur des ligamentum discussatum laterale. Dtsch. tierargtl Wschr., *69*:69–72, 1962.

Lustig-Lendva, E.: Displacement of os calcis and astragalus in a bitch. Vet. Jour., *99*:244, 1943.

Mackey, H. W. and McCune, R. F.: Surgical correction of congenital patellar luxation. Mod. Vet. Pract., *48*:52–56, 1967.

McManus, J. L., and Nimmons, G. B.: Ruptured anterior cruciate ligament in a cat. Canad. Vet. Jour., *7*:264, 1966.

Miller, M. E., Christensen, G. C., and Evans, H. E.: Anatomy of the Dog. Philadelphia, W. B. Saunders Co., 1964.

Nilsson, F.: Meniscal injuries in dogs. N. Am. Vet., *30*:509, 1948.

Obel, N.: Luxation of the canine hip. Nord. Vet. Med., *1*:62–69, 1949.

O'Donoghue, D. H., Rockwood, C. A., Frank, G. R., Jack, S. C., and Kenyon, R.: Repair of the anterior cruciate ligament in dogs. J. Bone Joint Surg., *48A*:503–519, 1966.

Ormrod, A. N.: Restabilization of femoro-tibial joint in the dog following rupture of the anterior cruciate ligament. Vet. Rec., *75*:375–377, 1963.

Paatsama, S.: Ligament injuries of the canine stifle joint: A clinical and experimental study. Dissertation, University of Helsinki, 1952.

Paatsama, S.: Regeneration of the canine meniscus. Nord. Vet. Med., *7*:953, 1955.

Pearson, P. T.: Alloy prosthesis to aid in correction of persistent patellar luxations. An. Hosp., *2*:191–198, 1966.

Pettit, G.: Use of the ischio-ilia (DeVita) pin in canine coxofemoral luxation. Calif. Vet., *9*:14–16, 1956.

Puget, E., and Cazieux, A.: Ruptures et distensions du ligament croisé antérior du grosset, chez le chien. Rev. Med. Vet., *112*:401–420, 1961.

Puget, E., and Cazieux, A.: La myoplastie des vasted les luxations traumatiques de la rotule du chien. Rev. Med. Vet., *114*:33–39, 1963.

Rathor, S. S.: Experimental studies and tissue transplants for repair of the canine anterior cruciate ligament. M.S.U. Vet., 20:128–134, 1960.

Rex, M. A. E.: Surgical treatment of three common orthopedic conditions of the dog's stifle. Aust. Vet. J., 39:268–274, 1963.

Ross, G. E., Jr.: Personal communication.

Roush, J. C., II, Hohn, R. B., and DeAngelis, M.: Evaluation of transplantation of the long digital extensor tendon for correction of anterior cruciate ligament rupture in dogs. J.A.V.M.A., 156:309–312, 1970.

Schebitz, H., and Zedler, W.: Contribution to the traumatic dislocation of the hip in dogs. Dtsch. tierargtl. Wschr., 67:369–375, 1960.

Schroeder, E. F.: Injuries in the region of the hip in small animals. J.A.V.M.A., 89:522–545, 1936.

Schroeder, E. F., and Schnelle, G. B.: The stifle joint. N. Am. Vet., 22:353, 1941.

Schuttleworth, A. C.: Dislocation of the patella in the dog. Vet. Rec., 15:765–774, 1935.

Singleton, W. B.: The diagnosis and surgical treatment of some abnormal stifle conditions in the dog. Vet. Rec., 69:1387–1396, 1957.

Singleton, W. B.: Differential diagnosis of stifle injuries in the dog. J. Small Animal Pract., 1:182–191, 1961.

Singleton, W. B.: Stifle joint surgery in the dog. Canad. Vet. Jour., 4:142–150, 1963.

Singleton, W. B.: The surgical correction of stifle deformities in the dog. J. Small Animal Pract., 10:59–69, 1969.

Singleton, W. B.: Observations based upon the surgical repair of 106 cases of anterior cruciate ligament rupture. J. Small Animal Pract., 10:269–278, 1969.

Stader, O.: The reduction of coxofemoral luxations in the dog. N. Am. Vet., 17:44, 1936.

Stader, O.: Dislocation of the hip joint. N. Am. Vet., 36:1026–1028, 1955.

Strande, A.: A study of the replacement of the anterior cruciate ligament in the dog by the tendon of flexor digitalis longus. Nord. Vet. Med., 16:820–827, 1964.

Strande, A.: Replacement of the anterior cruciate ligament in the dog. J. Small Animal Pract., 7:351–359, 1966.

Strande, A.: Repair of the Ruptured Cranial Cruciate Ligament in the Dog. Baltimore, Williams & Wilkins, 1967.

Titkemeyer, C. W., and Brinker, W. O.: Applied anatomy of the stifle joint. M.S.U. Vet., 18:84–88, 1958.

Vaughan, L. C.: A study of replacement of the anterior cruciate ligament in the dog by fascia, skin and nylon. Vet. Rec., 75:537–541, 1963.

Vaughan, L. C., and Bowden, N. L. R.: The use of skin for the replacement of the anterior cruciate ligament in the dog: A review of thirty cases. J. Small Animal Pract., 5:167, 1964.

Vierheller, R. C.: Surgical correction of patellar ectopia in the dog. J.A.V.M.A., 134:429–433, 1959.

Vierheller, R. C.: The canine stifle joint. Calif. Vet., 12:42–46, 1959.

Woolfe, D. T.: A practical method of fixation for recurrent dislocation of the hip in the dog. J.A.V.M.A., 126:458, 1955.

Zahm, H.: Operative treatment of crucial ligament injuries in dogs with synthetic material. Berl. Munch. tierarztl Wschr., 79:1–4, 1966.

Zakiewicz, M.: Recurrent hip luxation in the dog. Skin as a substitute ligament. Vet. Rec., 81:538–539, 1967.

Chapter 9

Luxations in the Pectoral Limb

SCAPULO-HUMERAL LUXATIONS (LUXATIONS OF THE SHOULDER)

This condition is extremely rare in the dog. Since there is no clavicle to give the shoulder joint solid support, it is difficult to dislodge the head of the humerus. The entire joint "rides with the blow" when force is applied.

Acute luxation results from a force or a blow centering on the cranial side of the humerus while the joint is in mild flexion. Chronic luxation results from torn or stretched ligaments and capsule and usually is of a recurrent type.

Although some of the literature indicates that the head of the humerus is displaced inward and backward, it has been the author's experience that the displacement is lateral with the head of the humerus coming to rest on the acromion. The capsule is stretched or torn, and in chronic cases there may be detachment of some of the scapular muscles, particularly the supraspinatus. In other instances the capsule, ligaments, and muscles may be intact following luxation.

Congenital luxations appear to be more common in Great Britain. These occur principally in the toy breeds. They are medial in direction and are characterized by a flattened humeral head and a shallow glenoid cavity.

The limb is carried abducted, extended, and rotated slightly outward. There is some elevation at the point of the shoulder. The glenoid cavity can be felt on the medial side of the upper arm by deep digital palpation. The diagnosis should be confirmed with a roentgenogram. The prognosis is good in acute cases but should be guarded in recurrent cases.

Usually reduction is easily achieved. The shoulder is extended and the limb is drawn medially while digital pressure is applied to the head of the humerus. Acute luxations usually glide into place and resist attempts to reluxate. Fixation is not necessary in such cases.

Chronic or recurrent luxations may require fixation for two weeks until the torn capsule and muscles have healed. The limb can be restrained by a

250

sling cast around the body or it can be held in a normally flexed position in a Thomas splint. When the Thomas splint is used, sufficient traction can be maintained by using skin traction instead of skeletal traction.

A number of clinicians (Vaughan, Ball, Campbell, Alexander, and Irwin) have described methods for open reduction and fixation of recurrent luxation of this joint. The methods are essentially the same but vary somewhat in the approach and the materials used.

In general, the skin incision begins at midpoint of the scapular spine and ends midway along the humerus. The line of the incision follows the spine of the scapula and the shaft of the humerus on the craniolateral side. The distal end of the scapular spine is uncovered by separating the supraspinatus and the infraspinatus so that a tunnel can be drilled through the spine close to the body of the scapula.

The crest of the greater tubercle of the humerus is drilled in a ventro-cranial direction.

Vaughn used whole thickness skin, $\frac{1}{8}$ inch wide, and threaded it through the tunnel in the humerus, behind the acromial part of the deltoideus muscle caudal to the joint, through the tunnel in the spine of the scapula, and down the cranial aspect of the joint to the point of beginning. The skin ends were fastened with sutures (Fig. 214).

Ball used $\frac{1}{4}$ inch nylon tape and placed one strand on the medial side of the humerus and scapula and the other on the lateral side. The purpose of this type of lacing was to prevent medial displacement of the humeral head (Fig. 215).

Campbell used both nylon and skin and laced these in three different ways.

Alexander prefers the use of $\frac{3}{8}$ inch wide teflon. This is threaded through the tunnel in the humerus in the caudal direction. The end is fastened to a screw cranio-lateral to the opening in the bone and sutured. The opposite end is passed under the supraspinatus and through a hole in the spine of the scapula. It is then passed beneath the acromion, where it is tied and sutured to itself near the point of entry into the scapular spine. The remainder of the strand then passes over the lateral side of the humeral head and is anchored to the screw (Fig. 216).

DeAngelis and Schwartz describe a method of fixation by using the tendon of the biceps brachii. The incision is craniomedial from the distal end of the scapula to a midpoint on the humerus. The fascia is separated over the greater tubercle and the acromial portion of the deltoideus reflected laterally. Further exposure is made by incising the aponeurosis over the greater tubercle and dividing the transverse humeral ligament. The tendon of the biceps lies beneath this ligament. It is necessary to open the joint capsule in order to free the tendon (Fig. 217).

The greater tubercle is cut with a drill so that the medial half can be removed along with its attachment to the supraspinatus muscle. A groove is made in the face of the cut across the humerus large enough to accommodate the tendon of the biceps brachii.

The tendon is moved laterally into the groove and the cut tubercle

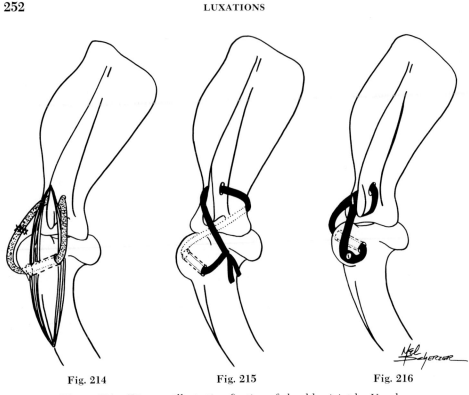

Fig. 214   Fig. 215   Fig. 216

Figure 214. Diagram illustrating fixation of shoulder joint by Vaughan.
Figure 215. Diagram illustrating fixation of shoulder joint by Ball.
Figure 216. Diagram illustrating fixation of shoulder joint by Alexander.

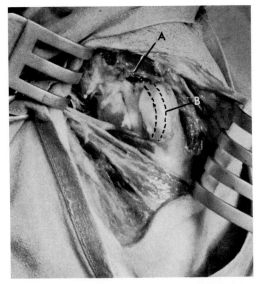

Figure 217. Use of tendon of biceps brachii to stabilize the shoulder joint. A, Normal
position of the tendon. B, Outline of new position.

replaced. It is fastened with two Stille nails. The joint capsule, fascial planes, and skin are closed in the usual way.

The limb is rested for nine days by binding it to the body in flexion. Gradual motion and stabilization return to the joint. A slight lameness may result in such cases.

HUMERO-RADIO-ULNAR LUXATIONS (LUXATIONS OF THE ELBOW)

Luxations of the elbow may involve all three bones of the joint, or there may be luxation of the radius with fracture of the ulna. Seldom does the radius luxate without some injury to the ulna. Actually there are three articulations in the region of the elbow. The humero-radial and the humero-ulnar are true hinge-type joints and are the principal articulations of the elbow. The proximal radio-ulnar articulation lies within the boundaries of the elbow joint, but since it contributes little to the movement of the joint it will not receive separate consideration. A fourth articulation, the distal radio-ulnar joint, lies near the distal end of the radius and ulna. This joint allows about 20° rotational movement of the foot. Slight supination will result from this movement, but it is not as pronounced as in man. Supination to any degree in the dog is indicative of fracture or luxation in the elbow region.

Luxations in dogs involve the elbow joint 8.75 per cent of the time. This type ranks third in frequency, yet the elbow is one of the most securely formed joints and therefore is not easy to luxate. In extension the ulna is locked in place by the interposition of the anconeal process in the olecranon fossa of the humerus. Only when the joint is flexed acutely is it free to luxate without fracture.

Etiology

Direct force is responsible for most luxations of this joint. The force is applied to the lateral side of the limb above the joint when the elbow is in acute flexion (45° or less) and the weight is on the forefoot. Indirect force in the form of twisting may also be a factor. Violent twisting with abduction or adduction is conducive to luxation. Johnson has reported a subluxation of the radial head apparently caused by rotation of the body while the limb is bearing weight. The body twist is toward the opposite limb.

Pathology

Displacement of the radius and ulna is lateral with disruption of both the medial and lateral collateral ligaments as well as the joint capsule. Swelling may be mild to severe, but hemorrhage is seldom serious. The ulnar nerve, which crosses the elbow joint just caudal to the medial epicondyle of the humerus, may be injured with resulting paralysis of some of the flexors of the digits, the deep digital flexors, and the flexor carpi ulnaris. This injury is usually not serious and the paralysis is temporary.

When the radius alone is luxated and the ulna is fractured, displacement may be dorsal but it is frequently lateral.

Signs

There is no weight bearing on the limb. The elbow is abducted and the forearm is rotated inward while being held in a fixed position. Usually there is mild flexion in all joints unless the ulnar nerve is injured. It is impossible to extend the elbow fully. The joint appears to be slightly swollen, but on palpation most of the protrusion proves to be the luxated coronoid process. Deep palpation on the medial side reveals the medial epicondyle of the humerus and perhaps the trochlear surface of the joint. During the examination a comparison should be made with the sound joint.

When the radius luxates with fracture of the ulna, the condition is more painful. The deformity may be somewhat variable since the radius may displace dorsally, although it usually does so laterally. Lateral deformity resembles a complete luxation. When the luxation is dorsal, the elbow cannot be flexed beyond 90° because the displaced radius is forced against the humerus. Palpation of the luxated radius is usually simple.

In subluxation of the radial head there is lameness. Palpation of the elbow joint elicits pain but swelling is not a constant sign. Usually there is increased pronation and suppination when the elbow and carpus are flexed at right angles. When the limb is supinated, the radial head can be felt to luxate laterally.

Diagnosis

A roentgenogram in the antero-posterior position is best for diagnosis (Fig. 218). Lateral views are deceiving and do not give a true perspective of the joint. The patient is placed in sternal recumbency and the foreleg is extended with the point of the elbow resting on the cassette. A perfect image can be made by slightly elevating the posterior end of the cassette and tilting the tube so that the beam is vertical to the cassette. Roentgenographic evidence is usually inconclusive in the case of subluxation of the radial head.

Prognosis

Ordinarily the prognosis is good. When the condition is chronic or complicated with fractures the results cannot be predicted accurately (Fig. 219).

Treatment

With the patient in lateral recumbency and under surgical anesthesia, the limb is flexed at all joints. It is important that the elbow angle be less than 45°, so that the anconeal process will clear the lateral condyle. The foot

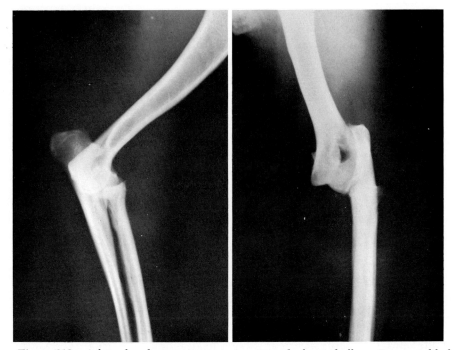

Figure 218. A lateral and an antero-posterior view of a luxated elbow. It can readily be seen that the A-P view is more diagnostic.

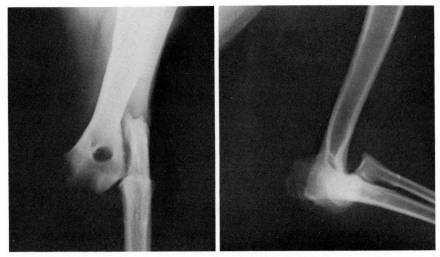

Figure 219. A chronic luxation of the elbow of two months' duration. This required an open reduction. Fibrosis can be seen in the periarticular areas.

is rotated outward so that the semilunar notch faces medially. Traction is then applied to the forearm to force it beyond the epicondyle, while at the same time the ulna and radius are forced medially. It is sometimes necessary, in order to obtain sufficient traction, to drill a full pin through the olecranon. This improves the leverage necessary to slide the olecranon over the lateral condyle in cases where there is muscle spasm or shortening. The pin is removed when reduction is completed.

A rocking motion may be helpful in a long-standing case. This is produced by alternately putting pressure on the olecranon and then on the foot. It has been referred to as "walking" the bone into position.

Some chronic luxations may require open reduction. The incision is made on the caudo-lateral aspect of the elbow for a distance of approximately 3 inches above and 3 inches below the point of the elbow. The joint is exposed by continuation of the incision through the aponeurosis of the triceps. Usually the anconeus muscle is ruptured, but if it is not, it will be necessary to separate this muscle to expose the joint.

Chronic luxations are characterized by fibrous growth in and around the joint. This must be carefully removed before repositioning the bones. In some instances it may be necessary to widen the tear in the capsule before reduction can be accomplished.

Recent luxations seldom require splintage, but if the rupture of the capsule and ligaments is great, some fixation may be required. Chronic luxations should always be splinted for at least one week. The leg is held in extension and a coaptation splint is applied.

Luxation of the radius with fracture of the ulna requires open reduction in most instances (Fig. 149). The best approach is from the lateral side of the forearm. A skin incision is made from a point 2 inches above the joint and extending halfway to the carpus. The radius is exposed by blunt separation of the lateral and common digital extensors. The heavy capsule is cut to allow the replacement of the radius while the leg is held in extension.

A stainless steel screw is placed through the radius and ulna about 1 inch distal to the joint. In drilling for this screw placement, the bit should be kept as close to the lateral edge of the radius as possible with the point slightly inclined in a lateral direction.

The joint capsule is sutured if possible, and the incision is closed in the usual manner. No external splintage should be necessary. The screw may be removed in six weeks or it may be allowed to remain.

A subluxation of the radial head usually responds to rest for one week to 10 days. The limb should be supported in flexion.

LUXATIONS OF THE CARPUS, METACARPUS, AND PHALANGES

Luxations involving the carpus are far less common than those in the tarsus. In our clinic they constitute only 1.5 per cent of all luxations.

Many of the injuries in this region are sprains with tearing of the interosseous ligaments. Dogs that perform violent exercise such as running and jumping are more prone to this type of damage.

Metacarpal and phalangeal luxations are infrequent. The usual injuries here are fractures.

Swelling, distortion, pain, and crepitus are all common signs. Lameness is evident when the animal is moving but usually some weight is borne when standing.

Reduction is effected by simple digital manipulation and pressure. Coaptation for two weeks is usually sufficient fixation to bring about healing.

REFERENCES

Alexander, J. E.: Open reduction and fixation of shoulder luxation. Small Animal Clin., 2:379–382, 1962.

Ball, D. C.: A case of medial luxation of the canine shoulder joint and its surgical correction. Vet. Rec., 83:195–196, 1968.

Bradley, O. C.: Topographical Anatomy of the Dog. 6th ed. London, Oliver & Boyd, 1959.

Brinker, W. O., and Sales, E. K.: Treatment of dislocation of the elbow in dogs. Vet. Med., 44:135, 1949.

Campbell, J. R.: Shoulder lameness in the dog. J. Small Animal Pract., 9:189–198, 1968.

DeAngelis, M., and Schwartz, A.: Surgical correction of cranial dislocation of the scapulohumeral joint in a dog. J.A.V.M.A., 156:435–438, 1970.

Gump, R. H., and Heiser, H. W., Jr.: Open reduction of a complete luxation of the elbow. Vet. Med., 50:183–184, 1955.

Hickman, J.: Veterinary Orthopaedics. Edinburgh, Oliver & Boyd, 1964.

Hoerlein, B. F., Evans, L. E., and Davis, J. M.: Upward luxation of the canine scapula. J.A.V.M.A., 136:258–259, 1960.

Hourrigan, J. L.: Medial luxation of the elbow joint in a collie. Vet. Med., 35:367, 1940.

Irwin, D. H. G.: Open reduction of scapulo-humeral dislocation in a dog. J. So. Afr. Vet. Med. Assoc., 33:397–399, 1962.

Johnson, L. A.: Traumatic subluxation of the radial head in the canine. J. Small Animal Pract., suppl. 4:9–11, 1963.

Kavit, A. U., and Pellegrino, R.: Surgical correction of scapulo-humeral luxation in a dog. J.A.V.M.A., 153:180–181, 1968.

Leighton, R. L.: Replacement of chronic luxation of the canine elbow. Vet. Med. Small Animal Clin., 62:766–773, 1967.

Miller, M. E., Christensen, G. C., and Evans, H. E.: Anatomy of the Dog. Philadelphia, W. B. Saunders Co., 1964.

Piermattei, D. L., and Greeley, R. G.: An Atlas of Surgical Approaches to the Bones of the Dog and Cat. Philadelphia, W. B. Saunders Co., 1966.

Pillet, B.: Une méthode de réduction d'une luxation du carpe. Canad. J. Comp. Med., 21:309, 1957.

Vaughan, L. C.: Dislocation of the shoulder joint in the dog and cat. J. Small Animal Pract., 8:45–48, 1967.

Vaughan, L. C. and Jones, D. G. C.: Congenital dislocation of the shoulder joint in the dog. J. Small Animal Pract., 10:1–3, 1969.

Chapter 10

Luxations of the Mandible and Spine

LUXATION OF THE MANDIBLE (TEMPORO-MANDIBULAR LUXATION)

The mandible articulates with the mandibular fossa of the temporal bone by means of the condyloid or articular process located about halfway along the caudal border of the ramus. It is a hinge-type joint. A thin articular disc separates the articulation into two joint cavities. The joint is surrounded by a strong capsule and is supported laterally by the temporo-mandibular ligament. The heavy temporal muscles afford the joint good protection from direct violence. Normally the mouth can be opened to about 70° without damage to the capsule.

The pterygoid and masseter muscles apply force in a rostral direction and slightly upward. The temporal muscle applies force in the caudal direction. This relieves the temporo-mandibular joint from undue pressure because it does not act as a fulcrum, but rather as a pivotal point for the forces exerted by these two sets of muscles (Fig. 220).

Mandibular luxations occur far less frequently than fractures, probably because the joint is so well protected. Indirect force is usually the cause. The three most common methods of producing luxation are biting on large solid objects, tugging at firmly embedded objects, and a blow on the chin while the mouth is open. Hunting dogs frequently tear roots from the ground and chew on large stones while pursuing burrowing types of game. This is probably the most common cause of mandibular luxations. Falls and blows in which the force is principally against the point of the jaw, particularly with the mouth ajar, are possible but less likely causes.

The ramus is displaced forward and upward. The condyloid process rests close to the posterior zygomatic process. Tearing of the capsule produces hemorrhage. Swelling is usually slight to moderate.

Frequently in this type of luxation, the mouth is open and the jaw

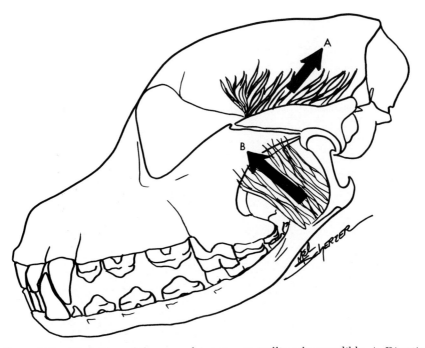

Figure 220. Illustration of the muscular action controlling the mandible. A, Direction of the force applied by the temporal muscle. B, Direction of the force applied by the masseter muscle.

appears paralyzed. Sometimes salivation is a prominent sign, so that on casual observation the condition may be mistaken for rabies. If the luxation is unilateral, the bite shifts toward the opposite side of the mouth. In bilateral luxations the jaw protrudes, and this may be noticeable even though the patient is unable to close his mouth. The eyes appear to bulge because of the pressure produced by the luxated rami.

Care should be taken to diagnose this condition correctly, because it can easily be confused with fractures of the rami or neck of the condyle (Fig. 221). A roentgenogram is important and should include views in several planes. Those who are equipped to do so may find it advantageous to take a laminograph, although ordinarily a simple flat picture is sufficient.

In recent luxations the prognosis is fairly good. Luxations several days old may not reduce easily and may also be difficult to keep reduced. Until correction has been achieved, the prognosis should be guarded.

Attempts at reduction should be made with the patient under anesthesia and in sternal recumbency. A wooden dowel or some other similar object that will not harm the teeth is placed transversely across the mouth at about the level of the last pre-molars. The mouth is then forced closed by applying pressure around the muzzle. At the same time the mandible is forced cau-

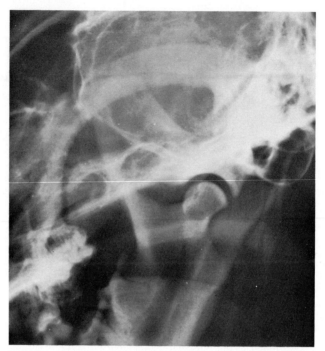

Figure 221.   Luxation of the mandible. The roentgenogram is taken at an oblique angle.

dally. If reduction does not occur fairly promptly, further examination of the injury should be made. It is quite likely then that the injury is a fracture.

Aftercare consists of feeding soft or liquid foods for two or three days. No fixation is required.

LUXATIONS OF THE SPINE

This injury seldom occurs without concurrent fracture of one of the articular processes. A common simultaneous fracture is that of the mammillary process. Luxation of the spine constitutes 7.5 per cent of all luxations seen in the dog and cat. Both complete luxations and subluxations are observed.

The cause is usually direct violence with displacement dorsally, ventrally, or laterally. Frequently the caudal segment is displaced ventrally. Subluxations can result when only the ligaments on one side are disrupted. If there is pressure on the cord from the vertebrae, hemorrhage, or swelling, the signs are identical with fracture of the spine. The forelimbs are extended, and the hindlimbs are paraplegic. Both sensory and motor paralyses are commonly present.

The back is arched at the point of injury and is extremely sensitive just cranial to the luxation. Lateral deviations of the spine are indicated by scoliosis. Depending upon the amount of pressure placed on the spinal cord, some luxations may show only pain without deformity or paralysis. Careful palpation of the spinous process will usually give some clue as to the difficulty.

Before the examination has proceeded very far, a roentgenogram should be taken to determine the exact location of the vertebrae on either side of the luxation. A lateral view in some cases will indicate whether the displacement is great enough to sever the cord (Fig. 222). In borderline cases it may be profitable to undertake reduction in the hope that the cord is not too badly damaged (Fig. 223).

In any event, a poor prognosis should be given. Greene has indicated that if reduction is carried out within eight hours after the injury the outcome is more likely to be good.

Open reduction must be used in most cases to obtain proper results. A skin incision is made over the dorsal spines for at least three vertebrae in either direction. The longissimus dorsi is separated from the spinous process so that the vertebrae are free to manipulate. The spinous process on either side of the luxation is grasped with heavy forceps and is distracted until the mammillary processes are longitudinally separated. While the vertebrae are thus distracted, the lower segment can be raised and the elevated segment depressed until the two are apposed.

Some sort of fixation should be applied in all cases. Internal fixation in the form of a bone plate is recommended (Fig. 224). This is applied in the

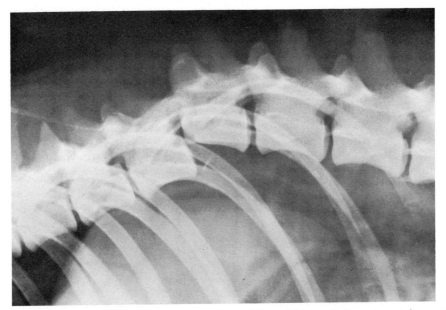

Figure 222. A spinal luxation between the twelfth and thirteenth thoracic vertebrae with severance of the spinal cord.

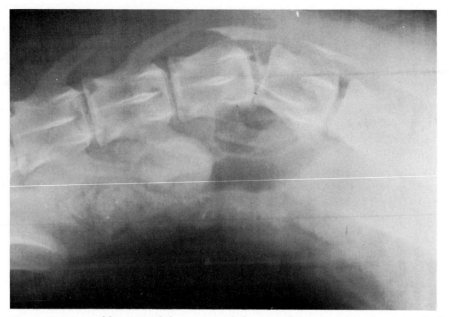

Figure 223. A subluxation of the spine with fracture of the transverse processes. In this case the cord damage was not severe.

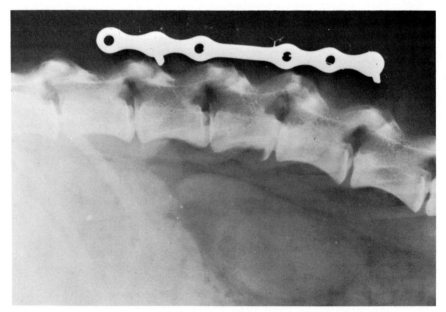

Figure 224. Repair of a spinal luxation by means of a bone plate attached with wires and screws.

same fashion as for spinal fractures. A body cast furnishes additional support and should be used if the injury is complicated by fracture of any of the articular processes.

Improvement should be noticeable in about two weeks. During the recovery period the patient should be kept fairly active in an exercise cart, and all possible measures should be taken to avoid decubital necrosis.

Geary, Oliver, and Hoerlein have described a slowly progressive sub-luxation of the atlanto-axial articulation. The ventral body of the axis rotates upward so that it presses the spinal cord against the dorsal arch of the atlas. This rotation is usually brought about as a result of fracture of the odontoid process or rupture of the transverse atlantal ligament.

Clinical signs may appear suddenly, but usually the onset is likely to be of a slow, chronic type. High cervical pain which can be intensified by flexing the neck is followed by knuckling of the paws, paresis, and paralysis. A lateral roentgenogram is necessary for positive diagnosis (Fig. 225).

Surgical repair consists of wiring the atlas and axis on the dorsal side (Fig. 226). This prevents rotation and tilting of the axis. Exposure is made on the dorsal midline, starting at the base of the skull and proceeding caudad until the atlas and axis can be reached easily. The aponeurosis is incised on the midline and dissected deep enough to expose the nuchal ligament. This ligament lies over the dorsal spinous processes. The incision should be continued lateral to the ligament and the muscles should be separated from the spinous processes to expose the dorsal arch of the atlas. The musculature is bluntly separated and retracted laterally from the dorsal arch of the atlas and the spinous process of the axis.

Heavy-gauge wire is passed around the dorsal arch of the atlas and passed through a hole drilled in the axial spinous process. When this wire is

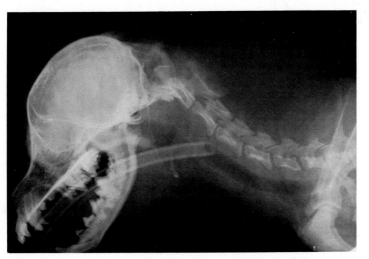

Figure 225.   Roentgenogram showing the rotation and tilting of the axis in a miniature poodle.

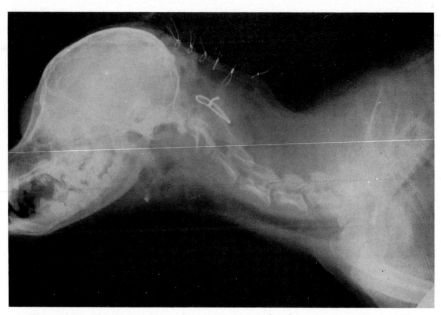

Figure 226. Roentgenogram taken postoperatively of case seen in Figure 225.

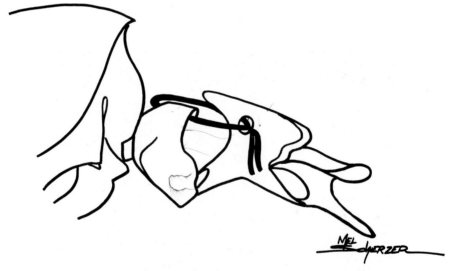

Figure 227. Diagram to illustrate the placement of the restraining wire in atlanto-axial subluxation.

tightened, the two vertebrae are brought into proper apposition and rotation of the axis is prevented (Fig. 227).

Failures of this method frequently occur because the wire breaks or because the wire gradually cuts through the relatively soft symphysis of the atlas. A suggested improvement would be the use of a Teflon strip placed around the dorsal arch of the atlas. The ends of the strip would be placed on either side of the spinous process of the axis. After reduction of the subluxation, the Teflon would be anchored to the axis by means of a bolt through the spinous process.

In those cases in which failure of the anchorage has not occurred, the subluxation has been corrected and the recovery has been complete.

REFERENCES

Bradley, O. C.: Topographical Anatomy of the Dog. 6th ed. London, Oliver & Boyd, 1959.

Bradley, I. W.: Repair of fracture-dislocation of lumbar vertebrae in a French poodle. Aust. Vet. Jour., 43:421–424, 1967.

Geary, J. C., Oliver, J. E., and Hoerlein, B. F.: Atlanto-axial subluxation in the canine. J. Small Animal Pract.,8:577–582, 1967.

Greene, J. E.: Reduction of vertebral luxation. N. Am. Vet. 31:816, 1950.

Miller, M. E., Christensen, G. C., and Evans, H. E.: Anatomy of the Dog. Philadelphia, W. B. Saunders Co., 1964.

Robinson, M.: The reflex controlled non-lever action of the mandible. Calif. Vet., 12:28–30, 1959.

White, C. A.: Bilateral forward mandibular luxation in a dog. N. Am. Vet., 30:777, 1959.

PART FOUR

Other Orthopedic Diseases

Chapter 11

Soft Tissue Repair
in Compound Fractures

An integral part of orthopedic surgery is the repair of all tissues in addition to bone that have been damaged and that might have a direct bearing on locomotion. The contaminated and lacerated soft tissues surrounding a fracture must be returned to as near normalcy as possible so that the restoration will not be interrupted. With a little help from nature, the restoration of muscles following laceration can usually be accomplished through simple suturing of the muscle sheath or the surrounding fascia. Such structures as nerves, blood vessels, and tendons require more exacting workmanship and more attention to detail. Since ligament repair has been extensively discussed under Luxations, this chapter will deal only with nerves, blood vessels, and tendons. The continuity of these tissues should be restored only after the wound has been completely cleaned and debrided.

The first step is wound débridement. Unless especially contraindicated, this should be performed under general anesthesia so that the patient is quiet and does not recontaminate the wound through struggling. General anesthesia also facilitates proper positioning so that the wound is easily accessible.

As soon as the patient is anesthetized, the wound is packed with dry sterile gauze sponges and the entire surrounding area is thoroughly clipped and cleansed. The wound is washed with generous amounts of sterile saline and is repacked. Other preparation is carried out with asepsis in mind.

When the preparations have been completed and the patient is fully draped, the packs are removed and débridement is begun. The skin margin is incised about 3 or 4 mm. from the wound edge, and this incision is carried completely around the wound with surgical scissors so that a completely fresh skin margin is created (Fig. 228). The separated skin should be turned toward the center of the wound so that the fresh edges do not become contaminated. Careful dissection of the tissues lining the wound should then be attempted. This is best accomplished by holding the contaminated tissue

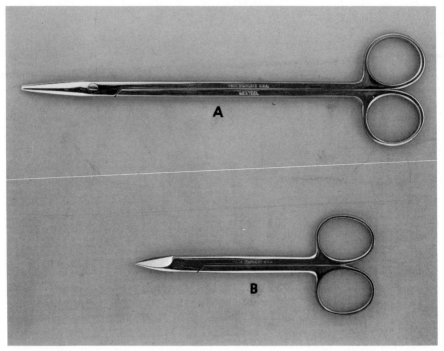

Figure 228. Metzenbaum surgical scissors (A). These are excellent for tissue cutting and separation. They should not be used to cut sutures; the scissors labeled B are used for this purpose, and they are shaped differently so that there will be no confusion between the two pairs of scissors.

with thumb forceps and separating the tissue beneath with scissors. If a portion of the soiled tissue separates from the rest, it should be removed from the area, but in many cases the entire contaminated lining of the wound can be separated and removed in one piece.

Small bleeding vessels are ligated and a complete survey of the wound is made to ascertain the extent of the damage and the amount of repair necessary before closure. The fracture is repaired by whatever method seems advisable, after which the repair of nerves, blood vessels, and tendons is undertaken.

NERVE REPAIR

The repair of nerves has met with poor success in most cases and therefore has not been undertaken to any extent in the dog and cat. The apposition of severed nerve trunks, even though carefully done, does not necessarily mean that the funiculi are properly aligned; in fact, they are quite likely not to be. If the nerve is badly traumatized but not separated, it is possible to suture soft tissue such as muscle around it to protect it during healing. In humans this is often done even when the nerve is divided. A delayed repair is then done about three or four weeks later.

If nerve repair is undertaken, it is necessary to uncover the divided ends for a distance of 2 cm. The ends must then be matched so that funiculi are aligned. A small blood vessel transversing the nerve may be of some value in matching the ends, and the general shape and position of the ends will also help. This part of the surgery is very exacting.

The nerve is sectioned transversely with a sharp knife so that uninjured nerve tissue will be exposed. When these important preliminary steps have been taken, the epineurium is sutured with fine stainless steel wire using two or three interrupted sutures and tying with a single knot.

VASCULAR REPAIR

In the dog and cat many of the blood vessels are too small for repair and must be ligated. One must rely on collateral circulation to maintain the blood supply in the distal parts of appendages under such circumstances. If the vascular damage is extensive, the blood supply may be inadequate, whereupon necrosis ensues. Seldom is vascular repair undertaken if collateral circulation will maintain the part affected. However, in certain instances the blood vessels may be large enough to warrant surgical repair. This applies more particularly to arteries than to veins because of their structure.

Vascular injuries which are extensive enough to cause complete interruption of the arterial supply to an extremity are usually caused by compound comminuted fractures with considerable tissue loss. Such an injury is characterized by total ischemia of the pendant portions of the limb. The signs of ischemia are lack of pulse, paralysis, and coldness distal to the injury.

Since total ischemia seldom occurs in the dog or cat at a high enough level on the limb that blood vessels are of sufficient size to make repair practical, the techniques which are described here will only occasionally be found useful to the veterinarian. In larger patients repairs can be made proximal to the stifle and the elbow, but in smaller patients the blood vessels, even in these areas, may be too diminutive for surgical repair.

The greatest hazard of blood vessel repair is clot formation within the lumen. This is brought about by the liberation of thromboplastic substances, usually through excessive trauma, rough uncoated suture material within the lumen, or extraneous bits of free tissue introduced into the lumen. If the intima is handled gently, the suture material is waxed or oiled, and the adventitia is stripped from the area to be sutured, there will be minimum stimulation of clot formation. The use of heparin has also been suggested as a means of preventing clotting. This may be placed directly in the sutured area or it may be given intravenously for its general effect during the

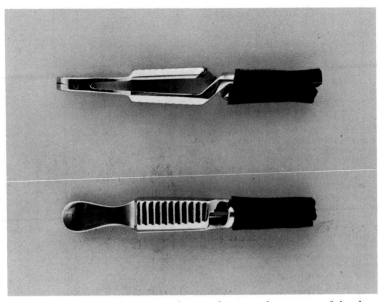

Figure 229. The small size serrafine used in vascular surgery of the dog.

operation. Markowitz recommends the subcutaneous use of heparin in Pit-
kin's medium. The release of heparin by this method is slow enough to
prolong the effect for 24 hours.

Arteries which are lacerated may be restored to use by a simple closure
of the rent. Trimming of the wound edges is seldom recommended unless
they are extremely uneven. Bulldog or serrafine clamps (Fig. 229) are
applied on either side of the wound. These should be rubber-shod. The
wound is flushed with normal saline and an intima to intima approximation
is made with 6-0 or 7-0 braided surgical silk that has been soaked in sterile
olive oil. The suture material should be swaged to a curved taper-point
needle so that trauma to the vessel wall is minimized. Either the BV-1
needle of Ethicon or the TE-1 D & G needle is satisfactory. Traction sutures
are first placed at either end of the wound and enough tension applied to
bring the wound edges into apposition (Fig. 230). The defect is then closed
with a continuous through and through suture, taking only small bites of
tissue on either side (2 mm.) and drawing the edges together so that they are
firm but not puckered. Before final closure a small amount of 0.01 per cent
heparin is instilled in the vessel on both sides of the serrafines to prevent
clotting. Following closure the tension sutures are removed and the distal
serrafine is released. Some oozing of blood from suture holes occurs when
the proximal serrafine is released, but this gradually subsides as clotting
takes place outside the vessel.

In injuries in which a large artery has been completely severed, it is
possible that an end to end anastomosis can be performed if there is not a
great loss of traumatized tissue. Two commonly used methods of end to end

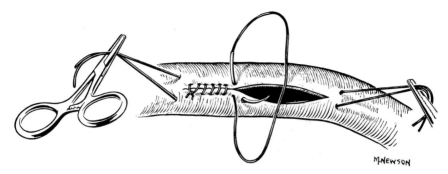

Figure 230.   Closure of a longitudinal wound in a blood vessel.

anastomosis are the Carrel technique and the Linton technique. The latter method employs splitting and trimming of the vessel ends so that a side to side technique is employed for an end to end joining.

Markowitz has recommended the Carrel technique in dogs, and this seems practical. The cut ends of the vessel are clamped with serrafines, leaving a reasonable length of vessel between the cut end and the clamp for easy manipulation during the suturing. The ends are then cut transversely with a sharp instrument so that the edges are even. As much of the vessel as possible should be preserved, and trimming should be very conservative.

The adventitia is grasped with a fine forceps and is stretched over the cut end of the vessel. The elongated adventitia stretching beyond the end of the vessel is detached with iris scissors. This will leave a narrow band at the end of the vessel devoid of adventitia so that this tissue will not be carried into the lumen during the suturing process. The cut ends of the vessel are then flushed with physiologic saline and are then covered with a film of sterile olive oil or paraffin oil.

Apposition of the two cut ends of the vessel is accomplished by placing three equally-spaced through and through stay sutures which are tied but not cut (Fig. 231). When tension is applied to these sutures a triangle will be formed. The traction should be great enough to evert the cut edges of the vessel. This can be achieved by weighting one suture with a hemostat and having an assistant pull lightly on the other two. On the other hand, the surgeon may prefer to apply traction on one suture with his free hand while suturing with the other.

Since each stay suture consists of a free end and an end with a needle attached, the closure is begun by placing a continuous through and through suture from the first stay suture to the second and there tying to the free end. These sutures should be placed evenly about 1 mm. apart and drawn tightly enough that there is intima to intima contact. The second needle is then used to close the second leg of the triangle in a like manner, and closure of the third leg is done with a needle attached to the third stay suture.

The distal serrafine is removed first. One should expect some seepage when the proximal serrafine is removed, but if the suturing has been done

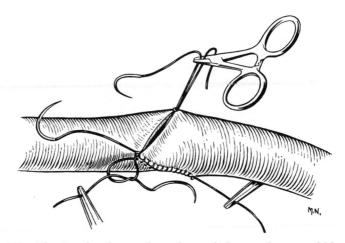

Figure 231. The Carrel technique for end to end closure of a severed blood vessel.

carefully this should soon subside. Gelfoam (Upjohn) may be packed around the blood vessel, and it is a good safeguard to support the repair by suturing muscle or fascia around it whenever possible.

Other methods of blood vessel repair could be described, but those set forth in this chapter seem to be the simplest to perform and have proved to be quite effective. The student who is interested in pursuing this phase of surgery further is referred to any good text on vascular surgery.

TENDON REPAIR

Tendon injuries occur most commonly in the region of the hock, the tarsus, or the carpus. Many times these injuries are not associated with fractures, but it is not unusual to encounter severance of a tendon in injuries of bone and soft tissue of the lower limbs. Many of these are caused by harvesting machinery. The most serious tendon injury is the division of the tendon of the gastrocnemius and the tendon of the superficial digital flexor.

Perhaps more important than the mechanics of repair of tendons is a knowledge of the healing of tendons. Surgical repair is comparatively easy once the healing process of this tissue is understood. The only cell present in tendons is the fibroblast; the remainder of the structure is composed of collagenous bundles which lie parallel and rather closely packed. The blood supply is limited and is mostly contained in the mesotendon, a synovial membrane which forms a fold between the tendon and the sheath. In some cases the mesotendon may stretch to form a bridge between the severed ends of a tendon. When this happens, healing may take place by granulation along the mesotendon, but the patient is left with a slack tendon.

Tendon tissue heals slowly because of its poor blood supply, but healing of the sheath is much more rapid. Proliferation begins about the fourth or fifth day and requires at least two weeks under optimum healing conditions. This growth resembles the growth of a callus in a fractured bone in many ways. Blood fills the space between the ruptured ends of the tendon. This is transformed into granulation tissue, which in turn is infiltrated by fibroplastic proliferation. The new tissue gradually assumes the appearance of tendon and becomes avascular. The change to tendinous tissue progresses more rapidly with mild use, but since early use of a tendon may lead to separation of the ends, it is generally recommended that movement of the tendon be delayed until the third week of healing.

Whenever the sheath is divided along with the tendon, there is a likelihood for scar tissue to form over the retracted ends, thereby setting up adhesions with the surrounding tissues and the tendon sheath. Such adhesions will not form in the presence of fatty tissue, and for this reason it is advisable to remove the sheath in the region of a tendon repair and to surround the sutured area with subcutaneous fat or muscle fascia. Such a healing response takes place whenever adhesions of the tendon and sheath are separated regardless of the aftercare. It is important, therefore, that some precaution be taken to prevent adhesions, whether the repair is primary or delayed, since an adhesion will nullify the action of a tendon distal to the lesion.

Of equal importance is the handling of tendon during the operation. Because this tissue is rather avascular, it is extremely easy to produce necrosis through excessive trauma. During the suturing it is best to grasp the end of the tendon firmly in a forceps. The bruised tip is then cut off with a sharp knife before the ends are joined.

For larger tendons, the Bunnell method of suturing (Fig. 232) or some modification (Fig. 233) is commonly used. The suture material can be cotton, silk, or stainless steel, and the knots are cut close and are slightly sunk in the tendon tissue. Either single or double armed suture is used; the needles should be straight taper.

In suturing the smaller tendons of the foot, a pull-out method is to be preferred. This requires a special suture made of stainless steel with a V-shaped barb in the middle, a straight taper needle on one end, and a half-circle cutting edge needle on the other (Fig. 234). The straight needle is used to suture through the tendon, starting about 0.5 cm. from the divided end, crossing the gap, and emerging about 0.5 cm. from the end of the

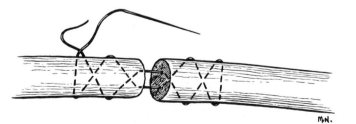

Figure 232. Bunnell method of suturing tendons.

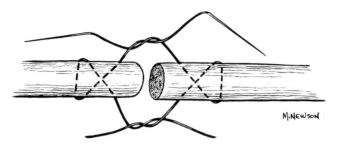

Figure 233. A modification of the Bunnell method in which the sutures are tied on both sides of the closure.

opposite tendon segment. A second suture is placed in a like manner but from the opposite direction. The curved needles in turn are pushed through the skin at a convenient spot and the needles are removed from the wire. These two ends are to serve as the pull-outs after healing is completed. The straight needles are next exteriorized fairly close to the point where they emerge from the tendon but a sufficient distance away so that the tendon ends will approximate when moderate tension is applied to the wires. A button is attached to each of these wires, and sufficient traction is applied to bring about end to end apposition of the tendon (Fig. 235). The skin is then closed and the buttons and pull-out wires are left in place under a bandage.

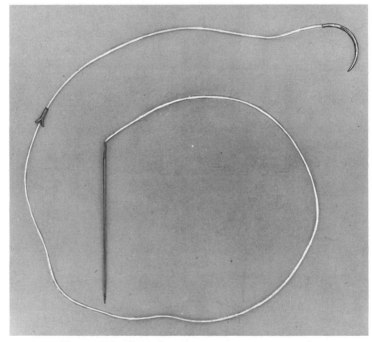

Figure 234. Special tendon repair suture material.

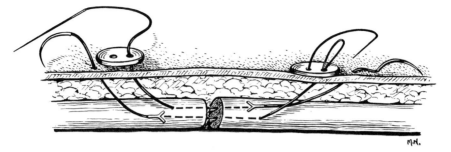

Figure 235. Application of the special tendon suture. The barbs hold the tendon while the buttons maintain the traction necessary for apposition of the ends.

Removal is accomplished simply by cutting the wire at the button and exerting traction on the pull-out.

Splintage is important in tendon repair because of the slow healing and the tendency for muscles to exert traction if not countered in some way. A simple rule to remember in this regard is to splint with the limb in flexion when the flexors are involved and in extension when the extensors are involved. In most instances a simple coaptation splint is sufficient, but if the patient will not allow this to remain in place, half pinning can be used if the bones are large enough, or a cradle may be applied if the small tendons of the feet are involved.

The part should be kept quiet for at least two weeks, after which a system of gradual testing and exercise in slowly increasing amounts should be instituted. More care needs to be given larger tendons during this period because they are subjected to greater strain.

REFERENCES

Armistead, W. W.: Canine Surgery. 4th ed. Evanston, Ill., American Veterinary Publications, 1957.

Bancroft, F. W., and Marble, H. C.: Surgical Treatment of the Musculo-Skeletal System. 2nd ed. Philadelphia, J. B. Lippincott Co., 1951.

Butler, H. C.: Canine Surgery. 1st Archibald ed. Santa Barbara, Cal., American Veterinary Publications, 1965.

Butler, H. C.: Tendon surgery in small animals. An. Hosp., 2:236-244, 1966.

Davis, L.: Christopher's Textbook of Surgery. 7th ed. Philadelphia, W. B. Saunders Co., 1960.

Dinsmore, J. R.: Canine Surgery. 4th ed. Evanston, Ill., American Veterinary Publications, 1957.

Linton, R. E.: Some practical considerations in the surgery of blood vessel grafts. Surgery, 38:817-834, 1955.

Markowitz, J., Archibald, J., and Downie, H. G.: Experimental Surgery. 4th ed. Baltimore, Williams & Wilkins Co., 1959.

Milch, H., and Milch, R. A.: Fracture Surgery. New York, Paul B. Hoeber, Inc., 1959.

Sterner, W.: Surgery of the tendons in dogs. Dtsch. tierarztl Wschr., 66:289-294, 325-329, 1959.

Chapter 12

Amputations

It has often been said in human surgical treatises on the subject that the aim of amputation is to save life and improve function. Much has been written and the skill of amputation is highly developed in human surgery. Prostheses are common. Many are very sophisticated, having mechanized and electronic parts which assist in moving the limbs.

In the dog and cat the primary purpose of amputation is somewhat different. To be sure, this type of surgery is done to save life in the case of injuries causing terminal necrosis, malignant tumors of the appendages, injuries from harvesting equipment or automobiles in which the distal portion is hopelessly damaged, or any condition of the limb which threatens the life of the patient. But more often amputation is performed to improve function by getting the useless appendage out of the way of the three remaining well-functioning limbs. In this respect the four-legged animal has the advantage. A major factor in amputation is cosmetic appearance. Frequently this becomes very important in the decision to amputate. This factor involves the client and not the patient. The veterinarian is often faced with a client who is horrified at the thought of amputation. Even after being convinced that the surgery should be done, he is quite likely to insist on preserving as much of the limb as possible. This is understandable because this is what is usually done in man, in whom the use of prostheses is common. In the dog and cat, a prosthesis is seldom used and a long stump is cumbersome, unsightly, and very frequently subject to abrasion, infection, and ulceration. It is therefore important to produce a good cosmetic effect provided the requirements of life and function can also be met.

AMPUTATION OF THE PELVIC LIMB

The level of amputation of the pelvic limb may vary somewhat with the circumstances, but it should be at least at the level of the stifle (Fig. 236). Sometimes it is necessary to amputate higher, and in such a case it is cosmetically helpful to save enough to cover the genitalia in the male, if at all possible (Fig. 237). In long-legged dogs the amputation can be slightly

278

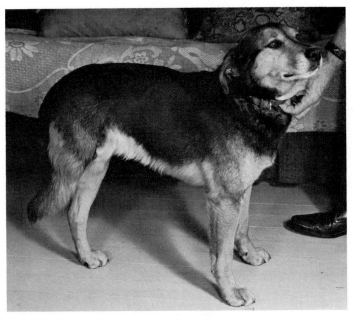

Figure 236. An amputation at the stifle, two years postoperative.

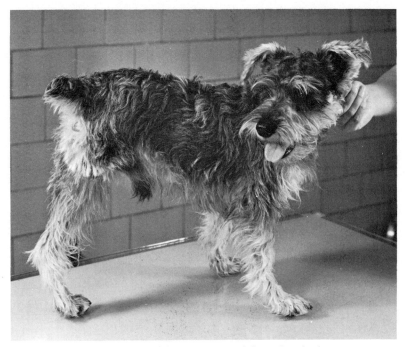

Figure 237. High amputation of the pelvic limb.

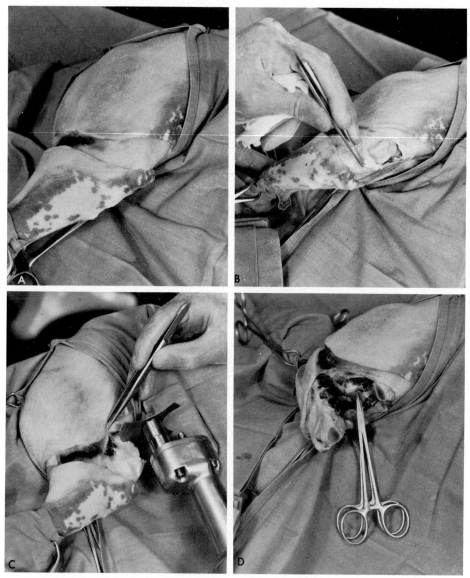

Figure 238A.   Skin incision just proximal to the stifle.
Figure 238B.   Tendon of the quadriceps transected and the joint capsule opened.
Figure 238C.   Cutting the femur with a Stryker saw.
     Figure 238D.   Blood vessels caudomedial to the femur are clamped ready for ligating. The femur has been divided.

(*Illustration continued on opposite page.*)

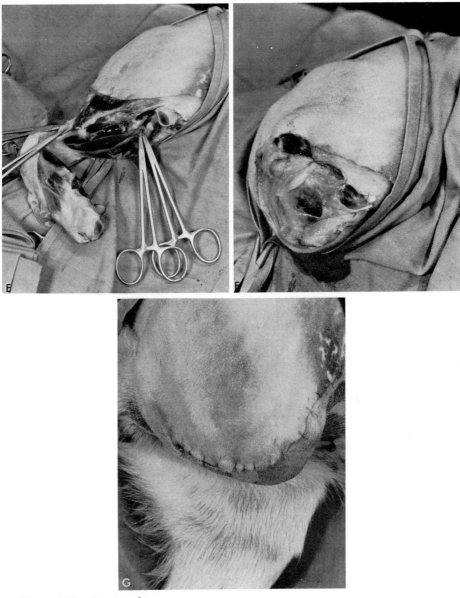

Figure 238. *Continued.*

Figure 238E. The gracilis, semimembranosus, and semitendinosus have been separated from the crural fascia along the tibia and the internal saphenous vessels clamped with hemostats.

Figure 238F. Muscle mass covering the stump of the femur.

Figure 238G. Skin closure with stainless steel sutures, showing length of final stump.

higher than in short-legged ones, because the femur is longer proportionately.

Probably the most common level used is just proximal to the stifle joint. The skin incision on the lateral side of the leg is made in an arc, with one end at the stifle and the other somewhat lower on the caudal side to conform with the contour of the leg (Fig. 238A). If there is doubt, it is always best to leave more skin than will be needed. An incision is next made on the medial side of the leg. This should connect with the lateral incision but should be fairly straight. The skin edges are reflected so that the underlying structures are plainly visible.

The distal shaft of the femur is exposed by nicking the fascia just proximal to the patella so that scissors can be inserted into the femoropatellar joint and the tendon of the quadriceps femoris cut just above the patella. Following this procedure, most of the musculature on cranial, medial, and lateral sides can be bluntly reflected from the bone (Fig. 238B). A saw is used to divide the bone just proximal to the origin of the gastrocnemius muscle on the caudal side of the femur. We prefer to use the Stryker saw (Fig. 238C) and cut carefully because the femoral and caudal femoral arteries and veins lie directly caudal to the bone. As soon as the bone is separated these vessels can be ligated and separated (Fig. 238D).

By transecting the fascial planes caudal and medial to the osteotomy, only four muscles remain. The abductor cruris caudalis is a narrow muscle on the medial side which can be transected without damage. The gracilis, semimembranosus, and semitendinosus must be dissected free from the crural fascia along the tibia. These muscles will separate from the muscle mass along the caudal aspect of the leg (Fig. 238E). The distal appendage has now been separated without transecting through the belly of any large muscle and with a minimum of hemorrhage.

The shorter muscle ends are sutured together. Then the caudal group of muscles are sutured to the tendon of the quadriceps. This forms a thick pad of muscle over the femur stump (Fig. 238F). If the bone end oozes excessively, it can be treated with bone wax either directly after cutting or before covering with the muscle mass.

The skin is trimmed so that the edges appose without tension or sagging. The lateral flap should be slightly longer than the medial. Interrupted stitches of stainless steel make a good closure and tend to discourage licking (Fig. 238G). The area should be well cleaned and a light dressing applied.

AMPUTATION OF THE PECTORAL LIMB

Amputation of the foreleg is performed more frequently than hindleg amputation. Presumably there are three reasons for this. Foreleg amputation is believed to be easier to perform. This supposition is not valid if in both cases a good cosmetic result is achieved. It is also believed that the dog can carry its weight better without a foreleg than it can without a hindleg.

Surprisingly enough, more weight is carried on the forelegs, and for a longer time, than on the hind legs. The third reason is that the client is less likely to object to the loss of a foreleg.

A common cause for loss of the foreleg is brachial or radial paralysis. Permanent damage to these nerves occurs much more frequently than similar deficits in the sciatic nerve. Paralysis of the forelimb leaves a shrunken, unsightly appendage which often becomes ulcerated and infected.

With few exceptions, the limb should be amputated at the shoulder joint to maintain a good cosmetic effect (Fig. 239). A stump is undesirable. The skin incision on the lateral side should begin at the point of the shoulder, follow the natural contour of the body, and end at the dorsal point of the skin fold between the arm and the thorax (Fig. 240A). On the medial side the skin incision should be a straight line between the two ends of the lateral incision (Fig. 240B).

After bluntly separating the subcutaneous tissues so that the musculature is plainly visible, the acromion is cut with bone cutters to free the attachment of the acromial part of the deltoideus muscles (Fig. 240C). When this muscle is reflected the tendons of insertion of the infraspinatus and the teres minor are exposed and transected (Fig. 240D). The other part of the deltoideus is divided by cutting through the tendinous sheath beneath the acromial deltoideus. The joint capsule is opened and with it the tendon of the biceps brachii and joint ligaments are cut (Fig. 240E).

At this point the brachial artery and vein should be ligated and divided

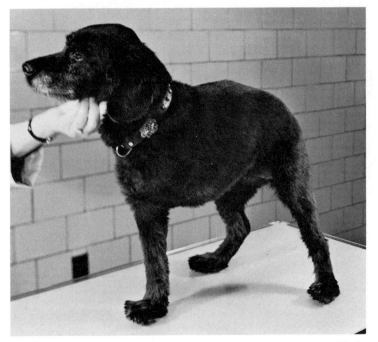

Figure 239. High foreleg amputation about one year postoperative. Notice the well-rounded effect conforming with the general lines of the body.

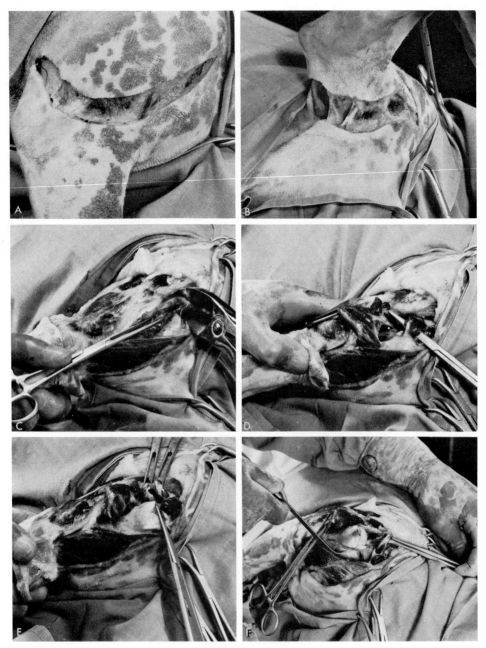

Figure 240A.   Lateral skin incision for foreleg amputation.
Figure 240B.   Medial skin incision for foreleg amputation.
Figure 240C.   Cutting the acromion so that the deltoideus can be reflected.
Figure 240D.   Transecting the tendon of insertion of the infraspinatus.
Figure 240E.   Opening the joint and transecting the tendon of the biceps brachii.
Figure 240F.   Exposure of the brachial artery and vein.

(*Illustration continued on opposite page.*)

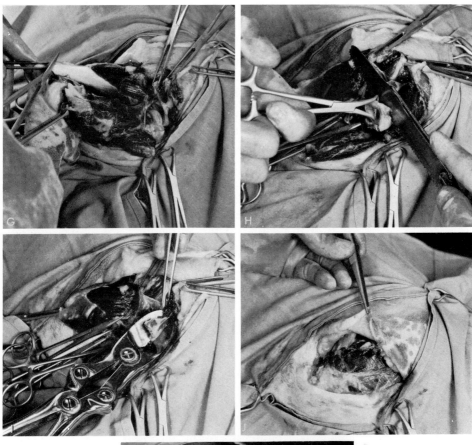

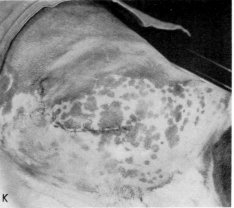

Figure 240. *Continued.*
Figure 240G.   Transecting the tendon of the long head of the triceps.
Figure 240H.   Sawing through the neck of the scapula.
Figure 240I.   Removing the distal portion of the scapular spine.
Figure 240J.   Musculature replaced to form a smooth covering over the stump of the scapula.
Figure 240K.   Closure of the skin.

separately. The site selected for ligation is important. It should be slightly below the level of the joint so that adequate circulation will be provided through the subscapular artery (Fig. 240F).

Separation of the muscles on the medial side is next in order. These are tendons of the coracobrachialis, the latissimus dorsi and teres major (one tendon), and subscapularis. The long head of the triceps is then bluntly dissected as far as the olecranon and transected through the tendinous portion. This completes the severance of the limb (Fig. 240G).

Because there is considerable atrophy of the shoulder muscles, it is necessary to remove some of the scapular spine to produce a good cosmetic effect. As a first step the glenoid cavity is removed by sawing through the neck of the scapula (Fig. 240H). The distal spine is then cut off with bone cutters (Fig. 240I). This reduces the bony prominence and gives the shoulder a smoother, more rounded appearance.

The small muscles at the center of the amputation are drawn together with interrupted stitches. This is followed by tacking the long head of the triceps over the shoulder joint area by drawing it dorso-cranially (Fig. 240J). The skin is trimmed so that the edges can be apposed without tension. Interrupted stitches of stainless steel complete the closure (Fig. 240K).

AMPUTATION OF THE DIGIT

The removal of a toe, if properly done, causes little or no impairment in the usefulness or strength of the foot. This type of surgery often becomes necessary following injury or because of infection or tumors. It is important that the foot be kept as compact as possible, because a "splay" foot is weak and often leads to lameness. Amputation of the second or fifth digit presents no problem concerning compactness because these toes are located on the medial or lateral side of the foot. However, amputation of the third or fourth digit leaves a space in the center of the foot if the stump is not closed in a way that will prevent spreading.

Preparation of the foot for aseptic surgery is a tedious task, but the healing results will pay for the time spent in meticulous preoperative clipping and cleansing. A tourniquet can be applied at the metacarpal or metatarsal region just prior to surgery.

If the second or fifth digit is to be removed, the skin incision should begin at the metacarpo- or metatarso-phalangeal joint and take an elliptical course around the toe and back to the beginning. This means that the incision will cut obliquely across the toe to the webbing between the toes and avoid the large metacarpal or metatarsal pad. There are three arteries to be ligated. These are the palmar or plantar proper arteries. The toe is then disarticulated at the metacarpo- or metatarso-phalangeal joint and the skin is closed with interrupted stitches placed so that the palmar or plantar surface is apposed to the dorsal surface.

When the third or fourth digit is removed, the skin incision is cut in a V, with the apex over the dorsal side of the joint (Fig. 241). The webbing is cut

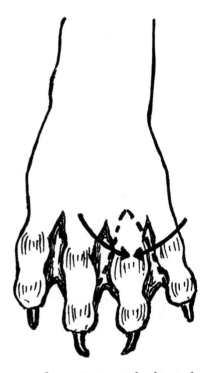

Figure 241. Diagram to illustrate closure after digit amputation.

close to the adjacent toe on either side. There are four arteries to be ligated, after which the toe can be disarticulated. Closure in this case is very important if one is to produce a compact foot. Interrupted stitches are placed on the palmar or plantar side across the gap left by the missing toe. This row of stitches is continued from the large pad forward until the halfway point is reached. Buried stitches are then placed from the dorsal side until the adjoining toes are drawn close together. A row of interrupted stitches on the dorsal skin from side to side completes the closure.

A light foot bandage kept in place for about one week is helpful in supporting the sutures and keeps the foot clean. This can be a stockinette-type of bandage, such as "Tubogauze," which allows air to circulate around the foot.

REFERENCES

Bechtol, C. O.: Amputations and artificial limbs. *In* Christopher's Textbook of Surgery. 7th Ed. Philadelphia, W. B. Saunders Co., 1960.

Brinker, W. O., and Jenkins, T. W.: Amputation of the foreleg in small animals. J.A.V.M.A., *130*:126, 1957.

Evans, H. E., and deLahunta, A.: Miller's Guide to the Dissection of the Dog. Philadelphia, W. B. Saunders Company, 1970.

Frick, E. J.: Amputation. *In* Canine Surgery. 4th ed. Evanston, Ill., American Veterinary Publications, 1957.

Lumb, W. V.: Amputations. *In* Canine Surgery. 1st Archibald ed. Santa Barbara, Cal., American Veterinary Publications, 1965.

Miller, M. E., Christensen, G. C., and Evans, H. E.: Anatomy of the Dog. Philadelphia, W. B. Saunders Co., 1964.

Chapter 13

Intervertebral Disc Disease (Enchondrosis Intervertebralis)

Disease in the intervertebral disc is a degenerative process which from an orthopedic standpoint is of no great consequence in itself. The orthopedist is primarily interested in the eventual effect this degeneration has on loco-motion. The sequence of events in this disease is degeneration of the annulus fibrosus, with or without degeneration of the nucleus pulposus; protrusion of the annulus; rupture of the annulus; extrusion of the nucleus; and, finally, calcification of the nucleus which has been extruded. The degeneration is therefore the primary disease and paresis or paraplegia is secondary.

Dexler first reported on this condition in the dog in 1896. The condition has also been reported as occurring in cats, but the incidence seems to be much lower and the clinical signs are far more infrequent. King et al. report that calcifications rarely occur in the cat. Since Dexler first indicated that protrusion of a degenerated disc brought about pressure on the spinal cord, thereby causing paralysis, it has been confirmed and enlarged upon by a number of investigators. Outstanding work in this field has been done by Riser, Hansen, Olsson, and Hoerlein.

Incidence

Although this condition appears to some extent in all breeds of dogs, it is mostly confined to a few breeds which Hansen designates as chondrodys-trophoid. He has indicated that the French bulldog, the dachshund, and the Pekingese are more disposed to disc troubles. To these breeds we would add the cocker spaniel and the beagle. Of the breeds mentioned, the dachs-hund seems to be afflicted most often.

A one-year survey by Hoerlein of the canine patients at our clinic indicated that 0.7 per cent were suffering from recognizable disc disorders. He also surveyed the routine autopsies during that period and found that 41.5 per cent showed disc lesions but no clinical signs immediately before death. This parallels the finding in humans. Most of the cases are seen in adult dogs between the ages of three and eight. The sexes are about equally affected, although some have credited the male with a higher incidence and have thought that this was due to his greater activity.

Etiology

Situated between the bodies of the vertebrae, the discs are subjected to considerable force and violence at times, particularly in those areas of the spine where the most bending occurs. The function of the disc is twofold: (1) It forms the amphiarthrodial articulation for the two adjoining vertebrae. (2) It acts as a shock absorber to reduce indirect force transmitted along the spine. Whether this intermittent aggravation is directly responsible or a contributing cause is not clear. Degeneration of the disc is apparent with advancing age. Hansen points out that this degeneration is particularly characteristic of certain types of dogs. The normal disc is composed of a gelatinous center (nucleus pulposus) surrounded by a fibrous capsule (annulus fibrosus). This makes an ideal cushion for dispersing a transmitted force in all directions. However, with the so-called chondrodystrophoid individual there is an early change in the nucleus from a gelatinous substance to one that is chondroid. The annulus also undergoes degenerative change, and the disc loses its elasticity. Sometimes the annulus degenerates and ruptures while the nucleus is still in a gelatinous state. This is likely to result in extrusion of the nucleus along the floor of the vertebral canal.

Force may play some part in the final disruption of the disc and it may be a factor in bringing about the changes within the disc, but the primary cause of protrusion and rupture is degeneration.

Pathology

Elasticity of the disc disappears as degeneration progresses. Degeneration may appear in devious forms. It is seen as a calcification, a dehydration, a fibrosis, or a necrosis, although there is some dispute as to the latter form. Degeneration of the annulus occurs with or without the deterioration of the nucleus. In general there are three principal results of decadence in the disc (Fig. 242):

PROTRUSION. In a strict sense, this is an extension of the annulus beyond its normal limits, so that it bulges, thereby putting pressure on surrounding tissues. Some of the fibers of the annulus are ruptured and the capsule is weakened, but the nucleus is still contained within the weakened and bulging annulus fibrosus. Through usage, however, this term has been broadened to include rupture of the annulus with extrusion of the nucleus beneath the dorsal longitudinal ligament and rupture of the annulus with extrusion of the nucleus through or around the dorsal longitudinal ligament, as well as protrusion or rupture of the annulus ventrally or laterally.

Hansen has classified these protrusions as: Type I, those that have spread along the canal for the length of a vertebra and occupy considerable

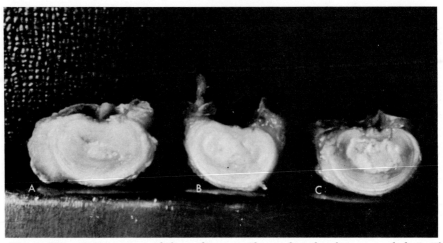

Figure 242. Cross-sections of three discs. A, The nucleus has been extruded. B, This nucleus is calcified but the annulus is still intact. C, A calcified nucleus with some protrusion. The dorsal annulus is degenerated.

space. They are rough and irregular and are adherent to the dura. They are most commonly seen in chondrodystrophoid dogs. Type II, those that produce a small bulge beneath the dorsal longitudinal ligament. They are smooth elevations which produce slight signs or none at all. These are seen in older dogs of all breeds.

Protrusions of the cervical discs produce pressure on the spinal roots rather than on the cord.

EXTRUSION.   When the annulus ruptures, the nucleus is released and extrudes through the opening. If the nucleus is soft and gelatinous it may be extruded with some force and spread for a considerable distance. Olsson has described these cases as resulting in total paralysis and death. He believes this to be due to the explosive nature of the rupture and some "dynamic" factor in the nucleus. Pressure does not seem to be involved, but the cord and its coverings are extremely inflamed. The cord is usually hemorrhagic and edematous for some distance and the nuclear material adheres to the dura mater.

When the extrusion is slow the lesion is usually circumscribed, is either smooth or rough, and varies considerably in size. Pressure from movement may be more important than pressure from size since some small lesions at times cause more severe signs than the larger lesions.

CALCIFICATION.   This seems to apply mostly to the nucleus and may occur either before or after extrusion. Sometimes an extruded nucleus is absorbed and there is spontaneous recovery from symptoms. At other times the material calcifies and becomes a constant source of irritation.

Some calcifications of the nucleus occur without protrusion. These are the result of degeneration and necrosis. They may cause subsequent rupture of the annulus because of their inelastic quality.

Hansen points out that calcification of the nucleus is the usual sign of degeneration seen in the chrondrodystrophoid breeds and may occur in dogs as young as one year old. According to some authors, calcification of the disc in older dogs may be associated with spondylosis. Dorsal spurring at the margins of the vertebral bodies may be mistaken at times for calcification of the disc or it may occur simultaneously with calcification (Fig. 243). A protruding disc that is calcified almost always produces clinical signs.

Some hemorrhage may be present in the cord and subdurally in chronic cases, but acute cases show severe cord hemorrhage as well as extradural hemorrhage in the area of the protrusion. When there is extreme pressure for some time, the cord caudal to the protrusion degenerates. This is an irreversible condition. When cord contusion is acute, hemorrhage and edema may ascend the cord, causing death.

There are 26 discs in the spine of the dog, starting between the second and third cervical vertebral bodies and ending between the seventh lumbar and first sacral. Some writers have named these in numerical order from 1 to 26, but the author prefers to designate them according to their anatomic position so that they are easily located. For example, the disc between the eleventh and twelfth thoracic vertebrae would be designated T11-12. In this chapter, therefore, this system of nomenclature will be used.

Protrusion of discs C2-3 through C7-T1 usually exerts only slight pressure on the cord, the more severe pressure being on the spinal roots, resulting in edema of these nerves. Protrusion or calcification of discs T1-2 through T9-10 is not likely to affect the cord since the heavy conjugal costarum ligament connecting the heads of the opposite ribs intervenes

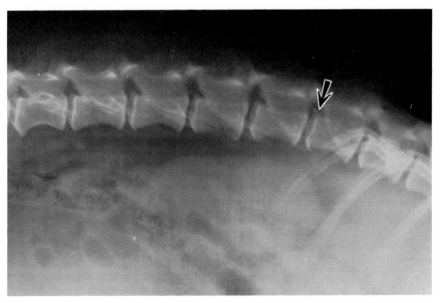

Figure 243.   Dorsal spurring or osteophyte formation at L 1-2.

between the discs and the dorsal longitudinal ligament. Most of the lesions in the cord are produced by protrusion or calcification of discs T10-11 through L4-5. The last two lumbar discs lie beyond the main body of the cord where the cauda equini traverses the spinal canal and where pressure is not easily exerted. Protrusions causing paresis and paraplegia occur most frequently between T11-12 and L2-3.

Signs

PROTRUSION OF THE CERVICAL DISCS. Pain is the most common symptom in cervical protrusions. Movement of the head will cause crying. The animal may be hypersensitive over most of the body. The neck is held rigid and contracted. The head is lowered with the nose depressed. One gets the impression of anxiety and fear of moving. The gait is cautious, with a slow stilted movement of the legs. When sitting or standing the foreleg on the affected side may be slightly flexed at the elbow. There may be some slowness in the placing reflex if the protrusion is pressing on the cord. Pinching of the forefoot (flexion reflex) and pressing against the pads of the forefoot (extensor thrust) may be slow if there is cord involvement over the caudal cervical discs.

PROTRUSION OF THORACO-LUMBAR DISCS. The onset may be slow. An arched back and reluctance to move quickly may be the only signs for several weeks. At other times the condition begins with a lameness in one hindleg or with slight incoordination. The dog refuses to climb stairs or get into a car. Some pain is present, but pain is not a prominent sign. There is gradual decline in muscular control from stumbling and knuckling of the hindfeet to paraplegia. Further progress of signs may cease at any point and the patient may recover without treatment. Such cases frequently have subsequent attacks. On the other hand, the patient may become a chronic paraplegic with or without incontinence.

If the patient is not apprehensive and can be examined in quiet surroundings, a good neurologic inspection may be helpful in locating the disc lesion. A depressed spinal reflex is seen in disc protrusion, especially on the side of the protrusion. The three most commonly used spinal reflexes are the flexion reflex, extensor thrust, and the patellar reflex. The flexor reflex is produced by pinching the toe, causing the normal animal to withdraw the foot by flexing the leg. The extensor thrust is produced by pressing against the sole of the foot, thereby causing extension of the the entire limb. The patellar reflex is produced by striking the patellar ligament sharply while the leg is relaxed; this produces a quick extension of the stifle joint. In the absence of reflexes or in diminished reflexes when paresis, paralysis, or paraplegia is present, one should suspect trouble with discs in the caudal lumbar region. If these spinal reflexes seem to be normal or exaggerated, the lesion will be found in the caudal thoracic or cranial lumbar region.

An active disc lesion can often be accurately located by the use of a skin prick test. The patient is placed in a comfortable position so that he is relaxed and the skin is pricked lightly with a hypodermic needle. Starting in the mid-thoracic region and proceeding toward the tail, a series of light probing thrusts are made lateral to the dorsal spines. When one side has been completed the other side is tested in a like manner.

Ordinarily the skin reaction to this stimulus is very slight. However, when the skin is pricked in the region of an active disc lesion there is a marked contraction or wrinkling. This may not always be exactly over the lesion, but it is reasonably near. Sometimes the skin reflex is more exaggerated just cranial to the lesion and depressed caudal to it. This test is very helpful in localizing the area to be roentgenographed.

Some cases begin dramatically by becoming paraplegic overnight or during severe exercise. The paralysis may involve the bladder and rectum, causing incontinence or retention. In males it may cause priapism. A flaccid paralysis of the hindlimbs may be present or it may be a paralysis in extension, depending on the location of the lesion. Middle and caudal lumbar lesions usually produce a flaccid paralysis, and those occurring in the thoracic and cranial lumbar region cause paralysis in extension (spastic) (Fig. 244).

A few cases show a rapidly developing paralysis which ascends the cord in the course of a few days and results in death. The onset is sudden with paraplegia and incontinence. This is soon followed by diaphragmatic breathing, extension of the forelegs, flaccid paralysis of the forelegs, prostration, and finally death within two or three days.

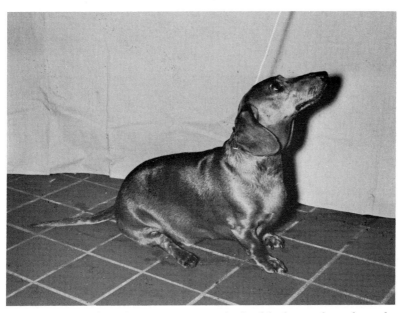

Figure 244. A case of paralysis in extension. The hind limbs are thrust forward in full extension.

Diagnosis

It is not usually difficult to recognize the signs of an active disc lesion, but since there are other conditions which produce some of the same signs, it is well to bear in mind that this condition must be differentiated from spondylosis, ossification of the dura (pachymeningitis), meningitis, demyelination of the cord, fractures and luxations of the spine, neoplasms in the spinal cord, and toxemias.

Examination of the blood, urine, or spinal fluid is of no diagnostic value in disc protrusions except in a negative way. The most valuable help in diagnosis is the roentgenogram. If this is preceded by a careful clinical examination, a flat spinogram will usually be sufficient. Investigators have used contrast media such as Pantopaque and Thorotrast in the subarachnoid space by injecting it into the cisterna magna, but the average clinician should not attempt this type of examination without instruction in the use of these materials, and then only when it is absolutely imperative that the cord be outlined (Fig. 245).

For routine spinograms the patient should be anesthetized so that all movement is controlled. The animal is placed in lateral recumbency with the feet slightly elevated so that an exact lateral roentgenogram is obtained. The lateral view is usually more diagnostic, although a ventro-dorsal view may be helpful. The tube should be centered over the area involved, as indicated by the clinical examination.

Reading of the spinogram should be done with the clinical signs in mind. Calcification of the disc means degeneration but not necessarily protrusion. At the same time, protrusion can occur without signs of calcification on the spinogram. A dorsal spondylosis of adjacent vertebral bodies does not necessarily mean disc protrusion, although the two are likely to be related in older dogs.

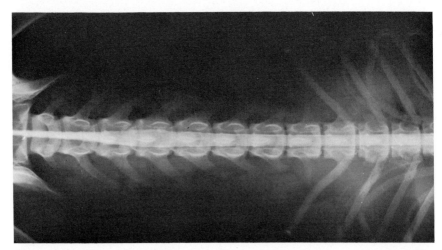

Figure 245. A normal spinogram using Pantopaque as a contrast medium to outline the arachnoid space.

Changes which may be seen on the spinogram which are of clinical importance are:

CALCIFICATION OF THE DISC (Figs. 246 and 247).   This assumes importance only if it appears above the level of the floor of the spinal canal. The calcification may spread over part of the canal floor. If it does not reach to the level of the canal floor it is probably a degeneration without protrusion. We see here the importance of having the feet elevated so that the spine is rotated to the exact lateral level. Calcified thoracic discs from T9-10 forward can be ignored, since they are quite unlikely to protrude into the canal. It is also unlikely that the last two lumbar discs produce clinical signs when calcified because the conus medullaris ends at L-5.

NARROWED INTERVERTEBRAL SPACE (Fig. 248).   It should be remembered that the spaces in the thoracic region are narrower than those in the lumbar region. For accurate interpretation the tube must be centered over the area to be studied, since the spaces that are off-center do not give a true perspective and appear to be narrowed. Comparison should be made with the space on either side of the suspected disc. A narrow space indicates protrusion or extrusion regardless of the presence or absence of calcification.

CALCIFICATION OF EXTRUDED MATERIAL (Fig. 249).   This frequently shows as a slightly opaque shadow along the floor of the spinal canal and indicates that an adjoining disc has ruptured. The pulp may spread for some

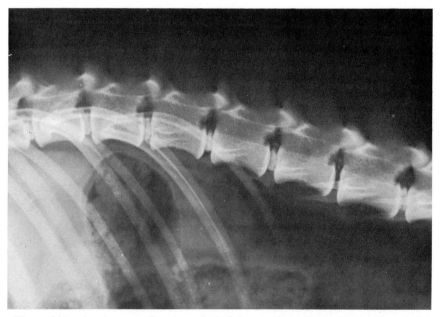

Figure 246.   A spinogram showing calcified discs at T 11-12, 12-13, T 13-L 1, L 1-2, 2-3, and 4-5. The clinical signs would be most helpful in this case to determine the offending disc. From the roentgenogram it would appear that L 2-3 is protruding. There is some calcification of the dura above L 3-4.

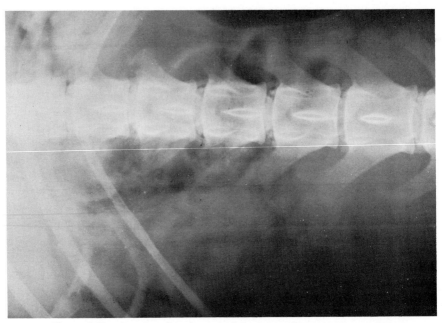

Figure 247. A ventro-dorsal view of the spine shown in Figure 246.

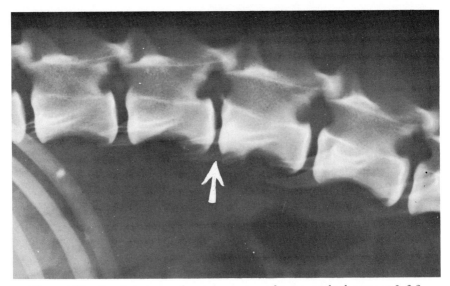

Figure 248. Roentgenogram showing a narrowed intervertebral space at L 2-3.

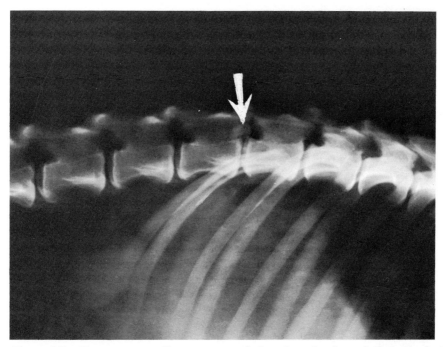

Figure 249. Roentgenogram illustrating extruded nucleus that has calcified. The lesion can be seen at T 13-L 1.

distance. Such a finding serves mainly as a sign that there is a disrupted disc somewhere in the vicinity.

SPONDYLOSIS (Fig. 250). The outstanding lesions in this condition are seen on the ventral edges of the vertebral bodies and may have no bearing on disc pathology. From time to time spondylosis is noted at the dorsal borders of the vertebral bodies in the form of a "lipping." This may cause signs of pressure on the cord but does not necessarily involve the disc.

Prognosis

Intervertebral disc protrusions in the cervical region can usually be given a good prognosis if they are treated surgically. Seldom is there extensive damage to the cord, so that early relief from symptoms follows release of pressure on the spinal nerves. Those treated medically may respond, but they should be given a guarded prognosis. There may be repeated episodes in these cases. The condition is less likely to recur in cases treated surgically.

A prognosis is much more difficult in protrusions involving the thoracic and lumbar discs. It depends largely on the type of lesion, the extent of the damage, and the method of treatment.

When the nucleus is extruded without severe pressure or irritation to the cord, the signs may gradually disappear over a period of several days and

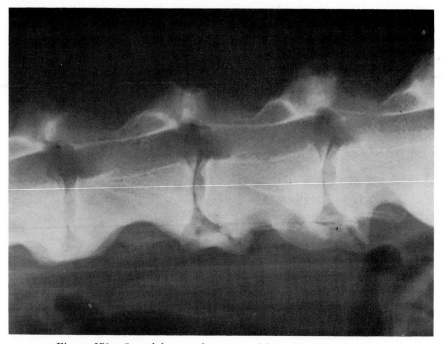

Figure 250. Spondylosis is the principal lesion in this spinogram.

the patient may be said to make a spontaneous recovery. In such a case, the cord compensates for the slight pressure, and the extruded material is absorbed without calcification because the lesion is not highly inflamed. An accurate prognosis cannot be made in such a situation.

If the onset is slow and the lesion is a calcification with protrusion, the prognosis is usually fair, particularly if surgical treatment is instituted before secondary complications set in (cystitis, decubital sores, etc.). Lesions of this nature seem to respond better when they are in the lumbar region. Some observers also feel that better response is seen in patients with flaccid paralysis than in those with paralysis in extension. Some of these patients also make a spontaneous recovery, but a recurrence is quite likely.

When the onset is sudden and the paralysis is progressive, the prognosis is grave. Most of these dogs die within three to four days. It is also grave in those cases where pressure has been exerted on the cord for long periods of time. In such a case the patient may not die, but recovery from the paralysis is doubtful.

All other things being equal, the prognosis is improved by surgery. The number of recurrences with medical treatment is rather high, but those seen following surgery are few. Because of the difficulty in making an accurate prognosis, it is best to delay until some signs of progress or regress are evident.

Medical Treatment

For many years the only treatment used on disc protrusions was medical. A surgical approach to this problem was unknown until it was suggested by Lindbloom and put into practice by Lindbloom, Olsson, Hansen, and Hoerlein. Many clinicians still prefer to treat medically in spite of the fact that the number of recoveries is smaller, the course is longer, and the possibility for recurrence is greater.

Probably the most common treatment is the use of one of the corticosterones. Another treatment that has gained favor is administration of vitamin B complex. Sedatives and antispasmodics are also commonly used. Thyroid and calcium or calcium gluconate has been used with reported success.

Physiotherapy plays an important role in the medical treatment. Heat, massage, diathermy, and the use of exercise carts have been recommended. Such treatment, no doubt, has a beneficial effect on circulation and the musculature of the paralyzed limbs.

Good nursing care plays a very important role in treatment, whether it is medical or surgical. The patient should be protected against decubital sores, and if they develop they should be dressed daily to promote healing. Ring pads fastened over them will prevent further pressure. Frequent bathing with mild soap and warm water will prevent urine burns; this should be augmented by frequent catheterization. Much can be added to the comfort of the patient by keeping the rear parts dry. Padding such as "Ensolite" (U.S. Rubber Co.) should cover the floor of the patient's quarters.

Whirlpool baths are extremely helpful in stimulating circulation and preventing decubital sores because they combine the beneficial effects of moist heat and gentle massage. The buoyancy of the water will help to support the body weight of the paraplegic. This relieves the pressure spots on the body and affords an opportunity for the patient to use its legs, thereby improving circulation and muscle tone.

The water in the tub should be deep enough to float the dog's body but still afford a foothold on the bottom of the tub. The temperature should be about 110° F. It may be necessary at this temperature to immerse the dog slowly until he becomes accustomed to the heat. Antiseptics or low-suds detergents may be added to the water if cleansing of the skin is required.

Treatment should last for 15 minutes and can be repeated several times daily if so desired. Whirlpool equipment may be purchased complete with tub and water turbine or the turbines may be obtained separately and used in an ordinary bathtub or tank.

The diet should be nutritious and high in proteins. Soft-boiled eggs, milk, casein, ground beef, and horse meat are excellent sources of protein.

Surgical Treatment

Both Redding and Greene have described the dorsal laminectomy. This method calls for exposure of the cord by removing the spinous processes and laminae.

General anesthesia is recommended. The patient is placed in sternal recumbency and a skin incision at least a hand's breadth in length is made directly over the dorsal spine. Blunt dissection is used to separate the muscles from the dorsal spines and the articular processes. A Frazer laminectomy retractor is inserted to keep the area exposed and the spine on either side of the disc is split to the roof of the canal. This may be done with bone cutters or saw. After the loosened bone is removed, the opening is enlarged with rongeurs (Fig. 70C).

The epidural fat is removed and the cord is gently retracted laterally so that the offending disc is exposed. With care to avoid the veins which are located laterally, the extrusion is cleared away with a hemostat or curet. Hemostasis must be maintained, as large clots may cause pressure on the cord postoperatively.

The bony opening may be closed by placing bone over it and anchoring with sutures or it may be left to granulate. The fascia is closed with interrupted sutures but the muscles are allowed to heal without suturing. The skin may be closed in any suitable fashion.

Light dressings are used, and healing is fairly rapid in spite of the traumatized muscles. Antibiotics may be given if there is reason to believe that the operative area has been contaminated.

Hemilaminectomy is performed in much the same way as laminectomy except that the approach is lateral to the dorsal spines. This calls for an exposure on one side only. After the articular processes have been exposed they are cut off with rongeurs, and a trephine opening is made into the canal. This can be enlarged with rongeurs so that the disc can be readily approached. Other phases of the surgery are practically the same as those given for dorsal laminectomy.

In 1951 Olsson suggested the fenestration operation for the relief of disc protrusion. It consists of opening the disc without invading the spinal canal. This operation provides for the removal of material ventral to the dorsal longitudinal ligament and for the relief of pressure within the capsule. It does not provide for the removal of material which might lie dorsal to the vertebral body within the spinal canal. The effectiveness of this type of operation was verified by Hoerlein in 1952.

The approach, which might be termed the dorsal approach, is the same as that used for hemilaminectomy. Blunt dissection is used to expose the articular process, the lateral process, the accessory process, the spinal nerves, and blood vessels. The disc will be found cranio-dorsal to the base of the lateral process and ventral to the accessory process. After the nerve and its satellite blood vessels are retracted, the disc is punctured with a 14 or 16 gauge needle. A core of material is removed for examination. If the material is abnormal, the opening is enlarged and the disc is curetted with the needle. Olsson prefers to use a small knife to penetrate the annulus and a narrow curet to remove the contents.

In 1952 Hoerlein, as well as Olsson and Hansen, described a method of fenestration for the cervical discs (Fig. 251). This consists of placing the dog

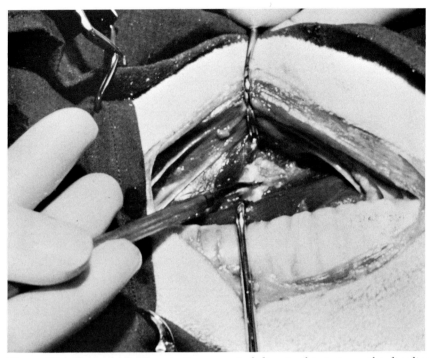

Figure 251. Exposure for fenestrating a cervical disc. In this instance the disc lies beneath the white band exposed between the two aneurysm hooks. The fenestration hook has been forced through the ventral longitudinal ligament and the annulus fibrosus.

in dorsal recumbency with padding under the neck to flex it dorsally. The skin incision is made along the ventral midline from the larynx to the thoracic inlet. The muscles are separated by blunt dissection and the trachea is held to one side by means of retractors (Fig. 252). The discs are easily exposed and the extra curvature of the neck makes them more accessible. The trachea and esophagus are reflected toward the operator. The attachment of the longus colli muscles is snipped with scissors to uncover the ventral longitudinal ligament covering the disc. This in turn is punctured with a scalpel (Fig. 253). It should be remembered that the cervical discs are not in a vertical position, so that the fenestration instrument should be directed slightly craniad (Fig. 254). If a hypodermic needle is used for this purpose, great care should be taken that it does not penetrate the dorsal annulus and damage the cord. A narrow-bladed tartar scaler is an ideal instrument, since it reduces the chance of overpenetration and has enough hook to facilitate removal of the calcified nucleus (Fig. 255).

The offending disc can always be located by establishing the wing of the atlas as a landmark and counting caudally from this point. The caudal border of the wing would be opposite the junction of the atlas and axis or C1-2. The first disc at C2-3 would appear as the next elevation caudal to this point.

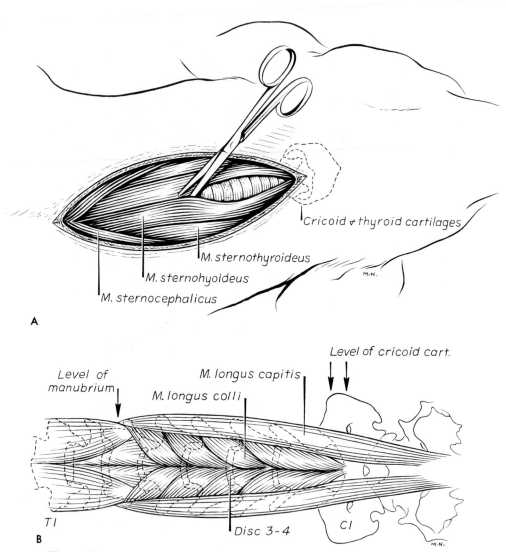

Figure 252. A, Exposure of the trachea by separation between the sternohyoideus muscles. B, Plan of the muscles on the ventral surface of the cervical vertebrae.

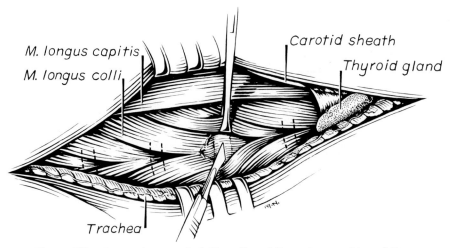

M. longus capitis

M. longus colli

Carotid sheath

Thyroid gland

Trachea

Figure 253. Approach to cervical discs. Dotted lines show position of discs.

It is the custom of some surgeons to fenestrate as many discs as can be handily reached through the original incision. The soundness of such a procedure might be questioned if the discs other than the protruded one appear to be normal. On the other hand, in the chondrodystrophoid breeds, or when the discs are degenerated, multiple fenestrations will prevent other protrusions in the area (Figs. 256 and 257).

In 1953 the author began using what might be termed a ventral approach for all fenestrations in the thoracic or lumbar regions. This seemed to be a logical method of exposing the discs without excessive tissue damage. The patient is positioned in lateral recumbency and suitable lung ventilation apparatus is applied if the chest is to be invaded. Thoracic discs and often the first two lumbar discs require a chest exposure. In such instances an incision is made directly opposite the lesion. This may be an intercostal incision or it may be far enough caudal to be a paracostal incision. The diaphragm is given no special consideration. If it interferes with good exposure it is incised. A Fraser laminectomy retractor (Fig. 258) is used to widen

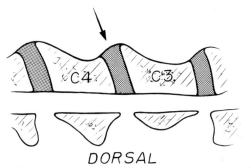

C4   C3

DORSAL

Figure 254. Longitudinal section showing discs slanting craniad. (Patient in dorsal recumbency.)

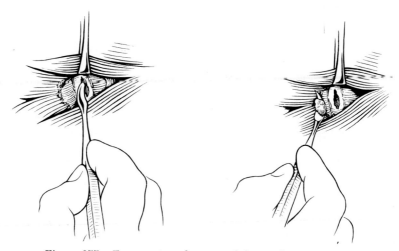

Figure 255.   Fenestration of a cervical disc with a tooth scaler.

the opening and sometimes an assistant uses a hand retractor to produce additional space.

For lumbar discs a paracostal incision is made on the left side (Figs. 259, 260, and 261). If it seems advisable, a retro-peritoneal approach can be made. This is particularly advantageous in the region of the kidney (Figs. 262 and 263).

The landmark for locating the offending disc is the thirteenth rib. This attaches near the cranial end of the thirteenth thoracic vertebra, and disc T12-13 lies immediately cranial to it. The disc can be palpated and recognized as the narrow space in an elevated portion of the spine where the bodies of the two vertebrae join. By counting these elevations forward or back, the proper disc can be located (Fig. 264).

The disc is uncovered by blunt dissection with scissors. Peritoneum or pleura, as the case may be, is pushed aside along with the sympathetic nerve trunk. The disc appears as a whitish band approximately 1/8 inch wide. A finger is placed on the aorta during fenestration to protect it from damage should the instrument slip.

A claw type tartar scaler is used after the ventral longitudinal ligament and the annulus fibrosus have been incised with the point of a scalpel (Figs. 265 and 266). Then with a hooking motion (upward and outward), the disc is cleared of all calcified and degenerated materials. Because of the curve of the hook and the presence of the dorsal longitudinal ligament, it is virtually impossible to damage the spinal cord. Since this approach is on the ventral side of the disc, the danger of injury to the spinal nerves is also lessened.

The pleura or peritoneum over the spine may be closed with a few interrupted sutures of catgut if the opening includes several discs. Chest closure can be facilitated by punching or boring three equally spaced holes in the two ribs adjacent to the incision and approximating them by lacing with monofilament wire. The pleura is opposed in an airtight fashion with-

(*Text continued on page 310.*)

Fig. 256

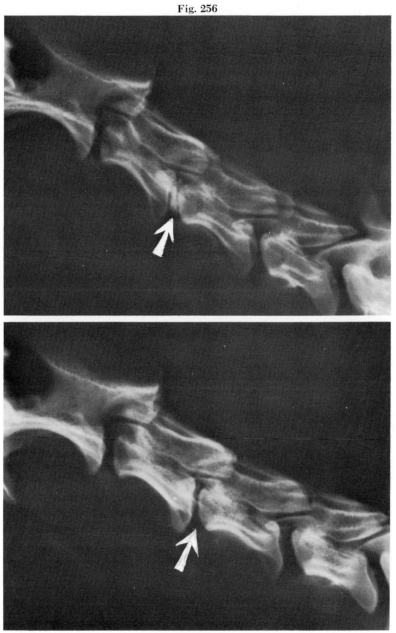

Fig. 257

Figure 256.   A calcified disc at C 3-4.
Figure 257.   A roentgenogram taken the day following fenestration of the disc shown in Figure 256.

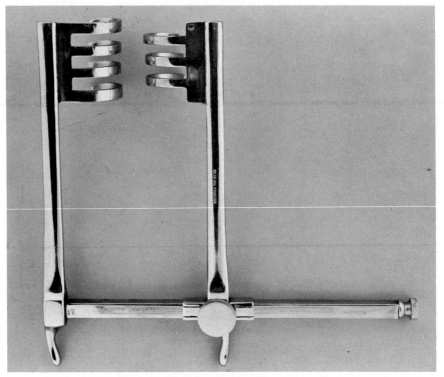

Figure 258. Frazer laminectomy retractor used to improve the size of the field in all fenestrations.

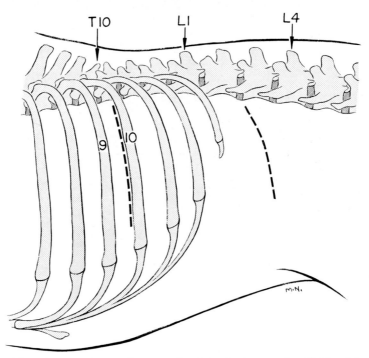

Figure 259. Diagram showing location of incision for thoracic disc 10-11 and lumbar discs 2-3 and 3-4.

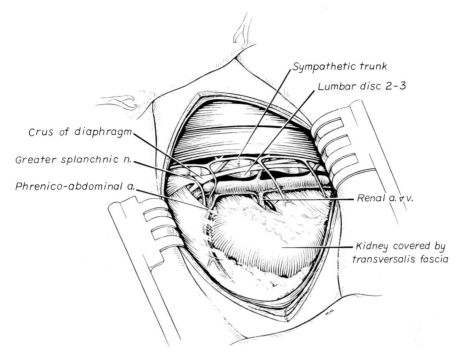

Figure 260. Paracostal incision with retroperitoneal approach for lumbar disc 2-3.

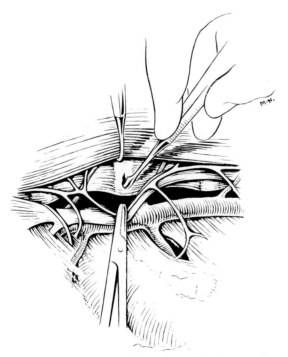

Figure 261. Fenestration of a lumbar disc. The sublumbar muscles have been elevated and the crus of the diaphragm, aorta, and sympathetic trunk have been depressed.

307

Fig. 262

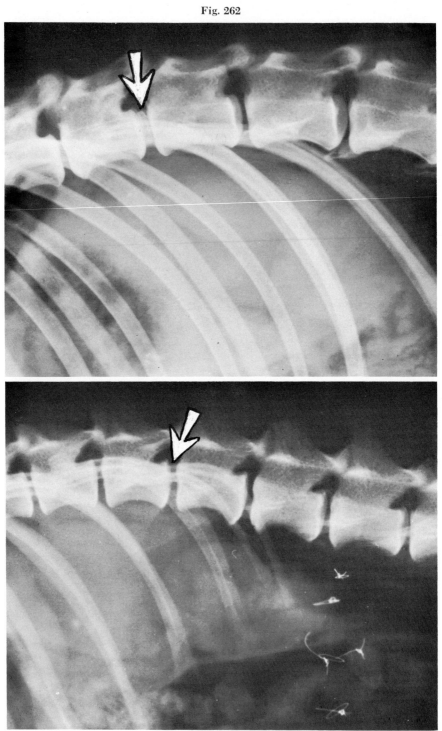

Fig. 263

(See legends on opposite page.)

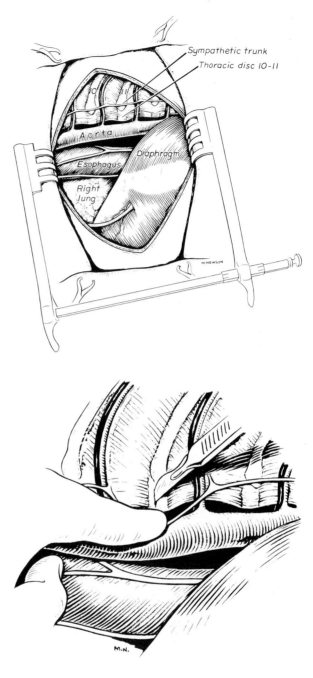

Figure 264. Exposure for thoracic disc 9-10, 10-11, or 11-12.

Figure 265. The aorta is depressed with the index finger and the ventral longitudinal ligament is penetrated with a scalpel.

Figure 262. Calcification of disc T13–L1. This was approached retroperitoneally through a paracostal incision. It could have been reached by opening directly through the diaphragm.

Figure 263. Postoperative roentgenogram showing fenestrated disc several months later. The stainless steel sutures are in the area of the original paracostal incision.

309

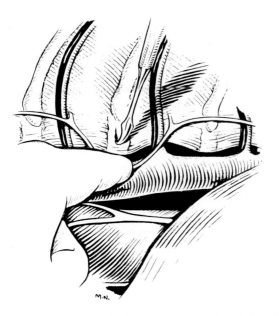

Figure 266. The hook is used with the point in the dorsal direction and the aorta protected by the finger.

out suturing and the incision is held firmly without cutting the intercostal vessels. Muscle, fascia, and skin are approximated in the usual fashion and the incision is covered with a gauze sponge held in place by liquid adhesive (Duo-adhesive).

Recovery varies considerably. Much depends on the condition of the patient at the time of surgery and the length of time the protrusion has existed. Perhaps the condition produced by the operation is just as important as any of the conditions existing prior to it. Much tissue damage and

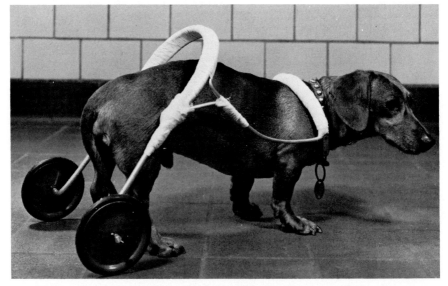

Figure 267. A simple orthopedic cart used for exercising paraplegic patients.

excessive hemorrhage produce the greatest delay in recovery. It is well therefore to conduct the operation carefully, paying great attention to hemostasis, particularly in the region of the cord. Gelfoam or gauze sponges soaked in thrombin are of great assistance in controlling capillary bleeding.

In addition to the usual nursing aftercare, it is advisable to have an ambulant patient as soon as possible. A custom-built exercise cart (Fig. 267) provides the best and easiest means of exercise with protection.

It is readily apparent from this discussion that fenestration is a superior method for dealing with degenerated discs so long as the material can readily be reached beneath the dorsal longitudinal ligament. If there has been extrusion into the canal, and especially if there has been subsequent calcification with irritation, a laminectomy must be performed in order to correct the lesion.

REFERENCES

Allison, C. C.: The intervertebral disc syndrome of the dog. Southwest. Vet., *14*:39, 1960.

Barnett, C. H.: The structure and functions of fibrocartilages within vertebrate joints. Jour. Anat., 88:363, 1954.

Brook, G. B.: The Spine of the Dog. Baltimore, William Wood & Co., 1936.

Bruder, C.: Radiological diagnosis of vertebral arthrosis in dogs. Thesis, Alfort (France), 1955.

Bruder, C.: Aspect radiologique des arthroses vertebrals des carnivores domestiques. Rec. Med. Vet., *131*:353, 1955.

Butler, W. F., and Smith, R. N.: The annulus fibrosis of the intervertebral disc of the newborn cat. Res. Vet. Sci., 4:454-458, 1963.

Butler, W. F., and Smith, R. N.: The nucleus pulposus of the intervertebral disc of the newborn cat. Res. Vet. Sci., 5:71, 1964.

Butler, W. F., and Smith, R. N.: Age changes in the annulus fibrosus of the non-ruptured intervertebral disc of the cat. Res. Vet. Sci., 6:280, 1965.

Cloward, R. B.: Anterior herniation of a ruptured lumbar intervertebral disc. A.M.A. Arch. Surg., 64:457-463, 1952.

Davidson, E. A., and Woodshall, B.: Biochemical alterations in herniated intervertebral disks. J. Biochem., *234*:2951, 1959.

Funkquist, B.: Studies on disk protrusion in the dog. Dissertation. Stockholm, 1952.

Funkquist, B.: Decompressive laminectomy for cervical disk protrusion in the dog. Acta Vet. Scand., 3:88-101, 1962.

Funkquist, B.: Thoraco-lumbar disc protrusion with severe cord compression in the dog. II. Clinical observations with special reference to the prognosis in conservative treatment. Acta. Vet. Scand., 3:317–343, 1962.

Funkquist, B.: Thoraco-lumbar disc protrusion with severe cord compression in the dog. III. Treatment by decompressive laminectomy. Acta. Vet. Scand., 3:344–366, 1962.

Funkquist, B.: Thoraco-lumbar myelography with water-soluble contrast medium in dogs. I. Technique of myelography, side effects and complications. II. Appearance of the myelogram in disk protrusion and its relation to functional disturbances and patho-anatomic changes in the epidural space. J. Small Animal Pract., 3:53, 67, 1962.

Funkquist, B., and Schantz, B.: Influence of extensive laminectomy on the shape of the spinal canal. Acta. Ortho. Scand., Suppl. 56, 1962.

Greene, J. E.: Surgical intervention for paraplegia due to herniation of the nucleus pulposus. N. Am. Vet., 32:411, 1951.

Hansen, H. J.: A pathologic-anatomical study on disc degeneration in dogs. Acta. Orthop. Scand., Suppl. 11, 1952.

Hansen, H. J., and Olsson, S. E.: The indications for disc fenestration in the dog. Proc. 15th Int. Vet. Congress, 2:938, 1953.

Hoerlein, B. F.: The treatment of intervertebral disc protrusions in the dog. Proc. 89th Ann. Meeting A.V.M.A., 1952, pp. 206-212.

Hoerlein, B. F.: Further evaluation of the treatment of disc protrusion paraplegia in the dog. J.A.V.M.A., 129:495, 1956.

Hoerlein, B. F.: Intervertebral disc protrusions in the dog. I. Incidence and pathological lesion. Am. J. Vet. Res., 14:260-283, 1953.

Hoerlein, B. F.: Various contrast mediums in canine myelography. J.A.V.M.A., 123:311, 1953.

Hoerlein, B. F.: Intervertebral disc protrusions in the dog. Vet. Scope., 4:9-14, 1959.

Hoerlein, B. F.: The modern treatment of traumatic spinal compressions in the dog. Canad. Vet. Jour., 5:216-218, 1960.

Hoerlein, B. F.: Cervical spinal surgery—ventral and dorsal approach. Proc. 100th Ann. Meeting A.V.M.A., 1963, pp. 103-104.

Hoerlein, B. F.: Canine Neurology, Diagnosis and Treatment. Philadelphia, W. B. Saunders Co., 1965.

Hurov, L. I.: Cervical disc disease—diagnosis and surgical treatment. Southwest. Vet., 19:37, 1965.

Jadeson, W.: Intervertebral disk lesions. J.A.V.M.A., 138:411-423, 1961.

Jadeson, W.: Rehabilitation of dogs with intervertebral disk lesions by physical therapy methods. J.A.V.M.A., 138:411, 1961.

King, A. S.: The anatomy of disc protrusion in the dog. Vet. Rec., 8:939, 1956.

King, A. S., and Smith, R. N.: Disc protrusion in the cat: Ventral protrusions and radial splits. Res. Vet. Sci., 1:301-307, 1960.

King, A. S., Smith, R. N., and Kou, V. M.: Protrusion of the intervertebral disc in the cat. Vet. Rec., 70:509, 1958.

Lawson, D. D.: Discussion on comparison of disorders of the intervertebral disc in man and animals. Proc. Roy. Soc. Med., 51:569, 1958.

Leonard, E. P.: Fenestration in the thoracolumbar region from the ventral approach. Proc. 100th Ann. Meeting A.V.M.A., 1963, pp. 168-169.

McGrath, J. T.: Neurological Examination of the Dog. 2nd ed. Philadelphia, Lea & Febiger, 1960.

Northway, R. B.: A ventrolateral approach to lumbar intervertebral disc fenestration. Vet. Med. Small Animal Clin., 60:884, 1965.

Olsson, S-E.: On disc protrusion in dog. Acta Orthop. Scand., Suppl. 8, 1951.

Olsson, S-E.: Studien über die bandscheiben-protrusion beim hund unter spezieller berucksichtigung der chirurgischen therapy. Wien. tierärztl. Wschr., 44:329, 1957.

Olsson, S.-E.: The dynamic factor in spinal cord compression. A study on dogs with special reference to cervical disc protrusions. J. Neurosurg. 15:308, 1958.

Olsson, S-E.: Diagnosis of canine spinal lesions. Mod. Vet. Pract., 45:39-44, 1964.

Olsson, S-E., and Hansen, H-J.: Cervical disc protrusions in the dog. J.A.V.M.A., 12:361-370, 1952.

Pettit, G. D.: The surgical treatment of cervical disc protrusions in the dog. Cornell Vet., 50:259, 1960.

Pettit, G. D.: Intervertebral disc protrusion: Selection of cases for surgery. Calif. Vet., 14:14–16, 1961.

Pettit, G. D. (ed.): Intervertebral disc protrusion in the dog. New York, Appleton-Century-Crofts, 1966.

Pettit, G. D., and Whitaker, R. P.: Hemilaminectomy for cervical disc protrusion in a dog. J.A.V.M.A., 143:379, 1963.

Redding, R. W.: Laminectomy in the dog. Am. J. Vet. Res., 12:123, 1951.

Rhodes, W. H., and Jenny, J.: A canine acetabular index. J.A.V.M.A., 137:97, 1960.

Riser, W. H.: Posterior paralysis associated with intervertebral disc protrusion in the dog. N. Am. Vet., 27:633, 1946.

Saunders, E. C.: Treatment of the canine intervertebral disc syndrome with chymopopain. J.A.V.M.A., 145:893, 1964.

Schnelle, G. B.: Radiography of the canine intervertebral disc. Sci. Proc. 100th Ann. Meeting A.V.M.A., 164, 1963.

Smith, R. N.: Anatomy and physiology of the intervertebral disc. In Intervertebral Disc Protrusion in the Dog. (G. D. Pettit, ed.) New York, Appleton-Century-Crofts, 1966.

Smith, R. N., and King, A. S.: Protrusion of the intervertebral disc in the dog. Vet. Rec., 66:2, 1954.

Vaughan, L. C.: Studies on intervertebral disc protrusion in the dog. Brit. Vet. J., 144:105-112, 203, 350, 355, 458, 1958.

Vaughan, L. C.: Some aspects of intervertebral disc protrusion in the dog. Vet. Rec., 70:764, 1958.

Vaughan, L. C.: Intervertebral disc. Parts I and III. Brit. Vet. Jour., 114:105-112, 350-355, 1958.

Chapter 14

Hip Dysplasia

Definition

Hip dysplasia is a term used to denote the abnormal development of the hip joint. The word dysplasia is derived from the Greek word plassein (to form) with the combining prefix "dys," meaning bad or disordered. Literally translated it means "badly formed." Actually the term applies to a poorly developed hip regardless of the cause. Any hip showing abnormal development could therefore be classified as dysplastic. Today the term is used in veterinary medicine to denote a hereditary developmental disease of the dog's hip which particularly affects the acetabulum and is sometimes called "subluxation of the hip" by laymen. It is a disease of large dogs. When dysplasia exists, all the components of the hip joint are subjected to unusual stress and unnatural wear, thereby bringing about tissue reaction both of a degenerative and regenerative nature. This creates, then, deformities varying in form, extent, and location, depending upon the nature, degree, and area of stress. Most osteoarthritis of the hip can usually be traced to some form of hip dysplasia.

A normal pelvis is shown in Figure 268 for purposes of comparison.

Distribution

This condition has been reported in dogs from various parts of North America and Europe. It is probably distributed worldwide. Many breeds — according to Schnelle, at least 40 — are affected. Apparently a high percentage of the German shepherd breed suffers from it, but because this is the breed in which most of the investigational work has been done, it is only natural that more cases have been brought to light. The author has found it especially prevalent in Gordon setters. Schnelle also mentions the Newfoundland, great Pyrenees, and English bulldog. As a matter of fact, most large breeds have been reported as affected to a greater or lesser degree.

Contrary to the findings in humans, there seems to be little sex difference in the incidence. Snavely states that there is a strong suggestion that

313

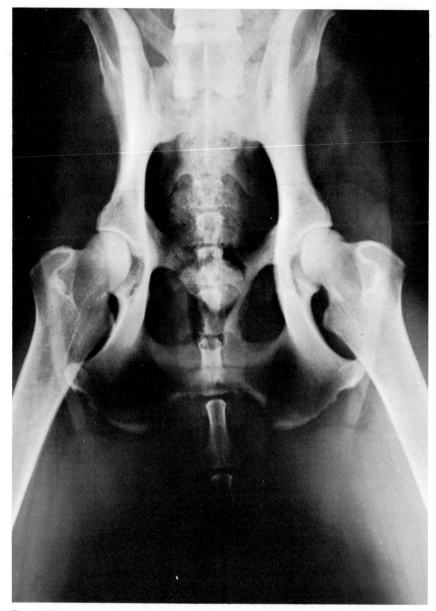

Figure 268. A roentgenogram of a normal pelvis. It does not necessarily follow that all pelves must look exactly like this to be normal, but the coxo-femoral articulation should form a smooth, well-rounded joint, the femur head should be globular, and the acetabular edges as well as the epiphyseal line at the femur head should be free of spurring.

the incidence is higher in females, but this has not been accepted by most investigators.

Etiology

It seems fairly well established that vascular changes take place in the bony structures of the hip at least, but whether the causes of these changes are prenatal or postnatal is not clear. In general, it is thought that hip dysplasia is hereditary in the dog, although opinions vary and little truly scientific work has been done to establish the genetic aspects of the disease (variously described as genetically conditioned, due to a recessive factor or due to a dominant factor with irregular penetrance). Some breeding has been done in an effort to clarify the genetic influence on hip dysplasia, but more work is needed in this field.

Pathology

In the young dog the joint capsule is enlarged and thickened. This thickening increases somewhat with age. The ligamentum teres is elongated, sometimes frayed, softened, and in a few instances completely ruptured. There is an increase in synovial fluid which is frequently discolored and blood-tinged. Some changes in the femur head begin to appear under one year. The head becomes flattened longitudinally and there may be some lipping at the epiphyseal line (Fig. 269). After one year the acetabular

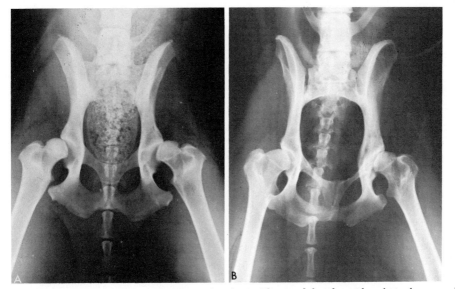

Figure 269. Flattening of the femur head. A, Flattened heads with relatively normal acetabuli in a young adult dog. The capsules are stretched as indicated by the bilateral subluxation. B, An adult dog with flattened femur heads and shallow acetabuli. Some arthritic changes are also present.

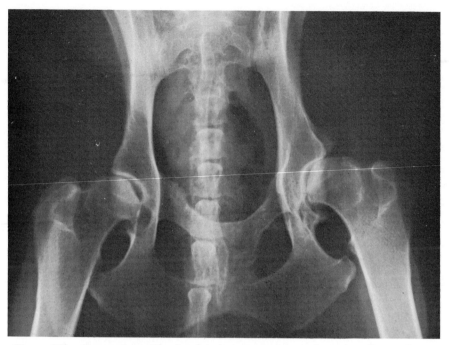

Figure 270. Coxa magna. The head is large proportionately with a flattened articular surface and lipping at the junction with the neck.

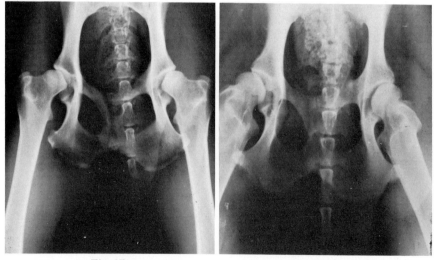

Fig. 271   Fig. 272

Figure 271. Coxa plana. The articular surface is flattened in the longitudinal direction, thereby producing a poor articulation.

Figure 272. Coxa valga. The neck is distorted so that it forms a straight line with the shaft. Note also the distorted femur heads.

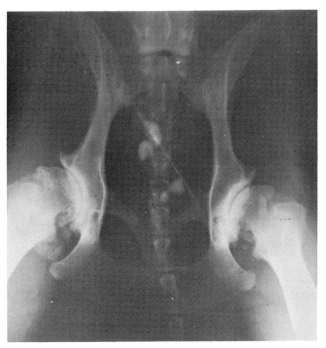

Figure 273. Osteochondrosis of the femur head and neck. This also shows the bony changes and flattening of the acetabulum.

changes become prominent. The cartilage is eroded, the socket is shallow and flattened, and arthritic changes begin to appear along the rim. The femur head becomes distorted, with some elevation at the epiphyseal line. There are areas of aseptic necrosis in the head which fill with cartilage. The neck frequently shortens because of the softening action of aseptic necrosis coupled with pressure from weight bearing.

Other abnormalities which appear as a result of the dysplasia are coxa magna (Fig. 270), coxa plana (Fig. 271), cox valga (Fig. 272), and coxa vara. Trauma resulting from the improper fitting of the hip joint frequently produces degeneration of the subchondral bone and cartilage (osteochondrosis) (Fig. 273), which is followed by regeneration and recalcification, producing various distortions of the head and neck of the femur as well as the acetabulum.

Signs

Dysplasia resulting in subluxation appears early in life, sometimes when the pup is only three to five months old, or the onset of signs is delayed until seven to nine months. We have found four to six months to be the usual time of onset of signs if the principal deformity is subluxation.

When the dysplastic result is coxa plana (Legg-Perthes' disease), the

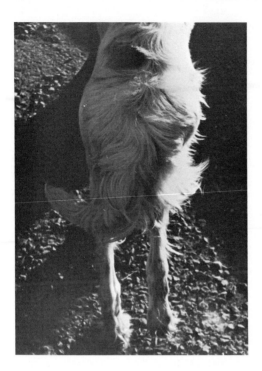

Figure 274. The hips as viewed from the rear. The contour is convex instead of straight or concave.

condition may appear to improve at 10 to 12 months, but this is probably due to compensation of some of the muscles in the pelvis and upper leg.

The hips are broader than usual, giving the pelvis a wide, flat appearance when viewed from the rear. Ordinarily imaginary lines drawn from the tuber coxae to the tuber ischii are straight parallel lines or perhaps slightly curved toward the midline over the hips. In cases of dysplasia, these lines have a definite lateral angulation over the hips (Fig. 274). The gait is clumsy, and in running the hindlegs are used in a hopping, rabbit-like manner. The stifles are frequently rotated outward, the trochanters are prominent, and there is atrophy of the thigh muscles as the deformity progresses.

In some cases pain is a prominent sign, as indicated by limping, wincing on pressure over the hips, and sitting in abnormal positions. At other times, there is difficulty in negotiating stairs. However, many animals exhibit no abnormalities of gait, particularly after the lesion has stabilized; neither do they indicate any evidence of pain.

Diagnosis

Clinically, hip dysplasia can often be diagnosed by the history coupled with the clinical signs, but it should always be verified by a roentgenogram. Many instances of unsuspected dysplasia are uncovered through a routine x-ray examination of the hips. The roentgenogram is therefore the best proof of dysplasia short of an autopsy, but even this may sometimes fail to distinguish adequately between the various forms which dysplasia may take.

The extent of the dysplasia sometimes governs the symptomatology, but this may be offset by compensation through the ability of structures around the joint to adapt themselves to the situation. It has been said that certain dysplastic dogs are able to gait well enough in the show ring to be judged good specimens.

Positioning for a roentgenogram is extremely important. The exposure should be made with the patient in dorsal recumbency. Schnelle recommends that the cranial spine be elevated with sand bags so that the pelvis will be parallel to the cassette. This produces a slight ventral angulation between the body and the legs. We prefer to allow the spine to be parallel to the film but the hindlegs elevated about 4 inches at the hocks. In either position, the legs should be extended caudally parallel to the midline and with very slight outward rotation of the stifles to simulate the normal vertical position of the leg in relation to its long axis. The shadow of the patella will fall within that of the lateral condyle of the femur. Schnelle also prefers to apply some traction to the legs in order to demonstrate the condition of the soft tissues (capsule and ligament) of the joint. We usually make our roentgenograms without traction (Figs. 275 and 276).

Our patients are anesthetized before the examination so that there is total relaxation. The pelvis is then braced on either side at the tuber coxae with weights. This ensures a reasonably symmetrical roentgenogram and avoids pelvic rotation.

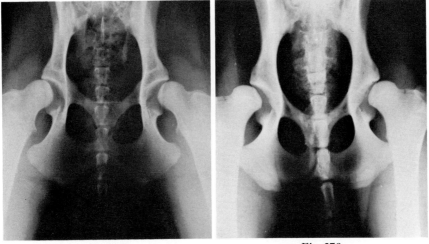

Fig. 275   Fig. 276

Figure 275. Subluxation taken without traction. The femur heads are still round and symmetrical.

Figure 276. Subluxation showing femur heads that are flattened. No traction was applied in this case.

Many breed clubs in the United States require certification of pelvic radiographs by the "Orthopedic Foundation for Animals" for breeding animals. Positioning in such a case should follow the instructions of the Foundation.

Schnelle has suggested a classification of dysplasia for diagnostic description as follows: Grade 1, slight (poor fit between head and acetabulum); Grade 2, moderate (acetabulum moderately shallow); Grade 3, severe (flat acetabulum); Grade 4, very severe (complete displacement at an early age). Other investigators feel that a positive or negative diagnosis is sufficient and that the condition is likely to be a progressive one in which the classification could change with the passage of time. Osteoarthritic changes seen in most dysplastic cases would also be a factor in classifying dysplasia according to the severity of the lesion.

Prognosis

Regardless of the prognosis, the owner should be discouraged from using the animal for breeding because of the danger of reproducing a deformed hip.

If subluxation is present, the prognosis is more uncertain because of the possibility of a permanent crippling effect. Schnelle regards the prognosis as poor in heavy breeds except in those cases classified as Grade 1. He also feels that the prognosis is reasonably good in retrievers, setters and shepherds in Grades 1 and 2 but poor in Grades 3 and 4. However, the age of the patient at the time of examination largely influences the prognosis since further regressive changes can conceivably take place.

In any case, the hip joint does not return to normal but rather compensates for the abnormality. Pain and discomfort usually remain or become worse in badly deformed hip joints, but the pain may subside or disappear in mild cases or as the animal matures.

Treatment

Nothing can be done medically for the dysplastic dog except to make him as comfortable as possible during the period of pain. Medication with aspirin, cortisone and butazolidine will help to keep the patient comfortable.

The weight level should be maintained at normal for the breed and mild exercise should be given regularly.

Gorman has recommended the use of his prosthesis to correct the crippled hip joint, but this would be a rather impractical method of correction in the average case. It could conceivably be of some help in a few carefully selected individuals.

Excision arthroplasty of the femoral head has been recommended by some who report satisfactory results. Details of the surgery will be found on page 110. However, this type of surgery in the very large individual places a tremendous strain on the already weakened and atrophied muscles of the thigh and may not succeed.

REFERENCES

Berge, E.: Die angeborene hüftgelenksdysplasie bein hund. Deutsche tierärztl Wchnschr., 64:509, 1957.

Henricson, B., and Olsson, S-E.: Hereditary acetabular dysplasia in German Shepherd dogs. J.A.V.M.A., 135:207-210, 1959.

Konde, W. N.: Congenital subluxation of the coxofemoral joint in the German Shepherd dog. N. Am. Vet., 28:595, 1947.

McClave, P. L.: Elimination of coxofemoral dysplasia from a breeding kennel. Vet. Med., 52:241, 1957.

Olsson, S-E.: Canine hip dysplasia in Scandinavian countries. Mod. Vet. Pract., 42:15, 1961.

Report of Panel on Canine Hip Dysplasia. J.A.V.M.A., 139:791-798, 1961.

Riser, W. H.: A new look at developmental subluxation and dislocation: Hip dysplasia in the dog. J. Small Animal Pract., 4:421-434, 1963.

Riser, W. H.: An analysis of the current status of hip dysplasia in the dog. J.A.V.M.A., 144:709-721, 1964.

Schales, O.: Genetic aspects of dysplasia of the hip joint. N. Am. Vet., 37:476, 1956.

Schales, O.: Hereditary patterns in dysplasia of the hip. N. Am. Vet., 38:152, 1957.

Schnelle, G.: Congenital dysplasia of the hip (canine) and sequelae. Proc. 91st Am. Meeting A.V.M.A., 1954.

Schnelle, G.: Congenital dysplasia of the hip in dogs. J.A.V.M.A., 135:235, 1959.

Snavely, J. G.: The genetic aspects of hip dysplasia in dogs. J.A.V.M.A., 135:201-207, 1959.

Legg-Perthes Disease (Legg-Calvé-Perthes Disease, Coxa Plana, Osteochondrosis, Osteochondritis)

Definition

Legg-Perthes disease is a deforming disease of the capital epiphysis and head of the canine femur. It derives its name from a disease in man to which it bears some similarity. It is characterized by a non-inflammatory avascular necrosis of the femoral head and neck and is frequently erroneously referred to as osteochondritis. In a broad sense it is a form of hip dysplasia, and for this reason it is often confused with the hereditary hip disease of larger dogs commonly known as hip dysplasia.

Distribution

The disease has been described in many parts of the world but particularly in Europe and North America. It is seen in the smaller breeds almost exclusively. Unlike the disease in man, this condition is distributed fairly evenly between the sexes.

Etiology

Although several theories have been advanced, the exact cause of Legg-Perthes disease is still somewhat obscure. Factors which have been postulated as causative are hereditary, inflammatory, traumatizing, hormonal, constitutional, nutritional, and circulatory. Ljunggren has investigated the etiology of this disease extensively and feels that the cause is hormonal. She has shown that hypergonadotropism brings about premature sexual maturity, excessive growth of endosteal bone, and closure of the growth plates. The result would be a circulatory deficit in the epiphysis. It is interesting to note,

322

however, that the femur heads are only affected bilaterally 12 to 16 per cent of the time.

Pathology

Early cases show little or no change in the gross appearance of the synovial fluid. There is hyperemia of the capsule and ligamentum teres. In later stages the density of the synovia increases and the capsule and ligamentum teres thicken. There is gradual cartilage destruction, fraying of the ligaments, and flattening or collapse of the femoral head. In some cases the articular cartilage of the femur head may be wrinkled or fractured; in others it may be replaced with fibrous tissue. In the late stages there may be some exostoses along the acetabular rim, but this is usually not extensive. The lesions for the most part are confined to the femoral head and neck. The head will be found in various stages of necrosis and collapse or will be completely absent.

Signs

The principal sign is lameness. It varies considerably in degree from slight to complete disuse of the limb. This lameness persists for four months to one year. In some cases the soreness is severe, but in others it gradually subsides although it rarely disappears entirely. There is muscular atrophy over the hip and prominence of the trochanter major.

Palpation and manipulation of the joint reveals pain, especially on abduction, and a noticeable reduction in mobility. In unilateral cases the leg appears to be shortened and frequently cannot be extended fully. Crepitus is a variable sign.

Diagnosis

Legg-Perthes disease is seen in the small breeds between the ages of five and 11 months. Larger dogs or dogs over one year can usually be eliminated as suspects. A positive diagnosis is made with a roentgenogram with the patient in a ventro-dorsal position and the hindlimbs extended horizontally.

RADIOGRAPHIC DIAGNOSIS. The femoral head shows a slight decalcification at the capital epiphyseal line in the very early stages. Sometimes lameness appears in advance of this very early radiographic sign. Decalcification progresses until there is fragmentation and deformity of the head. The joint space is widened and small spots of decreased density begin to appear in the head. As the disease advances, some spurring on the acetabular rim may appear. Usually only the most severe cases show flattening of the acetabulum, however.

As the disease advances the conformation of femur head changes. It becomes flattened and rarefaction becomes more noticeable, spreading to the neck (Fig. 277). Finally the head becomes fragmented (Fig. 278), followed by indications of remodeling (Fig. 279) or resolution.

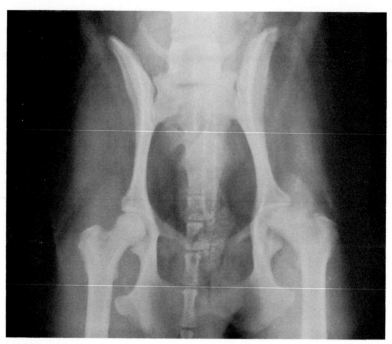

Figure 277. Legg-Perthes disease of the left hip joint. Both femur head and neck are rarefied. The head is flattened.

Paatsama recommends a radiograph at six to eight months for the diagnosis of Legg-Perthes disease and at four to six months for hip dysplasia. Borderline cases of hip dysplasia may require roentgenograms as late as one year or older in our experience.

Prognosis

Frost optimistically states that most cases will regain almost complete use of the leg after six to eight months from the onset. Ljunggren, on the other hand, found that only 24 per cent of 62 cases treated conservatively recovered and only 6 per cent recovered within two months. Some of this discrepancy may be due to a lack of a standard definition of recovery. Most cases treated conservatively remain slightly lame, and many retain some atrophy of the hip muscles, especially the gluteal muscles.

If properly done, an excision arthroplasty will relieve the pain and thereby restore reasonable function to the limb. Most of the time, these patients regain a reasonable amount of use but the motion is still limited and the joint is not as stable as a normal joint. Nevertheless, surgical intervention provides a fairly satisfactory outlook with about 15 per cent chance of failure.

Treatment

Medical treatment consists of resting the leg and reducing the pain and discomfort. Most of the time small dogs will carry the leg if it is uncomfort-

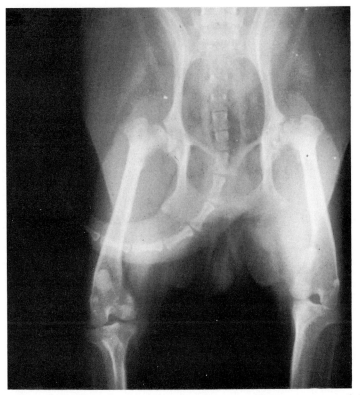

Figure 278. Bilateral lesions of Legg-Perthes disease with fragmentation of the femoral heads.

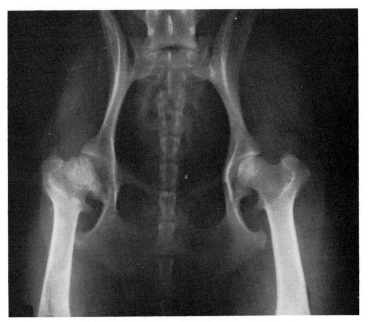

Figure 279. Remodeling of the femoral head.

325

able to use it. It is, therefore, better if the limb is left unfettered by bandages, casts, or other forms of immobilization. If the patient is confined to small quarters he will do a very fine job of resting the leg. It should be borne in mind that confinement must be continued for at least three months. When pain is severe, it should be controlled with appropriate drugs.

Surgical treatment consists of excision arthroplasty as described by Spruell. Each surgeon follows his own approach to the hip for this operation but we prefer the dorsal or Brown approach (see Figure 87-2). It is important that the neck be cut parallel to the long axis of the femoral shaft so that the stump does not protrude (see Figure 88). A long stump will produce pain from contact with the acetabulum and lameness will continue until it is removed. A clean, smooth amputation will heal without secondary signs.

Mild exercise is recommended following surgery and the period of hospitalization should be fairly short. The leg should not be splinted. There may be a slight shortening of the leg and some atrophy of the hip muscles may remain. There should be no pain and most cases resume a fairly normal gait. Complete functional recovery should be obtained in about two months.

REFERENCES

Anderson, W., and Schlotthauer, C. F.: Legg-Perthes disease (coxa plana) in the dog. J.A.V.M.A., 122:115, 1953.

Formston, C., and Knight, G. C.: Affections of the hip joint in the dog with special reference to the differential diagnosis. Vet. Rec., 54:481, 1942.

Frost, C.: Osteochondritis of the hip in the dog. Vet. Rec., 71:687, 1959.

Hickman, J., and Spickett, S. R.: Avascular necrosis of the femoral head in the dog. Proc. Roy. Soc. Med., 58:366-369, 1965.

Hulth, A., Norberg, I., and Olsson, S-E.: Coxaplana in the dog. J. Bone Joint Surg., 44A:918, 1962.

Lee, R., and Fry, P. D.: Some observations on the occurrence of Legg-Calvé-Perthes' disease (Coxaplana) in the dog, and an evaluation of excision arthroplasty as a method of treatment. J. Small Animal Pract., 10:309-317, 1969.

Ljunggren, G.: Legg-Perthes Disease in the Dog. Acta Orthop. Scand., Suppl. 95, 1967.

Ormrod, A. N.: Treatment of hip lameness in the dog by excision of the femoral head. Vet. Rec., 73:576-577, 1961.

Paatsama, S., Rissanen, P., and Rokkanen, P.: Some aspects of hip dysplasia and coxa plana in dogs. J. Small Animal Pract., 7:477-481, 1966.

Paatsama, S., Rissanen, P., and Rokkanen, P.: Legg-Perthes disease in the dog. J. Small Animal Pract., 8:215-220, 1967.

Paatsama, S., and Rokkanen, P.: The canine hip joint: post-natal development, dysplasia and Legg-Perthes' disease. Finsk. Vet. Tidskr., 73:273-281, 1967.

Spruell, J. S. A.: Excision arthroplasty as a method of treatment of hip joint diseases in the dog. Vet. Rec., 73:573-575, 1961.

Chapter 16

Elbow Dysplasia

Definition

Elbow dysplasia is a general term used to denote the abnormal development of the elbow joint. It has been variously referred to as "ununited anconeal process," "ectopic sesamoid bones," "free processus anconeus," and "congenital detachment of the processus anconeus." Elbow dysplasia is used loosely as a term covering all of the abnormalities of the humero-radio-ulnar joint which develop as a result of the failure of the anconeal process to fuse with the olecranon.

Distribution

The condition has been reported in several areas of the United States and Canada as well as the United Kingdom and Germany. It is probably found wherever extensive dog breeding is common. There is evidence to indicate that this condition has existed in dogs since 1936, at least, and probably has gone unrecognized for many years. It has been seen most frequently in German Shepherds but has also been reported in Saint Bernards, Labrador retrievers, basset hounds, bloodhounds, Irish setters, Great Danes, Newfoundlands, Weimaraners, Doberman pinschers, and mongrels.

Etiology

There are three centers of ossification in the ulna. The diaphysis, which includes the shaft and the olecranon, develops from one center which is ossified at birth. Another center is in the distal epiphysis and the third is in the proximal epiphysis. This center appears during the second month and is finally united with the diaphysis between the eighth and tenth months. The anconeal process does not have a separate center of ossification, and therefore its failure to fuse with the olecranon would tend to indicate embryological anomaly.

The processus anconeus has no ligament attaching it to the humerus, and under ordinary circumstances it is a protuberance on the cranial aspect of the olecranon. It lies within the joint capsule and moves in the olecranon fossa of the humerus during flexion and extension of the limb. When the process fails to fuse with the olecranon the two are connected by fibrous tissue which varies in amount but never produces a firm bond. As a result, the stabilizing effect of the anconeal process firmly interlocked between the condyles of the humerus during extension of the joint is lost.

While the primary lesion is believed to be inherited, the secondary lesions result from the inflammation produced in the unstable joint.

Pathology

The joint usually shows evidence of degeneration and attempts at regeneration. There is erosion of the articular cartilage in the area of the semilunar notch. Proliferative alterations are evident at the line of separation as well as along the margins of the humeral condyles and occasionally even on the cranial border of the humero-radial articulation. Severe cases show inflammation and swelling of the joint capsule and the olecranon bursa. The process is usually quite free and is only attached to the joint capsule in these cases. On the other hand, some mild cases will show very slight or no inflammatory reactions. Some minute separations in dogs under five months of age may fuse without producing any tissue reaction.

Signs

Lameness is a common sign and this may be either a standing or a swinging leg lameness or it may be both. Usually the lameness, while not severe, increases with exercise and the gait is shortened. The pain is often increased by forced extension or flexion. The elbow is abducted, giving the dog a "bowed leg" appearance. Sometimes the joint is swollen and tender to palpation. In rare instances, manipulations of the joint may produce crepitus.

Diagnosis

A roentgenogram is the only means of making a definite diagnosis. A lateral view with the limb in complete flexion produces the best definition of the lesion. Other views may be helpful in portraying secondary or accessory lesions in various parts of the elbow joint.

A line of separation of varying magnitude can be seen on the cranial side of the olecranon (Fig. 280). This line runs parallel to the caudal aspect of the ulna and penetrates to the trochlear notch. There is often some evidence of exostosis along the line of cleavage and lipping at the proximal edge is common. Osteophyte formation is sometimes seen on the cranial side of the joint as well.

Prognosis

Ordinarily a good prognosis can be given if the condition is treated surgically. A guarded prognosis should be given when osteoarthritis is extensive. Cases of long standing usually show some improvement following

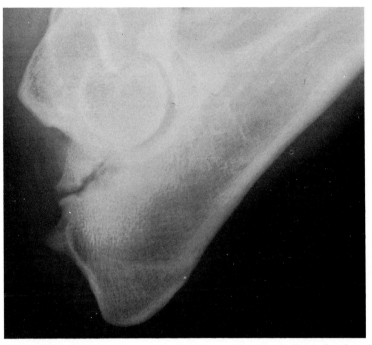

Figure 280.   Roentgenogram showing a typical lesion of elbow dysplasia.

surgery but often retain some signs of lameness. There may even be some regression. In those instances in which the anconeal process is removed shortly after signs appear, recovery is frequently complete.

Treatment

Surgical removal of the anconeal process usually relieves the lameness quite promptly. Directly following surgery the lameness appears to be unabated, but during the second week of convalescence there is a gradual improvement in the gait. Although some abduction of the elbow may remain, the patient often returns to a normal gait within a month.

Surgery is performed under general anesthesia with the patient in lateral recumbency and the affected limb uppermost. Draping should cover all but the elbow. This can be done by wrapping the lower limb or encasing it in sterile stockinette followed by a longitudinal drape beneath the limb and two cross-drapes covering the body and shoulder.

The skin incision should be approximately 10 cm. in length. It should be about equidistant above and below the lateral epicondyle and just caudal to it. The location can usually be established by palpating the condyle and the ulna. Immediately beneath the skin incision lies the investing fascia; along its caudal border and continuous with the fascia will be the cranial edge of the lateral head of the triceps muscle. An incision through the fascia will expose the anconeus muscle. This is a thin muscle overlying the joint capsule. A crescent-shaped incision is made through the anconeus and the joint capsule to expose the joint.

At this point the elbow is flexed acutely so that the anconeal process is fully exposed. In so doing, the lateral head of the triceps may interfere slightly, but it can be held aside with a simple retractor. The line of cleavage is fully visible and a chisel or periosteal elevator is inserted to widen the gap or break down any fibrous attachment which may exist. Often the segment is free along this border. As the bone fragment is lifted by prying it will be found that it is attached to the joint capsule and the anconeus muscle at its caudal extremity. Using scissors, it should be carefully dissected free.

The incision through the joint capsule and the anconeus muscle is closed with interrupted stitches of #2–0 chromic catgut. The fascia is closed in a like manner. A row of supporting sutures should be placed in the subcutaneous tissues so that very little strain will be placed on the suture line in the skin.

Moderate exercise following surgery is beneficial but it should be controlled for the first week to 10 days.

REFERENCES

Bradney, I. W.: Non-union of the anconeal process in the dog. Aust. Vet. Jour., 43:215-216, 1967.

Carlson, W. D.: Veterinary Radiology. Philadelphia, Lea & Febiger, 1961.

Carlson, W. D., and Severin, G. A.: Elbow dysplasia in the dog, a preliminary report. J.A.V.M.A., 138:295-297, 1961.

Cawley, A. J., and Archibald, J.: Ununited anconeal processes of the dog. J.A.V.M.A., 134:454-458, 1969.

Corley, E. A., Sutherland, T. M., and Carlson, W. D.: Genetic aspects of canine elbow dysplasia. J.A.V.M.A., 153:543-547, 1968.

Flipo, J.: Joints of the pectoral limb. In Canine Surgery. 1st Archibald ed. Santa Barbara, Cal., American Veterinary Publications, 1965.

Hare, W. C. D.: Radiographic anatomy of the canine pectoral limb. Part II. Developing limb. J.A.V.M.A., 135:305-310, 1959.

Hare, W. C. D.: The ages at which centers of ossification appear roentgenographically in the limb bones of the dog. Amer. J. Vet. Res., 22:825-835, 1961.

Hare, W. C. D.: Congenital detachment of the processus anconeus in the dog. Vet. Rec., 74:545-546, 1962.

Hickman, J.: Veterinary Orthopaedics. London, Oliver & Boyd, 1964.

Ljunggren, G., Cawley, A. J., and Archibald, J.: The elbow dysplasia in the dog. J.A.V.M.A., 148:887, 1966.

Loeffler, K.: Der isolierte processus anconeus bein deutschen schaferhund. Dtsch. tierärztl Wschr., 70:317-321, 1963.

Miller, M. E., Christensen, G. C., and Evans, H. E.: Anatomy of the Dog. Philadelphia, W. B. Saunders Co., 1964.

Mulnix, J. A., Corley, E. A., and Carlson, W. D.: Serum and synovial alkaline phosphatase levels in canine elbow dysplasia. Am. J. Vet. Clin. Path. 2:49-54, 1968.

Piermattei, D. L., and Greeley, R. G.: An Atlas of Surgical Approaches to the Bones of the Dog and Cat. Philadelphia, W. B. Saunders Co., 1966.

Seer, G., and Hurov, L.: Elbow dysplasia in dogs with hip dysplasia. J.A.V.M.A., 154:631-637, 1969.

Stiern, R. A.: Ectopic sesamoid bones of the elbow (patella cubiti) of the dog. J.A.V.M.A., 128:498-501, 1956.

VanSickle, D. C.: The relationship of ossification to canine elbow dysplasia. An. Hosp., 2:24-31, 1966.

VanSickle, D. C.: The postnatal osteogenesis of the anconeal process in the Greyhound and the German Shepherd dog. Diss. Abst., 2713:3763, 1967.

Vaughan, L. C.: Congenital detachment of the processus anconeus in the dog. Vet. Rec., 74:309-311, 1962.

Chapter 17

Osteochondritis Dissecans

Osteochondritis dissecans was the term applied to a type of epiphyseal ischemic necrosis, seen in the weight-bearing bones of man, by König in 1888 and described first by Alexander Monro. In veterinary literature the term is used primarily to describe a lesion appearing in the proximal epiphyses of the humerus of the dog and possibly in swine. This condition has been reported in Europe, Great Britain and the United States.

Incidence

Although a few cases have been reported in smaller dogs, such as the Cocker spaniel, the majority of the dogs so affected appear to be the larger breeds, such as the Great Dane, German shepherd, German short-haired pointer, German wirehaired pointer, Great Pyrenees, greyhound, Newfoundland, Saint Bernard, Vizsla, springer spaniel, English setter, Irish setter, Labrador, golden retriever, Dalmatian, boxer, Afghan, standard poodle, old English sheepdog, Irish wolfhound, collie, and large mongrels.

This is primarily a disease of young dogs that are under one year of age at the onset. Reports vary as to the sex distribution, some indicating that it is seen more frequently in males and others finding the condition equally distributed.

Etiology

While the exact cause of osteochondritis dissecans has not been established, it is a common observation that the condition occurs in joints subjected to force and pressure. The most common site in man is the medial condyle of the femur. This is a weight-bearing joint which is subjected to traumatizing forces. By the same token, the shoulder joint in the dog receives a similar degree of pressure and traumatizing force. More weight is carried on the forelegs and the contact time is longer than the back legs. In the larger breeds, the slower-maturing epiphysis and the greater body weight expose the articular cartilage and the subchondral bone of the hu-

331

meral head to a greater degree of insult than other joints. Craig and Riser believe that excessive force on the articular cartilage with the limb in the extended position produces a lesion in the caudo-central portion of the humeral head by fracturing the subchondral spongiosa or the articular cartilage or both.

Pathology

The lesion occurs on the caudo-central portion of the humeral head and may be either unilateral or bilateral. In very mild cases the lesion may be a very tiny red spot with slightly thickened cartilage. Such a lesion would probably be subclinical and pass unnoticed if it developed no farther. More advanced lesions show separation of cartilage and absorption of bone (Fig. 281). Where the cartilage plaque has completely separated from the subchondral bone, the defect fills with fibrocartilage. Since the cartilage is nourished by synovial fluid it may continue to grow and change shape somewhat, even after becoming detached. The pieces are known as "free bodies," "joint mice," or "ossicles," and usually lodge in the caudal pouch of the joint capsule.

According to Craig and Riser, the subchondral bone beneath the lesion first resorbs to form a crater and then fills with remodeled bone.

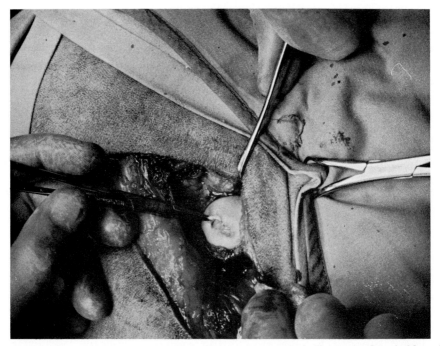

Figure 281. Osteochondritis dissecans lesion illustrating the loose cartilage held in the forceps.

Signs

The patient may show a mild swinging leg lameness or the condition may be severe enough that he refuses to use the limb. Often there is a pronounced limp which increases with exercise and decreases with rest. Even when both shoulders are involved there may be lameness only in one. The limp is likely to increase in severity over the first three to four weeks. There is a tendency to lie rather than stand or sit. The affected leg often is abducted slightly.

Pain is not severe on palpation and the patient generally does not resist examination. However, full extension of the limb usually causes enough pain that the dog shows signs of discomfort. There is no evidence of swelling or fluid around the joint. In long-standing cases the supraspinatus and infraspinatus muscles are atrophied. The movement of the joint is usually within normal limits unless there is interference from a free body.

Diagnosis

A roentgenogram produces the best clinical evidence of osteochondritis dissecans. Both shoulder joints should be radiographed from the mediolateral direction with the limb extended fully and the lateral side against the cassette.

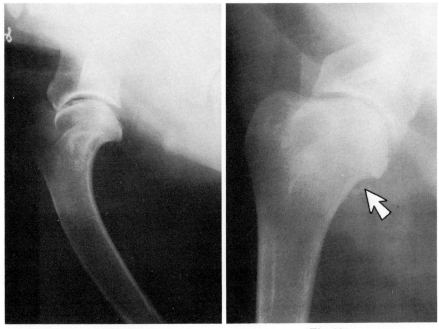

Fig. 282   Fig. 283

Figure 282. Osteochondritis dissecans of the humeral head with typical flattening and cavitation at the caudal edge.

Figure 283. Typical roentgenogram of osteochondritis dissecans showing a free body in the caudal pouch of the joint.

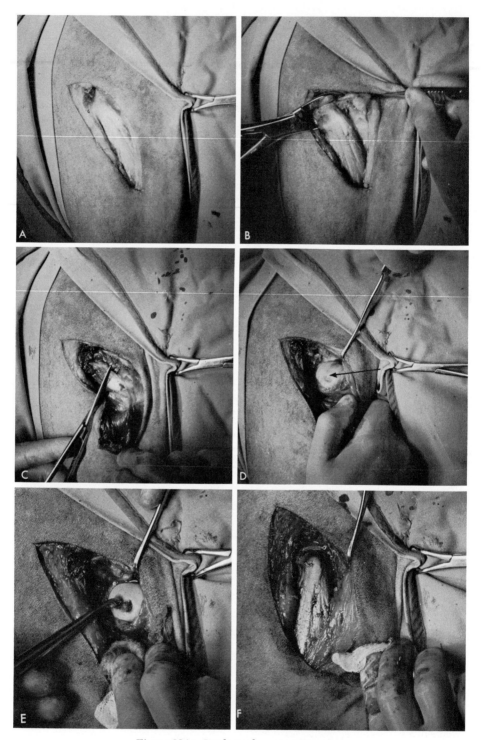

Figure 284.   *See legend on opposite page.*

The major joint changes will be seen in the caudo-central portion of the articular surface of the humeral head. In early cases there is an area of rarefaction in the subchondral bone. This appears as an inverted equilateral triangle with the base next to the articular cartilage.

In cases of four to eight weeks' duration the bone beneath the lesion may have become denser and the cartilage may appear as a plaque above the spot. The convex surface at the caudal edge may be flattened or slightly concave (Fig. 282).

Vaughan and Jones report a high percentage of joint mice. We have not been able to demonstrate these very often on our roentgenograms. Mostosky suggests that they do not radiograph well until they have ossified. This would mean that they would only be visible in long-standing cases (Fig. 283).

Chronic cases usually reveal osteophyte formation along the caudal border of the glenoid cavity and at the epiphyseal junction of the head and neck.

Prognosis

The prognosis is fair in 80 per cent of the cases but should be guarded in chronic situations when osteoarthritis is already in evidence. Many cases return to normal without clinical signs and others with very conservative treatment. Such individuals can be given a good prognosis. The prognosis should be more conservative if treatment requires invasion of the joint.

Treatment

Conservative treatment consists of rest, mild exercise, or intra-articular medication. Wherever the lameness is slight or only follows exercise, the patient should be confined and rested as much as possible. A leash should be used if the dog is to be moved. Heavy dogs should be kept on adequate bedding so that they are able to lie comfortably most of the time. Short walks on leash may be started after two months. Gradually, more vigorous exercise may be instituted.

When the lameness is more severe it becomes necessary to administer intra-articular corticosteroids. On the average, about 20 mg. of methylprednisolone acetate per joint per dose is given. Some may require a 50 per cent increase in dosage. The second dose will be required in about one week.

Figure 284A. Skin incision for exposure of shoulder joint.
Figure 284B. Cutting the acromion to free the deltoideus.
Figure 284C. Transecting the tendon of insertion of the infraspinatous muscle.
Figure 284D. The joint capsule is opened and the limb rotated to expose the lesion. See arrow.
Figure 284E. Curetting the lesion.
Figure 284F. The acromion replaced and wired.

Usually the interval between doses will increase until signs of lameness are gone or reasonably abated.

Needless to say, aseptic precautions must be taken and some kind of sedation provides the greatest safety and comfort for the patient. After the skin is properly prepared, the acromion process is palpated. The needle is thrust into the joint capsule on the cranial aspect of the shoulder just distal to a line level with the acromion process. A small amount of synovial fluid should be aspirated to assure proper location of the needle before injection.

Surgical treatment consists of arthrotomy, curettage of the lesion, and removal of any free bodies. This treatment is usually reserved for nonhealing lesions with large plaques or free bodies in the joint. The approach to the joint suggested by Piermattei gives the best exposure. An adequate exposure is very important in the larger breeds.

The skin incision begins at about the midpoint of the scapular spine and follows an arc over the lateral aspect of the shoulder to uncover the proximal third of the humerus (Fig. 284A). The acromial branch of the deltoideus muscle is uncovered by separating the omobrachial fascia. The acromial part of the deltoideus is dissected free at its upper end. A hole is drilled through the acromion and the process is cut proximal to the hole (Fig. 284B). The deltoideus can be reflected distally with the acromion attached. The tendon of the infraspinatus muscle is divided about 1 cm. from its attachment to the lateral aspect of the humerus and dissected away from the joint capsule (Fig. 284C).

A cranio-caudal incision is made in the joint capsule and the elbow is rotated away from the body to expose the caudal portion of the humeral head and the lesion (Fig. 284D). The lesion is thoroughly curetted so that the edge and the crater are completely freshened (Fig. 284E). Saline is used to flush the joint capsule of all debris and any free body is removed. The capsule is closed with chromic catgut.

The tendon of the infraspinatus is sutured with stainless steel, using a mattress-type stitch. Before replacing the deltoideus, the infraspinatus is freed for a short distance along the scapular spine so that a hole can be drilled through the spine. A stainless steel suture is then threaded through the hole in the acromion and through the hole in the spine. The ends are tied tightly, thereby drawing the acromion back into apposition with the spine (Fig. 284F). The incised fascia is repaired and the skin incision closed.

The patient should be rested for a week. This can be followed by mild exercise for one month. The normal gait should gradually return following such a postoperative routine. Corticosteroids should be avoided during the early healing period.

REFERENCES

Aegerter, E., and Kirkpatrick, J. A., Jr.: Orthopedic Diseases. Philadelphia, W. B. Saunders Co., 1963.
Birkland, R.: Osteochondritis dissecans in the humeral head of the dog. Nord. Vet. Med., 19:294-306, 1967.

Carlson, W. D.: Veterinary Radiology. Philadelphia, Lea & Febiger, 1961.

Craig, P. H., and Riser, W. H.: Osteochondritis dissecans in the proximal humerus of the dog. J. Am. Vet. Rad. Soc., *VI*:40-49, 1965.

Griffiths, R. C.: Osteochondritis dissecans of the canine shoulder. J.A.V.M.A., *153*:1733-1735, 1968.

Hutton, W. C., Freeman, M. A. R., and Swanson, S. A. V.: The forces exerted by the pads of the walking dog. J. Small Animal Pract., *10*:71-77, 1969.

Leighton, R. L.: Canine osteochondritis dissecans. Veterinary Scope, *XIII*:14-16, 1968.

Miller, M. E., Christensen, G. C., and Evans, H. E.: Anatomy of the Dog. Philadelphia, W. B. Saunders Co., 1964.

Mostosky, U. V.: Osteochondritis dissecans of the canine shoulder. Proc. 13th Gaines Vet. Symposium, 16-19, 1964.

Mostosky, U. V.: Osteochondritis dissecans of the canine shoulder. *In* Current Veterinary Therapy (R. W. Kirk, ed.). Philadelphia, W. B. Saunders Co., 1966.

Piermattei, D. L., and Greeley, R. G.: An Atlas of Surgical Approaches to the Bones of the Dog and Cat. Philadelphia, W. B. Saunders Co., 1966.

Sawyer, D. C.: The arthritides. *In* Current Veterinary Therapy (R. W. Kirk, ed.). Philadelphia, W. B. Saunders Co., 1966.

Vaughan, L. C., and Jones, D. G. C.: Osteochondritis dissecans of the head of the humerus in dogs. J. Small Animal Pract., 9:283-294, 1968.

Chapter 18

Hypertrophic Pulmonary Osteoarthropathy (Marie's Disease, Acropachia, Hypertrophic Osteoperiostitis)

Definition

This is a disease in which the secondary or tertiary lesions are seen in the bones but the primary lesion is situated elsewhere. It is characterized by a clubbing effect in the extremities due to subperiosteal proliferation of the long bones.

Distribution

It is seen in various parts of the world, but it seems to be more prevalent where chronic lung disease is common. The dog is only one species of many affected; in fact, it is described more frequently in man than in the dog. The disease has also been described in a number of other mammals. It is seen more commonly in the larger breeds of dogs and especially in those used for hunting.

Etiology

Although the exact cause is not known, many theories have been advanced. Such factors as congenital heart disease, circulatory disturbances, increased peripheral blood flow, foreign bodies in the lung, pulmonary or cardiac tumors (Fig. 285), metastasis of tumors to the lungs, as well as chronic pulmonary infections such as tuberculosis, have been held responsible for the bone changes. Hypoxemia could conceivably be the cause. It is quite possible that the blood is shunted around a lesion in such a fashion that it returns to the general circulation without proper ventilation, according to Brodey et al. Lord has further indicated the possibility that the degree of hypoxemia influences the extent of the bony proliferation. The

338

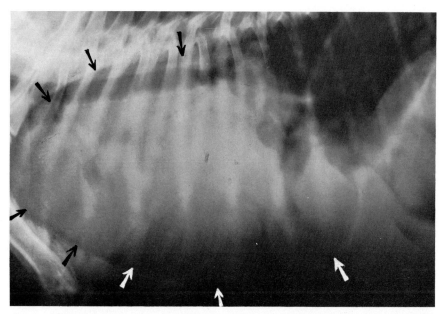

Figure 285. A tumor in the chest of a dog afflicted with hypertrophic pulmonary osteoarthropathy. The heart is entirely obscured and only a small amount of normal lung tissue can be seen.

general consensus at the present time seems to be that reduced oxygen tension in the blood is the primary cause. This results from interference with the oxygen–carbon dioxide exchange in the lungs due to the presence of tumors or tuberculosis.

The tumor in the lung may be primary or it may be the result of metastasis from tumors in other organs. These tumors have been described as fibrosarcomas, giant cell tumors, adenocarcinomas, and osteosarcomas. The primary tumor has been found in the liver, the kidney, and the bones as well as in the lungs. In general, the primary lesion in young dogs is tuberculosis and in older dogs it is a tumor. However, when the primary lesion is tuberculosis the bone lesion is not tuberculous.

Pathology

There is extensive subperiosteal proliferation of bone (Fig. 286). These rough accumulations along the shaft of the long bones are usually thickest in the epiphyseal region and at the points of tendon insertion. Although the distal extremities of the limbs are usually involved, it is possible for all bones to be affected. Lesions are first seen in the phalanges, metacarpals, and metatarsals. From these sites they gradually progress upward. The joint capsule is thickened, but the articular surface is seldom involved. In some instances the joint is ankylosed but usually it is freely movable. Bone changes include thickening of the periosteum, thinning of the cortical bone with osteoporosis, and occasionally pathologic fractures.

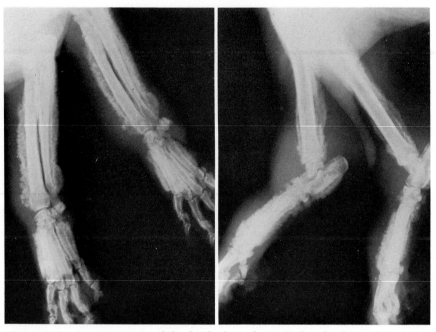

Figure 286. Roentgenogram of the forelimbs and rear limbs of a dog with hypertrophic pulmonary osteoarthropathy. There is considerable proliferation along the long bones, but the joints are relatively free.

There is an increased vascularity of the extremities, with a swelling of the subcutaneous tissues. This is probably due to increased arterial pressure.

Signs

The signs are variable and may appear at any age. In some cases the patient may be asymptomatic at first, the only detectable lesion being discovered by a roentgenogram. At other times the signs may be primarily those of pulmonary disease. Ordinarily the condition is first indicated by a swelling of the lower appendages. Usually there is pain on palpation and tenderness over the long bones and joints. The pain may even precede roentgenographic changes in some instances. There is not full agreement on this sign, since Poley and Taylor state that there is little or no pain.

Lameness with some limitation of joint movement is often observed, and in rare instances the patient may be unable to stand. The gait is stiff, and flexion is often restricted because of the thickening around the joint, which usually extends over the tarsals and carpals nearly to the stifle and elbow.

On palpation, the skin feels thickened and the underlying tissues are hard and unyielding.

The course is frequently long if the primary lesion is tuberculosis and somewhat shorter if a tumor is the cause.

Prognosis

The prognosis is always poor.

Treatment

No satisfactory treatment has been found, since the primary cause is frequently a malignant disease. Some cases have been recorded in which temporary relief has been afforded by surgical removal of the pulmonary lesion. In most instances the osteoarthropathy has recurred in eight to 10 weeks because of the recurrence of neoplastic tissue in the lungs. It is true, however, that definite improvement is seen whenever the pulmonary lesion can be removed and controlled.

REFERENCES

Bloom, F.: Pathology of the Dog and Cat. Evanston, Ill., American Veterinary Publications, 1954.

Brodey, R. S., and Wind, A. P.: Surgical management of hypertrophic pulmonary osteoarthropathy in the dog. J.A.V.M.A., 130:208, 1957.

Brodey, R. S., Craig, P. H., and Rhodes, W. H.: Hypertrophic osteoarthropathy in a dog with pulmonary metastases arising from a renal adenocarcinoma. J.A.V.M.A., 132:231, 1958.

Brown, J. M.: Hypertrophic pulmonary osteoarthropathy in dogs. J. S. Africa Vet. Med. A., 25:35, 1954.

Cordy, C. R., and Dinsmore, J. R.: Pulmonary hypertrophic osteoarthropathy in a dog. N. Amer. Vet., 31:30, 1950.

Innes, J. R. M.: The pathology and pathogenesis of tuberculosis in animals compared to man. Vet. J., 96:96, 391, 1940.

Leighton, R. L., and Stoyak, J. M.: Hypertrophic pulmonary osteoarthropathy resulting from metastasis to the lungs in dogs. J.A.V.M.A., 123:437, 1953.

Lord, G. H.: Hypertrophic osteoarthropathy in a dog—a clinico-pathological report. J.A.V.M.A., 134:13, 1959.

Lumb, W. V., and Carlson, W. D.: Pulmonary lobectomy for a malignant mixed cell tumor with hypertrophic osteoarthropathy in a dog. J.A.V.M.A., 128:185, 1956.

Mather, G., and Low, D.: Chronic pulmonary osteoarthropathy in the dog. J.A.V.M.A., 122:167, 1953.

Mendlowitz, M.: Clubbing and hypertrophic osteoarthropathy. Medicine, 21:269–306, 1942.

Poley, P. P., and Taylor, J. S.: Hypertrophic pulmonary osteoarthropathy associated with a bronchiogenic giant cell tumor in the left lung of a dog. J.A.V.M.A., 100:346, 1942.

Rex, M. A.: The effect of surgical intervention in a case of chronic pulmonary osteoarthropathy in a dog. Vet. Record, 71:409, 1959.

Rumney, W. J., and Schoefield, F. W.: Hypertrophic pulmonary osteoarthropathy (Marie's disease). Canad. J. Comp. Med., 14:385, 1950.

Schlotthauer, C. F., and Millar, J. A. S.: Hypertrophic pulmonary osteoarthropathy in association with pulmonary neoplasm in dogs. J.A.V.M.A., 119:442, 1951.

White, E. G.: Osteoarthropathy in dogs. J.A.V.M.A., 101:202, 1942.

Index

Acetabulum, fracture of, 89, 194
Acropachia, 338
Acute luxations, 199
Adhesion, in tendon repair, 275
Adventitia, in artery repair, 273
Aire-Cast, 39, 47, 130
  in vertebral fractures, 187
Airplane cast, 210
Alcohol, as skin disinfectant, 24
Alexander method of shoulder fixation, 251,
  252
Alkaline phosphatase, 12
Alumafoam splint, 37
Aluminum, padded, 196
Aluminum rod, 42
Aluminum sheeting, 33
Amman's method for treating mandibular
  fractures, 178
Amputation, of the digit, 286, 287
  of the pectoral limb, 282–286
  of the pelvic limb, 278–282
Anastamosis, vascular, 272–274
Anderson splint, 51
Angulation, in closed reduction, 31
Annulus fibrosis, 289
"Anterior drawer sign," 228, 231
AO, 68
  application of, 69–74
  equipment for, 70
Armistead and Lumb method of fracture
  fixation, 123
Arthrodesis, 245, 247
Arthroplasty, in Legg-Perthes disease, 326
  of femoral head, 111
Artificial ligamentum teres, 216, 217
Arwedsson method of arthrodesis, 245
Aseptic necrosis, 98, 99
Aseptic surgery, 17
Astragalus, luxation of, 242
Atlanto-axial subluxation, 263, 265

Auburn type spinal plates, 188
Autogenous bone grafts, 15
Avascular necrosis, 98, 99
Avulsion, of tibial tuberosity, 128

Ball method of shoulder fixation, 251, 252
Basswood, 33
Beaded wire, Thomson, 54
Beaver knife, 232, 242
Biceps brachii, 251, 252
Bicycle spoke, 52–54, 112, 126
  in pelvic fractures, 195
Blood vessel, repair of, 271
Bone, 3
  canaliculi, 8
  cancellous, 7
  circulation in, 8
  collagen in, 6
  compact, 7
  composition of, 6
  cortical, 7
  formation of, 6
  graft, 15, 84
  healing of, 10
  lacunae, 8
  lamellae, 8
  marrow, 8
  medullary, 8
  membranous, 10
  mineral, 6
  mucopolysaccharides in, 6
  nerve supply in, 9
  organic matrix in, 6
  water in, 6
Bone clamp, 67
Bone cutters, 81
Bone peg, 84

Bone plates, 65–76
   in vertebral fractures, 188
   in vertebral luxations, 261, 262
Bone rongeurs, 81
Bone saw, Stryker, 84
Bone screws, 65–76, 137
Bone tongs, 54, 55
Bone transplant, 15
Brown prosthesis, 77–83, 113
   installation of, 79
   size of, 78
Bulldog clamp, 272
Bunnel method of tendon repair, 275
Butler method of stabilizing stifle, 238
Butterfly cast, 210

Calcification, 6
   of disc, 290, 295
   of extruded material, 295
Calcium mobilization, 12
Cameron method of stabilizing stifle, 238
Campbell method of shoulder fixation, 251
Canaliculi, 8
Cancellous bone, 7
Cancellous transplants, 15
Capital fractures, 97
Carpal and metacarpal fractures, 171
Carpal luxation, 256
Carrel technique of vascular repair, 273
Cart, orthopedic, 299, 310
Cartilage, 3, 10
   composition of, 3–5
   elastic, 3, 4
   hyaline, 4, 11
Cast, application of, 32
Cast scissors, 39
Caudal coxo-femoral luxation, 205
   diagnosis of, 207
Caudal cruciate ligament, 226, 228
Cavitation, of humeral head, 333
Cell proliferation, 10
Centers of ossification, 6, 7
Central tarsus, 242
   fracture of, 139, 142
Cervical disc, protrusion of, 292
Chemical sterilization, 19
Childers method of stabilizing stifle, 238
Chondroblasts, 10
Chondrodystrophoid breeds, 288
Chronic dislocations, 199
Circulation of the hip joint, 98
Circumferential wiring of the mandible, 180
Clamp, bulldog, 272
Classification of fractures, 90
Closed fracture, 90
Closed reduction, 30
Coaptation, 32–45
   cotton in, 32, 33
   in humeral fractures, 150

Coaptation (Continued)
   in radial fractures, 166
   in tibial fractures, 132
   with Aire-Cast, 39, 41
   with Alumafoam, 37
   with meta splints, 37
   with plaster of Paris, 38, 40
   with plastic, 33
   with tongue depressors, 33, 36
Coat hanger splint, 42
Collagen, 4, 6
Collateral ligaments, 228–230
"Colles" fracture, 163
Comminuted fracture, 90
Compact bone, 7
Compact transplants, 15
Complete fracture, 90
Composition of bone, 6
Composition of cartilage, 3–5
Compound fracture, 90
Compound luxation, 199
Compression fracture, 91
   of vertebrae, 185, 186
Compression plating, 68–76, 118
Condyle clamp, 157, 158
Condyle pin, in intercondylar fractures, 157
   in supracondylar fractures, 155, 157
Congenital luxation, of shoulder, 250
   of patella, 223
Cortical bone, 7
Cotton, application to limbs, 33, 34
Cotton padding, 32–36
Coxa magna, 316
Coxa plana, 316
Coxa valga, 316
Coxa vara, 316
Coxo-femoral joint, luxation of, 203–211
   caudal, 205
   cranial, 204
   diagnosis of, 207
   dorsal, 205
   etiology of, 203
   open reduction of, 215
   pathology of, 204
   prognosis in, 207
   reduction of, 209, 210
   signs of, 206
   skeletal traction in, 211
   treatment of, 209
   subluxation of, 200
Cranial cruciate ligament, 226–228, 230, 231
Craver operation, 221
Crepitus, 94
Cruciate repair, 231–241
Cutters, bone, 81
   for pins, 49

DeAngelis and Schwartz method of shoulder
   fixation, 251, 252
Débridement, 269

Degeneration, of disc, 291
Delayed union, 12
Depression fracture, 91
Desmotomy, 220
DeVita method of fixation, 212, 214
Diagnosis, of coxo-femoral luxation, 207
  of dislocations, 201
  of fractures, 94
Diaphysis, 6
Disc degeneration, 291
Disc disease, 288–311
  diagnosis of, 294
  etiology of, 289
  incidence of, 288
  medical treatment of, 299
  naming of, 291
  number of, 291
  pathology of, 289
  prognosis in, 297
  roentgenography of, 294–297
  signs of, 292
  surgery in, 299–311
    ventral approach in, 303–311
Dislocations, 199
  compound, 199
  coxo-femoral, 203
  diagnosis of, 201
  treatment of, 201
Distracted fracture, 91, 92
Distribution of fractures, 89
Dobbelaar method of fixation, 218
Dorsal coxo-femoral luxation, 205
Dorsal laminectomy, 300
Dorsal longitudinal ligament, 289
Dorsal luxation, diagnosis of, 207
Dorsal spurring, 291
Drapes, 17
  plastic, 25
Draping, of patient, 22, 23
  to incision, 26
"Drawer sign," 228, 229
Dueland method of stabilizing stifle, 236
Dysplasia, of elbow, 327
  of hip, 313–321

Ectopic sesamoid bones, 327
Ehmer cast, 210–212
Ehmer reduction gear, 52
Elastic cartilage, 3, 4
Elbow dysplasia, 327
  treatment of, 329
Elbow luxation, 253–256
  reduction of, 254
Endosteum, 9, 10
Ensolite, 299
Epiphyseal fracture, 97, 98
  of femur, 121, 122, 124, 125
  of tibia, 129
Epiphysis, 6

Ethyl alcohol, 24
Examination, for fractures, 94
Excision, of femoral head, 111
Exercise cart, 299, 310
Extension, by weights, 95, 96
Extensor thrust, 292
External fixation, 32
Extracapsular fracture, 97, 100
Extrusion, of disc, 290

Fascia bank, 218
Femoral head, arthroplasty of, 111
  fracture of, 97
  fragmentation of, 324, 325
  prostheses for, 76–83, 103
  rarefaction of, 324
  remodeling of, 325
Femoro-tibial luxation, 226
Femur, fracture of, 97
  distal segment of, 120
  epiphyseal, 121
  middle segment, 113
  neck of, 97
  open reduction of, 116
  proximal segment of, 113
  surgical approach to, 115, 116
  traction for, 118, 119
  treatment of, 114, 122
Fenestration, of cervical discs, 300–303
  of discs, 300–311
Fibroblasts, 10
Fibrocartilage, 4, 11
Fibula, fracture of, 128
Fibular tarsal, fracture of, 139
Fissure fracture, 91, 93
Fixation, external, 32
  internal, 55
  of luxated shoulder, 251
  with intramedullary pins, 59–65
Flat bones, healing of, 11
Flexion reflex, 292
Forces, in fractures, 89
Formula, for Thomas splint, 43
Fracture, capital, 97
  classification of, 90
  closed, 90
  "Colles," 163
  comminuted, 90
  complete, 90
  compound, 90
  compression, 91
  definition of, 89
  depression, 91
  diagnosis of, 94
  distracted, 91, 92
  distribution of, 89
  epiphyseal, 97, 98
  examination of, 94
  extracapsular, 97, 100

Fracture (*Continued*)
  fissure, 91, 93
  green stick, 91, 93
  hematoma, 11–14
  immobilization of, 32
  impacted, 91, 92, 196
  in pectoral limb, 145
  in pelvic limb, 97
  incomplete, 91
  intracapsular, 97
  intracondylar, 152
  longitudinal, 90
  malleolar, 135
  non-union, 165
  oblique, 31, 90, 91
  of acetabulum, 194
  of carpus and metacarpus, 171
  of central tarsus, 139, 142
  of coccygeal vertebrae, 188
  of femoral head, 97
  of femoral neck, 97
    diagnosis of, 101
    prognosis in, 101
    signs of, 100
    treatment of, 102
  of femur, 97
    in distal segment, 120
      definition of, 120
      diagnosis of, 122
      etiology of, 121
      incidence of, 120
      pathology of, 121
      prognosis in, 122
      signs of, 121
      treatment of, 122
    in middle segment, 113
      definition of, 113
      diagnosis of, 114
      etiology of, 113
      incidence of, 113
      pathology of, 114
      prognosis in, 114
      signs of, 114
      treatment of, 114
    in proximal segment, 111
      definition of, 111
      diagnosis of, 112
      etiology of, 111
      incidence of, 111
      pathology of, 112
      prognosis in, 112
      signs of, 112
      treatment of, 112
  of fibula, 128
  of fibular tarsal, 139
  of humerus, coaptation of, 151
    in middle segment, 148
    in proximal segment, 147
    treatment of, 150
  of ilium, 192, 193
  of ischium, 192, 193

Fracture (*Continued*)
  of mandible, 175, 177
  of mandibular ramus, 183
  of metatarsus, 138, 142
  of olecranon, 168
  of parietal bone, 174
  of patella, 127, 128
  of pelvis, 191
  of phalanges, 138, 142
  of radius and ulna, 163
  of ribs, 189, 191
  of scaphoid, 139, 142
  of scapula, 145
  of sesamoids, 172
  of skull, 173
  of spine, 184
  of sternum, 189, 190
  of tarsus, 138, 141
  of tibia, 128–136
    in distal segment, 135
      definition of, 135
      diagnosis of, 136
      etiology of, 135
      incidence of, 135
      pathology of, 135
      prognosis in, 136
      signs of, 135
      treatment of, 136
    in middle segment, 131
      definition of, 131
      diagnosis of, 132
      etiology of, 131
      pathology of, 131
      prognosis in, 132
      signs of, 131
      treatment of, 132
    in proximal segment, 128
      definition of, 128
      diagnosis of, 130
      etiology of, 128
      pathology of, 130
      prognosis in, 130
      signs of, 130
      treatment of, 130
  of trochanter major, 112
  of tuber calcis, 139, 141
  open, 90
  pathological, 89
  patterns of, 89
  simple, 90
  spiral, 90, 91
  supracondylar, 120, 152
  supramalleolar, 135
  transverse, 90, 91
  treatment of, 95
Fragmentation, of femur head, 324, 325
Frazer laminectomy retractor, 306
Free bodies, 332
Free processus anconeus, 327
Frost aluminum splint, 166
Full pin splintage, 52

Galvanic activity, of metals in body, 55
Gay prosthesis, 77
Gibbens method of stabilizing the stifle, 236
Gigli saw, 110
Gloves, surgical, cream for, 21
    donning, 26, 28
    powder for, 20
    preparation of, 20
Gordon extender, 209
Gorman prosthesis, 76, 78, 113
Gown, surgical, donning, 27
    folding, 20
Graft, autogenous, 15, 84
  heterogenous, 15
  homogenous, 15
  inlay, 84
  onlay, 84
Green stick fracture, 91, 93, 163

Half pin fixation, of coxo-femoral luxation,
  212
Half pin insertion, 48
Half pin splint, 45, 47, 115, 118
  application of, 46, 48–51, 122, 125, 126
  in femur fractures, 115
  in mandibular fractures, 179
  in pelvic fractures, 195, 197
  in radial fractures, 166
  in supracondylar fractures, 155, 157
  in tibial fractures, 132
Hall air drill, 223, 224
Haversian canals, 7
Healing of bone, 10
Hematoma of fracture, 12
Hemilaminectomy, 300
Heparin, 271, 272
Heterogenous bone grafts, 15
Hexachlorophene, 26
Hip dysplasia, 313–320
  classification of, 320
  definition of, 313
  diagnosis of, 318
  distribution of, 313
  etiology of, 315
  pathology of, 315
  prognosis in, 320
  signs of, 317
  treatment of, 320
Hip joint, caudal approach to, 108, 109
  circulation of, 98
  cranial approach to, 104, 105
  dorsal approach to, 104, 106, 107
  medial approach to, 108, 110
  surgical approach to, 104, 110
  ventral approach to, 108, 110
Hip prosthesis, cranial approach for, 80
Hirschhorn compression device, 75
Hirschhorn modification, for compression
  plating, 69, 72–76

Hock joint, luxation of, 242
Hohn method of stabilizing the stifle, 238,
  240
Homogenous bone grafts, 15
Humeral condyle, repair of, with condyle
    pin, 155
  with half pin, 157
  with screw, 159
  with wires, 155
Humero-radio-ulnar luxation, 253–256
Humerus, fracture of, 147
  surgical approach to, 149
Hyaline cartilage, 4, 11
Hypergonadotropism, 322
Hypertrophic osteoperiostitis, 338
Hypertrophic pulmonary osteoarthropathy,
  338
Hypoxemia, 338

Ilium, fracture of, 192, 193
Imbrication, 238
Immobilization, 13, 32, 95
Impacted fracture, 91, 92, 196
Incision site, for fenestration, 306, 307, 309
Incomplete fracture, 91
Insertion of half pins, 48
Installation of Brown prosthesis, 79
Instruments, cleaning of, 18
Intercondylar fracture, 152
Intermaxillary wiring, 181, 182
Internal fixation, 55
Intervertebral disc disease, 288–311
Intervertebral space, narrowing of, 295
Intracapsular fracture, 97
Intramedullary pin, 56–65, 114, 122
Intramedullary pinning, of femur, 122, 123,
  126
  of humerus, 150
  of mandible, 180
  of pelvic fractures, 196, 197
  of radius, distal, 168
  of tibia, 130, 132, 134, 136, 137
  of tibio-tarsal luxations, 244, 245
Intramembranous ossification, 6
Intrapelvic luxations, diagnosis of, 207
Ischium, fracture of, 192, 193
Isopropyl alcohol, 24

Jacob's chuck, 60
Jenny method, for repair of intercondylar
    fractures, 154, 157
  of applying plaster, 39, 40
Johnson method of stabilizing the stifle, 238
Joint mice, 332
Jonas splint, 62

Kirschner condyle pin, 155
  in supracondylar fractures, 157
Kirschner half pins, 112
Kirschner intramedullary pin, 58–60, 114,
  122, 130, 136
Kirschner splint, 51
Kirschner wire, 112
  in pelvic fractures, 195
  in skull fractures, 177
  in supracondylar fractures, 154, 155, 157
Knowles method of stabilizing the hip, 216
Kuentscher nail, 57, 60, 61, 112, 113, 115

Lacunae, 8
Lacroix method of patellar desmotomy, 220
Lamellae, 8
Laminectomy, 300
Lane bone plate, 66
Lawson method of arthrodesis, 245
Legg-Perthes disease, 322–326
  treatment of, 324
Leighton shuttle pin, 64
  in radial fracture, 167
Ligament, caudal cruciate, 226–228, 230, 231
  collateral, 228, 230
  cranial cruciate, 226–228
  dorsal longitudinal, 289, 304
  meniscal, 226, 227
  ventral longitudinal, 301, 304, 309
Ligamentum teres, artificial, 216, 217
Longitudinal fracture, 90
Longitudinal ligament, 289
Luxation(s), 199
  acute, 199
  carpal, 256
  chronic, 199
  compound, 199
  coxo-femoral, 203
  diagnosis of, 201
  femoro-tibial, 226
  hock joint, 242
  humero-radio-ulnar, 253, 256
  mandibular, 258
  metacarpal, 256
  metatarsal, 247
  patellar, 218
  phalangeal, 247, 256
  scapulo-humeral, 250
    congenital, 250
    fixation of, 251
  spinal, 260–265
  tarsal, 242, 245
  tarso-metatarsal, 242
  tibio-tarsal, 242–244
  treatment of, 201

Malleolar fracture, 135
Mandibular luxation, 258
  reduction of, 259

Mandibular symphysial fractures, treatment
  of, 178
Mannitol, use in brain edema, 176
Marie's disease, 338
Marrow, 8
Mason meta splint, 33, 37
Measurements for Thomas splint, 44
Medial desmotomy, 220
Medullary bone, 8
Membranous bone, 10
Meniscal ligaments, 226, 227
Meniscus, 227, 228, 232
Meta splint, 33, 37
Metacarpus, luxation of, 256
Metatarsus, fracture of, 138, 142
  luxation of, 247
Methods and materials, 30
Method, of Alexander, for shoulder fixation,
  251, 252
  of Armistead and Lumb, for epiphyseal
    fractures of femur, 123
  of Ball, for shoulder fixation, 251, 252
  of Butler, for stabilization of stifle, 238
  of Cameron, for stabilization of stifle, 238
  of Campbell, for shoulder fixation, 251
  of Childers, for stabilization of stifle, 238
  of DeAngelis and Schwartz, for shoulder
    fixation, 251, 252
  of Dueland, for stabilization of stifle, 236
  of Gibbens, for stabilization of stifle, 236
  of Hohn, for stabilization of stifle, 238, 240
  of Johnson, for stabilization of stifle, 238
  of Ormrod, for stabilization of stifle, 237
  of Rathor, for stabilization of stifle, 239
  of Singleton, for stabilization of stifle, 237
  of Strande, for stabilization of stifle, 239,
    240
  of Vaughan, for shoulder fixation, 251, 252
  of Zahm, for stabilization of stifle, 238
Methyl methacrylate, 103
Mineralization, 6
Mobilization of calcium, 12
Modification of Ross for stabilization of stifle,
  239
Modified Bunnel method, for tendon repair,
  276
Modified Thomas splint, 42–46
Mold for Thomas splint, 45
Monteggia fracture-dislocation, 170
Mostosky method, for repair of humeral
  condyles, 159–163
Mucopolysaccharides, 6

Necrosis, aseptic, 98, 99
  avascular, 98, 99
  of femoral head, 98, 99, 324, 325
Nerve repair, 270
Non-union, 12, 165
  prevention of, 13
  treatment of, 14

Normal healing, 10
Normal pelvis, 314
Nucleus pulposus, 289

Obel method of hip fixation, 211
Oblique fracture, 31, 90, 91
Olecranon, fracture of, 168
Open fracture, 90
Open reduction, 32
   of coxo-femoral luxation, 215
   of femur, 116
   of radius, 170
Operating gloves, 20, 26, 28
Operating gown, 20, 27
Ormrod method, of stabilizing stifle, 237
Orthopedic cart, 299, 310
Orthopedic Foundation for Animals, 320
Ossicles, 332
Ossification, 6
   centers of, 6, 7
   endochondral, 6
   intramembranous, 6
Osteoblastic activity, 11
Osteoblasts, 3, 10
Osteoclastic activity, 11
Osteoclasts, 3
Osteochondritis dissecans, 331
Osteochondrosis, of femur head, 317
Osteocytes, 9
Osteophyte formation, 291
Osteotomy of femur, 221
Overriding, 31, 91

Paatsama operation, 231–235
Padded aluminum, 196
Pantopaque, 294
Paralysis in extension, 293
Patella, fracture of, 127, 128
   luxation of, 218
      treatment of, 220
Patellar reflex, 292
Patellectomy, 221
Pathological fracture, 89
Patient, draping of, 22, 23
   positioning for surgery, 24
Pearson implant, 224
Pelvic fractures, treatment of, 194
Pelvic roentgenography, 319
Pelvis, normal, 314
Perichondrium, 4
Periosteum, 6, 9, 10
pH of tissue fluids, 12, 13
Phalanges, fracture of, 138, 142
   luxation of, 247, 256
Phylogenetic reduction, 128
Physiotherapy, in disc disease, 299

Pin(s), bicycle spoke, 53, 112
   chisel pointed, 57, 58
   condyle, 155, 157, 158
   cutter, 49
   double pointed, 57
   insertion of, 48, 59
   intramedullary, 56
      in femoral fractures, 114, 116, 122–124
      in femoral neck fractures, 102
      in humeral fractures, 150
      in mandibular fractures, 177
      in olecranon fractures, 169
      in supracondylar fractures, 154
      in tibial fractures, 130, 134
      in tibio-tarsal luxations, 245
   Kirschner, 54, 58, 104, 114, 122, 130
   Kuentscher, 57, 60, 62, 112, 113
   Leighton shuttle, 64, 167
   migration of, 60
   Rush, 61, 63, 167
   Thomson beaded, 54, 57, 132, 156, 181, 183
   threaded, 58, 59
   types of, 57, 58
Plaster of Paris, 38–40, 130
   in vertebral fractures, 187
   Jenny method of application, 39, 40
Plastic drape, 25
Plastic sheet splintage, 33
Plate(s), benders, 66
   spinal fusion, 188, 189
Positioning patient, 24
"Posterior drawer sign," 228
Preparation for surgery, 17
   of bicycle spoke, 53
   of materials, 17
   of patient, 21
   of skin, 24
   of surgeon, 26
Pressure cooker, 21
Prostheses, 76–83
   femoral head, 103, 113
   Gay, 77
   Gorman, 78, 113
Protrusion, of disc, 289
Pull out tendon suture, 275–277

Quaternary ammonium compounds, 26

Radius, fracture of, definition, 163
   diagnosis of, 165
   etiology of, 164
   green stick fracture of, 163
   incidence of, 163
   open reduction of, 170
   pathology of, 164
   signs of, 165
   treatment of, 165

Rarefaction, of femur head, 324
Rathor method of stabilizing the stifle, 239
Reduction, closed, 30
    gear, Ehmer, 52
    of coxo-femoral luxation, 209, 210
    of elbow luxation, 254
    of mandibular luxation, 259
    of shoulder luxation, 250
    open, 32
Remodeling, of femur head, 325
Repair, of blood vessels, 271
    of cruciates, 231–241
    of nerves, 270
    of soft tissue, 269
    of stifle joint, 231–241
    of tendons, 274
Retrograde pinning, 115
Richards Plasti-Coat splint, 196
Richards plate, 74
Richards plating technique, 72–76
Roentgenogram, of elbow dysplasia, 329
    of osteochondritis dissecans, 333
    of pelvis, 319
Roentgenography, of the spine, 294–297
    to diagnose Legg-Perthes disease, 323
Rongeurs, bone, 81
Ross modification, for stabilizing the stifle,
    239
Rush pin, 63, 126
    in radial fractures, 167

Sacro-iliac separation, 193
Scaphoid, 242
    fracture of, 139, 142
Scapula, fracture of, 145
Scapulo-humeral luxation, 250
Scissors, cast, 39
    surgical, 270
    suture, 270
Screw, in the humeral condyle, 159
    in the radius and ulna, 170
    transfixion, 68, 69
Screw driver, 68
Scrubbing, for surgeon, 26
Separation, epiphyseal, 98
Serrafine clamps, 272
Sesamoids, fracture of, 172
Sherman bone plate, 66
Shoulder, luxation of, 250
Shuttleworth operation, 221
Signs, of coxo-femoral luxation, 206
Simple fracture, 90
Singleton method, of stabilizing the stifle,
    237
Skeletal traction, 32, 122
    in coxo-femoral luxation, 211
Skin preparation, 24
    prick test, 292
    reflex, 293
    traction, 32

Soft tissue, repair of, 269
Spastic paralysis, 293
Spinal fixation, 188
    fractures, 184
    fusion plates, 188, 189
    reflexes, 292
Spine, luxation of, 260–265
Spinograms, 294
Spiral fracture, 90, 91
Splint, Anderson, 51
    formula, 43
    Kirschner, 51
    Mason meta, 33, 37
    modified Thomas, 32
    mold, 45
    Thomas, 42, 46, 147
    Tower, 51, 52
Splintage, full pin, 33, 52
    half pin, 45, 122
    in tendon repair, 277
    with Aire-Cast, 39, 41
    with plaster of Paris, 38–40
    with tongue depressors, 33, 36
Spondylosis, 297, 298
Spread cast, 210
Stader operation for luxated patella, 221, 222
Stainless steel, 56
Steel formula, 65
Sterilization, chemical, 19
    of instruments, 19
    with ethylene oxide, 19
Sterilizing tubing, 19
Stifle joint repair, 231–241
Strande method for stabilizing the stifle, 239,
    241
Stryker bone saw, 84, 280
Subluxation(s), 199
    of coxo-femoral joint, 200, 319
    of spine, 262
Supracondylar fracture, 120, 152
    treatment of, 154
Supramalleolar fracture, 135
Surgeon, preparation of, 26
Surgery, aseptic, 17
    for osteochondritis dissecans, 334, 336
    of the disc, 299–311
Surgical approach, preparation, 17
    scissors, 270
    to femur, 115, 116
    to hip joint, 104–110
Suture scissors, 270

T fracture, of humerus, 159, 161
T splint, 155
Tarsal arthrodesis, 244–246
Tarsal luxation, 242, 245
Tarso-metatarsal luxations, 242
Tarsus, fracture of, 138, 141
Temporo-mandibular luxation, 258

Tendon repair, 274
Thomas splint, 32, 42
 aluminum rod for, 42
 application of, 117
 construction of, 43–46
 dimensions of, 43
 for coxo-femoral luxations, 211
 for epiphyseal fractures, 122
 for femoro-tibial luxations, 233
 for femur fractures, 119, 120, 122
 for forelimb, 147
 for hip fixation, 196, 213
 for humeral fractures, 155, 156
 for pelvic fractures, 196
 for supracondylar fractures, 125, 126
 for tibial fractures, 132
 formula for, 43
 measurements for, 44
 padding of, 45, 46
 shaping of, 43, 45
 traction with, 211
Thomson beaded wire, 54, 57, 132
 in mandibular fractures, 181, 183
 in pelvic fractures, 195
 in supracondylar fractures, 155, 156
Thoraco-lumbar discs, protrusion of, 292
Thorotrast, 294
Tibia, fracture of, 128
  in distal segment, 135
  in middle segment, 131
  in proximal segment, 128
Tibial crest, translocation of, 223, 225
Tibial tuberosity, separation of, 129, 131
Tibio-tarsal fixation, 244, 245
Tibio-tarsal luxation, 242–244
Toggling, 31
Tong, bone, 54, 55
Tongue depressors, as splints, 33, 36
Tower splint, 51, 52
Traction, in femur fractures, 118, 119
 in spinal fractures, 189
 skeletal, 32, 122
 skin, 32
Transfixion screw, 68, 69
Translocation, of tibial crest, 223, 225
Transolecranon approach to the elbow, 159–163
Transplants, cancellous, 15
 compact, 15
Transverse fracture, 90, 91
Treatment, of dislocations, 201
 of elbow dysplasia, 329
 of femur fractures, 114

Treatment (Continued)
 of fractures, 95
 of luxations, 201
 of patellar luxations, 220
 of skull fractures, 176
 of tibial fractures, 130, 132
 of vertebral fractures, 187
Trochanter major, fracture of, 112
Trochlear implant, 24
Tuber calcis, fracture of, 139

Ulna, fracture of, 163
Union, delayed, 12
Ununited anconeal process, 327

Vanadium steel, 55
Vascular repair, 271
Vaughan method, of shoulder fixation, 251, 252
Ventral approach to discs, 303–311
Vertebral luxations, 260–265
Vitallium, 56, 65, 78
Volkman canals, 9

Weights, for extension, 95, 96
Whirlpool bath, 299
Wilson spinal fusion plates, 188, 189
Wiring the mandible, 178
Wolff's law, 11

X-ray, in elbow dysplasia, 329
 in Legg-Perthes disease, 323
 in osteochondritis dissecans, 333
 of pelvis, 319
 of spine, 294–297

Y fracture of humerus, 159, 161
Yarborough method of hip fixation, 214, 215

Zahm method for stabilization of the stifle, 238